MORE 4U!

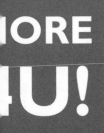

theclinics.com

This Clinics series is available online.

e's what get:

■ Full text of EVERY issue from 2002 to NOW

■ Figures, tables, drawings, references and more

■ Searchable: find what you need fast

Search [All Clinics ▼] for [ ] [GO]

■ Linked to MEDLINE and Elsevier journals

■ E-alerts

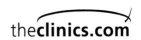

Robert A. Smith, DVM, MS
CONSULTING EDITOR

VETERINARY CLINICS
OF NORTH AMERICA
Food Animal Practice

Bovine Theriogenology

GUEST EDITOR
Grant S. Frazer, BVSc, MS, MBA

July 2005 • Volume 21 • Number 2

SAUNDERS

An Imprint of Elsevier, Inc.
PHILADELPHIA   LONDON   TORONTO   MONTREAL   SYDNEY   TOKYO

W.B. SAUNDERS COMPANY
A Division of Elsevier Inc.

Elsevier, Inc., 1600 John F. Kennedy Blvd., Suite 1800, Philadelphia, PA 19103-2899

http://www.vetfood.theclinics.com

VETERINARY CLINICS OF NORTH AMERICA: Volume 21, Number
FOOD ANIMAL PRACTICE   ISSN 0749-072
July 2005   ISBN 1-4160-2850-
Editor: John Vassallo

The ideas and opinions expressed in *Veterinary Clinics of North America: Food Animal Practice* do not necessarily reflect those of the Publisher. The Publisher does not assume any responsibility for any injury and/or damag to persons or property arising out of or related to any use of the material contained in this periodical. Th reader is advised to check the appropriate medical literature and the product information currently provide by the manufacturer of each drug to be administered to verify the dosage, the method and duration of ad ministration, or contraindications. It is the responsibility of the treating physician or other health care profes sional, relying on independent experience and knowledge of the patient, to determine drug dosages and th best treatment for the patient. Mention of any product in this issue should not be construed as endorseme by the contributors, editors, or the Publisher of the product or manufacturers' claims.

Veterinary Clinics of North America: Food Animal Practice (ISSN 0749-0720) is published in March, July, an November by Elsevier, Inc. Corporate and editorial offices: Elsevier, Inc., 1600 John F. Kennedy Blvd., Suit 1800, Philadelphia, PA 19103-2899. Accounting and circulation offices: 6277 Sea Harbor Drive, Orlando, Fl 32887-4800. Subscription prices are $115.00 per year for US individuals, $182.00 per year for US institu tions, $58.00 per year for US students and residents, $137.00 per year for Canadian individuals, $238.0(per year for Canadian institutions, $160.00 per year for international individuals, $238.00 per year for in ternational institutions and $80.00 per year for Canadian and foreign students/residents. To receive stu dent/resident rate, orders must be accompanied by name of affiliated institution, date of term, and th *signature* of program/residency coordinator on institution letterhead. Orders will be billed at individua rate until proof of status is received. Foreign air speed delivery is included in all *Clinics* subscription prices All prices are subject to change without notice. POSTMASTER: Send address changes to *Veterinary Clinic of North America: Food Animal Practice*, Elsevier, Customer Service Department, 6277 Sea Harbor Drive Orlando, FL 32887-4800, USA; phone: (+1) (877) 839-7126 [toll free number for US customers], or (+1) (407 345-4020 [customers outside US]; fax: (+1) (407) 363-1354; e-mail: usjcs@elsevier.com

Reprints. For copies of 100 or more, of articles in this publication, please contact the Commercial Reprint Department, Elsevier Inc., 360 Park Avenue South, New York, New York 10010-1710. Tel.: (212) 633-3813 Fax: (212) 462-1935; e-mail: Reprints@elsevier.com

Veterinary Clinics of North America: Food Animal Practice is covered in *Current Contents/Agriculture, Biolog and Environmental Sciences, Index Medicus,* and *Excerpta Medica.*

Printed in the United States of America.

CONSULTING EDITOR

ROBERT A. SMITH, DVM, MS, Diplomate, American Board of Veterinary Practitioners; Veterinary Research and Consulting Services, LLC, Greeley, Colorado

GUEST EDITOR

GRANT S. FRAZER, BVSc, MS, MBA, Diplomate, American College of Theriogenologists; Associate Professor, Large Animal Theriogenology, College of Veterinary Medicine, The Ohio Sate University, Columbus, Ohio

CONTRIBUTORS

CAROLE A. BOLIN, DVM, PhD, Department of Veterinary Pathobiology and Diagnostic Investigation, Michigan State University College of Veterinary Medicine, East Lansing, Michigan

ROBERT H. BONDURANT, DVM, Diplomate, American College of Theriogenologists; Professor and Chair, Department of Population Health and Reproduction, School of Veterinary Medicine, University of California, Davis, California

ROBERT A. DAILEY, PhD, Davis-Michael Professor of Animal Sciences and Reproductive Physiology, Division of Animal and Veterinary Sciences, College of Agriculture, Forestry, and Consumer Sciences, West Virginia University, Morgantown, West Virginia

MICHAEL L. DAY, MS, PhD, Professor, Department of Animal Sciences, The Ohio State University, Columbus, Ohio

JAMES M. DEJARNETTE, MS, Reproduction Specialist, Select Sires, Inc., Plain City, Ohio

J.P. DUBEY, MVSc, PhD, Agricultural Research Service, Animal and Natural Resources Institute, United States Department of Agriculture, Beltsville Agricultural Research Center, Beltsville, Maryland

JAMES D. FERGUSON, VMD, MS, Professor, Clinical Nutrition, School of Veterinary Medicine, University of Pennsylvania, New Bolton Center, Kennett Square, Pennsylvania

GRANT S. FRAZER, BVSc, MS, MBA, Diplomate, American College of Theriogenologists; Associate Professor, Large Animal Theriogenology, College of Veterinary Medicine, The Ohio Sate University, Columbus, Ohio

PAUL M. FRICKE, PhD, Associate Professor, Department of Dairy Science, University of Wisconsin, Madison, Wisconsin

DANIEL L. GROOMS, DVM, PhD, Diplomate, American College of Veterinary Microbiologists; Department of Large Animal Clinical Sciences, Michigan State University College of Veterinary Medicine, East Lansing, Michigan

DAVID E. GRUM, MS, PhD, Research Associate, Department of Animal Sciences, The Ohio State University, Columbus, Ohio

E. KEITH INSKEEP, PhD, Professor; Chair, Program in Reproductive Physiology, Division of Animal and Veterinary Sciences, College of Agriculture, Forestry, and Consumer Sciences, West Virginia University, Morgantown, West Virginia

G. CLIFF LAMB, PhD, Associate Professor, North Central Research and Outreach Center, University of Minnesota, Grand Rapids, Minnesota

ROBERT L. LARSON, DVM, PhD, Diplomate, American College of Theriogenologists; Diplomate, American College of Animal Nutrition; Diplomate, American College of Veterinary Preventive Medicine; Associate Professor, Department of Veterinary Medicine and Surgery; Director, Veterinary Extension and Continuing Education, College of Veterinary Medicine, University of Missouri, Columbia, Missouri

CHEYNEY MEADOWS, VMD, Department of Veterinary Preventive Medicine, College of Veterinary Medicine, The Ohio State University, Columbus, Ohio

PEDRO MELENDEZ, DVM, MS, PhD, Assistant Professor, Department of Large Animal Clinical Sciences, Section of Food Animal Reproduction and Medicine Service, College of Veterinary Medicine, University of Florida, Gainesville, Florida

CARLOS A. RISCO, DVM, Diplomate, American College of Theriogenologists; Professor, Section of Food Animal and Reproduction Medicine Service, Department of Large Animal Clinical Sciences, College of Veterinary Medicine, University of Florida, Gainesville, Florida

DONALD E. SANDERS, DVM, Diplomate, American College of Theriogenologists; Urbana Veterinary Clinic, Inc., Urbana, Ohio

BILLY I. SMITH, DVM, MS, Assistant Professor of Medicine, Department of Clinical Studies, Section of Field Service, University of Pennsylvania School of Veterinary Medicine, New Bolton Center, Kennett Square, Pennsylvania

JEFFREY S. STEVENSON, PhD, Department of Animal Sciences and Industry, Kansas State University, Manhattan, Kansas

JEFF W. TYLER, DVM, PhD, Diplomate, American College of Veterinary Internal Medicine; Professor, Department of Veterinary Medicine and Surgery; Section Head, Food Animal Medicine and Surgery; Director, Clinical Research, College of Veterinary Medicine, University of Missouri, Columbia, Missouri

CONTENTS

high rates of fertility requires management of rations throughout the nonlactating and lactating periods. Feed management that encourages high consumption is as important as provision of well-balanced rations. Body condition and body condition loss, incidence of periparturient problems, proportion of cows ovulating before 40 days postcalving, and milk urea nitrogen (MUN) are all important considerations in monitoring nutritional effects on reproduction.

Breeding Strategies to Optimize Reproductive Efficiency in Dairy Herds

Jeffrey S. Stevenson

This article discusses various programmed artificial insemination breeding schemes for dairy cattle. Protocols discussed for lactating cows are Targeted Breeding, Modified Targeted Breeding, Ovsynch, Presynch + Ovsynch, and potential uses of the intravaginal progesterone-releasing controlled internal drug release (CIDR) insert. Protocols for virgin replacement heifers include those that use CIDR inserts, orally active melengestrol acetate (MGA), gonadotropin hormone-releasing hormone (GnRH), and prostaglandin (PGF2α.). Methods to resynchronize estrus in previously inseminated cattle, including traditional estrus-detection technologies, are also discussed.

Breeding Strategies to Optimize Reproductive Efficiency in Beef Herds

Michael L. Day and David E. Grum

Our ability to synchronize estrus in beef cattle has increased substantially with enhanced understanding of reproduction physiology in cattle, and new technologies and approaches. Pregnancy rates of 50% to 70% in timed artificial insemination (AI) programs for well-managed herds with compact calving seasons can be achieved; however, unsatisfactory results (<50%) still occur. Reasons for poor pregnancy rates within a single herd can range from reproductive diseases to the use of semen of inadequate fertility. A common limitation of some programs appears to be the incidence of anestrus in the group of females to be synchronized. Whether AI will be performed based on detected estrus or at a set time influences the synchronization program that is selected, and the conception and pregnancy rates achieved.

Venereal Diseases of Cattle: Natural History, Diagnosis, and the Role of Vaccines in their Control

Robert H. BonDurant

With the large majority of beef cattle and increasing numbers of dairy cattle in North America bred by natural service, venereal disease is still prevalent. Several agents can be transmitted by coitus, but the classical two are still *Campylobacter fetus venerealis* and *Tritrichomonas foetus*. Their epidemiology is essentially identical, and indeed much of the pathophysiology is very similar, so the two should be considered simultaneously in most diagnostic situations. In this article, means of diagnosis, treatment (where appropriate), and prevention are discussed at both the individual and herd level. A brief mention is made of other potential venereal agents, including *Haemophilus somnus, Ureaplasm diversum,* and *Leptospira borgpetersenii.*

authors, much of the loss of potential offspring in cattle is concentrated in the embryonic period, the first 42 days after breeding. This article covers the impact of embryonic mortality on success of pregnancy in cattle, and some of the hormonal factors involved in pregnancy losses during the embryonic period. To establish the relative importance of embryonic death in the final outcome of mating, brief consideration is given to conception rate and fertilization rate.

Determining a cause of reproductive loss in cattle can be difficult. With proper use of diagnostic tools and strategies, the chance of getting a more definitive diagnosis increases significantly. Bovine viral diarrhea virus and *Leptospira* are two common pathogens associated with reproductive losses in cattle. By understanding the disease pathogenesis and the diagnostic tools available, strategies to diagnose and control these important reproductive pathogens can be developed.

Neospora caninum is a coccidian parasite of animals. It is a major cause of abortion in cattle in many countries. Domestic dogs and coyotes are the only known definitive hosts for *N caninum*. It is one of the most efficiently transmitted infections of cattle, and up to 90% of cattle in some herds are infected. Transplacental transmission is considered the major route of transmission of *N caninum* in cattle. There is no proven vaccine to prevent *N caninum* abortion.

Appropriate management of the transition period is of paramount importance to optimize fertility in dairy cattle. Physiologic goals are a strong immune system, maintenance of normocalcemia, positive energy balance, prevention of calving-related diseases, and a rumen adapted to a postpartum high-energy diet. These goals can be met by feeding an appropriate diet, by providing cow comfort, and by proper calving assistance. If these goals are met on a continued basis, they will provide the foundation necessary for a successful reproductive program. Assurance of proper management of transition cows can be achieved by periodic monitoring and evaluation.

GOAL STATEMENT

The goal of the *Veterinary Clinics of North America: Food Animal Practice* is to keep practicing veterinarians up to date with current clinical practice in food animal medicine by providing timely articles reviewing the state of the art in food animal care.

ACCREDITATION

The *Veterinary Clinics of North America: Food Animal Practice* will be offering continuing education credits, to be awarded by a school of veterinary medicine, contract pending.

The aforementioned school of veterinary medicine is a designated provider of continuing veterinary education. Veterinarians participating in this learning activity may earn up to 6 credits per issue up to a maximum of 18 credits per year. Credits awarded may not apply toward license renewal in all states. It is the responsibility of each participant to verify the requirements of their state licensing board.

Credit can be earned by reading the text material, taking the examination online at *http://www.theclinics.com/home/cme*, and completing the program evaluation. Each test question must be answered correctly; you will have the opportunity to retake any questions answered incorrectly. Following successful completion of the test and the program evaluation, you may print your certificate.

TO ENROLL

To enroll in the *Veterinary Clinics of North America: Food Animal Practice* Continuing Education program, call customer service at 1-800-654-2452 or sign up online at *http://www.theclinics.com/home/cme*. The CME program is available to subscribers for an additional annual fee of $49.95.

FORTHCOMING ISSUES

RECENT ISSUES

The Clinics are now available online!

Access your subscription at:
www.theclinics.com

Vet Clin Food Anim 21 (2005) xiii–xiv

VETERINARY
CLINICS
Food Animal Practice

Preface

Bovine Theriogenology

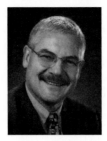

Grant S. Frazer, BVSc, MS, MBA
Guest Editor

When Dr. Bob Smith honored me with an invitation to serve as guest editor for an issue on cattle reproduction, my initial reaction was to say, "Thanks, but no thanks." It occurred to me, however, that this might be a good opportunity to promote the name of my veterinary specialty— theriogenology. The meaning of the word is still not widely appreciated, despite the fact that it is the name of a prestigious international scientific journal. When there are reproductive issues in human medicine, women visit an obstetrician and gynecologist, whereas men tend to seek out the advice of a urologist. Because veterinarians work with diverse reproductive problems in both genders, a new, all-encompassing term was proposed. The word theriomorphic means "thought of as having the form of a beast or animal," and was used to refer to certain Greek gods. Genesis is well-known to mean creation, coming into being, the beginning or origin. The suffix "-logy" refers to the science or study of, a branch of learning. The name theriogenology was adopted because it means "the study of the coming into being of the beast," that is, animal reproduction. The veterinary specialty of theriogenology embraces all aspects of animal reproduction (physiology, pharmacology, pathology, and surgery), including veterinary obstetrics, genital diseases, and the more recent "assisted reproduction" technologies. It is common practice to place the name of the relevant species with the term; thus the title of this issue of *Veterinary Clinics of North America: Food Animal Practice* is "Bovine Theriogenology."

My hope is that readers will find this issue to be a very helpful addition to their personal library. The goal was to provide a broad update that would be

doi:10.1016/j.cvfa.2005.03.003
vetfood.theclinics.com

of use to private practitioners, faculty and students in veterinary schools, animal scientists, and extension specialists. To my colleagues who contributed to this endeavor, I offer my sincere thanks. I take no credit for the quality of this issue. Its merits are due to the expertise and diligence of the authors. As is the case with any publication of this type, the articles reflect the opinions of the authors—supported, as necessary, by pertinent scientific references. Some of the material in this issue does challenge widely accepted dogma. I fully expect that my own article will be controversial, and have endeavored to support my rationale by extensive referencing of the scientific literature. If it causes some clinicians to reconsider their approach to postpartum uterine therapy, and stimulates my scientific colleagues to pursue further research in this important area, then I will have achieved my objective. Perhaps the following quote will place my approach in the correct context...

> *"Perhaps the sentiments contained in the following pages are not yet sufficiently fashionable to procure them general favor; a long habit of not thinking a thing wrong gives it a superficial appearance of being right, and raises at first a formidable outcry in defense of custom. But the tumult soon subsides. Time makes more converts than reason."*
> –Thomas Paine, *Common Sense*, February 14, 1776

I would like to thank John Vassallo from Saunders/Elsevier for his encouragement and patience during this issue's gestation, and for helping to prevent the occasional impending abortion. Lastly, a special thanks to my wife of 25 years. Lou's love and support have permitted me to achieve more in my professional career than I ever thought possible.

Grant S. Frazer, BVSc, MS, MBA
College of Veterinary Medicine
The Ohio State University
1920 Coffey Road
Columbus, OH 43210

E-mail address: frazer.6@osu.edu

ELSEVIER
SAUNDERS

VETERINARY
CLINICS
Food Animal Practice

Vet Clin Food Anim 21 (2005) 289–304

Troubleshooting Poor Reproductive Performance in Large Herds

Donald E. Sanders, DVM

Urbana Veterinary Clinic, Inc. 985 Norwood Avenue, Urbana, OH 43078, USA

When veterinary scholars and students discuss factors involved in diagnosing a disease or condition, they often speak in terms of examining individual animals. Like most veterinarians, this author was trained to examine an individual animal, make a diagnosis, and prescribe appropriate therapy.

But when a health condition involves a herd, the diagnostic process becomes complex and convoluted because of the interplay of determinants such as nutrition, housing and environment, diseases, management, and employee protocols. This certainly is true when examining a dairy herd set back by inefficient reproductive performance—one of the greatest challenges to a veterinarian's diagnostic skills.

This article inventories and examines many of the parameters that should be considered when investigating poor reproductive performance of a herd. Succeeding articles in this issue continue the discussion in greater depth.

Interview the herd manager and key individuals

Regardless of the sincerity, commitment, and skill of the investigator, the evaluation will likely fail without the wholehearted support of the herd's owner and manager. Oftentimes, the solution to reproductive inefficiency requires significant changes by the management. Seldom will a vaccination program or an additional nutrient "make it all better." Continuing follow-up is almost always necessary, either by the principal investigator or an attending veterinarian, on-site or through regular visits, to monitor implemented management changes and pregnancy examinations. Weekly

The author has a contract with Arm & Hammer Nutrition Group to provide his dairy management books and produce educational DVDs for use by their technical service staff.
E-mail address: dsanders@urbanavc.com

doi:10.1016/j.cvfa.2005.02.004   *vetfood.theclinics.com*

pregnancy examinations—with greater frequency in extremely large herds—are encouraged. If the principal investigator is not on-site, it is essential that an ongoing dialog be maintained between the respective experts and management.

Early in the investigation, the manager and key employees must be interviewed in order to gain an understanding of their perceptions of the problem. If the manager believes there is no problem, then the investigation will be very difficult. In other instances, the manager may acknowledge that a problem exists, but may need outside expertise to identify the changes required to manage it.

Records

Veterinarians have numerous parameters to measure in identifying and quantifying reproductive inefficiency. Accurate records are essential. The old axiom, "If you can't measure it, you can't manage it," certainly applies. If the problem is one of a low pregnancy rate [1], important factors to consider are the voluntary waiting period, interval to first service, heat detection methods and rate, and conception rate.

Other considerations: is the herd using reproductive protocols for follicle recruitment and timed insemination [2–4]? Is pregnancy wastage a problem? Early embryonic death? Abortions? Stillbirths? Does the herd use artificial insemination or natural service?

Pregnancy diagnosis

Also significant are the stage of pregnancy and frequency of diagnosis, and the method of diagnosis and skill of the diagnostician. The accuracy of diagnosis depends upon whether the procedure was rectal examination, ultrasonography, blood test [5], or milk test [6].

Routine health surveillance

By continually collecting information about a herd through the practice of routine health surveillance, a veterinarian has at his disposal a valuable bank of data for diagnosing inefficient reproductive performance. For example, when there is no obvious cause for an abortion, the veterinarian should routinely conduct a necropsy of the fetus and placenta, with diagnostic tests for virology, microbiology, and toxicology. It is important that this be incorporated with serological studies of aborting dams and several herdmates. Veterinarians rarely recommend pursuing such a practice, this author believes, because of the potentially low yield of diagnostic information, but it is important to remember that routine health surveillance is as much about building a data bank of information for managing a herd as it is about making a diagnosis of an individual case.

Various epidemiological tools should be included as a part of routine health surveillance. Naïve sentinel animals running with the herd are often very useful for detecting circulating bovine viral diarrhea virus (BVDV) [7]. BVDV can be a surreptitious enemy that often causes significant economic losses in a herd before the problem is discovered. Blood collected through an ongoing Johne's disease serology testing program can provide serum for excellent surveillance of BVDV and other diseases such as brucellosis, neosporosis, anaplasmosis, and leptospirosis (with the exception of *Leptosprira hardjo*).

Types of reproductive inefficiency

Infertility

Once reproductive inefficiency has been identified in a herd, the investigation should focus on determining the cause. Heat detection is a fundamental contributor to good reproductive performance. Conversely, in this author's observation, failure to detect heat is often a key contributor to infertility within a dairy herd.

Heat detection failure can be classified into several subsets. Cows may be in true anestrus, or they may cycle with unobserved estrus, which is often termed "silent heat." True anestrus may occur because of low body-condition scores, resulting in the ovaries failing to produce follicles. In "silent," or unobserved, estrus, the cows have follicular development and go through an estrus but do not exhibit visible signs. Sometimes the signs are not visible when cows are bothered by sore feet, slippery footing, or hot and humid environmental conditions. In other instances, those responsible for heat detection either do not observe the estrus or fail to recognize the signs.

Some persons responsible for heat detection may make inaccurate conclusions regarding a cow that is in heat. This is understandable, because cows often provide their caretakers little opportunity to observe estrus. It has been suggested by some experts that the average dairy cow either stands to be ridden or rides other cows for only 3 seconds seven to nine times during an average 7-hour estrus [8].

Low conception rates are another cause of reproductive inefficiency. Although low conception rates may be caused by an inherent problem within the cows, other common contributors to the problem are inadequately trained artificial insemination (AI) technicians and faulty thaw box thermometers or nitrogen tanks. This author has observed on many occasions low conception rates in herds infected by infectious bovine rhinotracheitis (IBR) or BVDV. It takes months after resolution of such infections before conception rates return to normal. In the case of BVDV, the problem often is not resolved until all persistently infected animals are identified and removed from the herd.

Low conception rates often are found in herds that have profound micronutrient deficiencies. As is discussed in the article by Ferguson elsewhere in this issue, trace minerals and vitamins, such as selenium, copper, zinc, and vitamins A, D and E, must be included in an investigation. Low conception rates also are characteristic of cows enrolled in follicle recruitment programs, because such cows are usually inseminated with the assumption that a dominant follicle has developed and is ready for ovulation [2]. Lower conception rates are offset because every cow is serviced at the end of the voluntary waiting period upon being enrolled in an insemination protocol.

Pregnancy loss

Pregnancy loss is divided into losses from early embryonic death (EED), abortions, and stillbirths. The article by Inskeep and Dailey on embryonic death elsewhere in this issue covers early embryonic loss in depth, but several observations are worth noting now. Any of these types of losses may have a complex etiology, which may require an intensive investigation should the initial preliminary diagnostic work-up prove unremarkable. EED losses may occur due to unskilled palpation technicians, nutritional deficiencies, mycotoxins in the feed, or diseases such as BVD and leptospirosis. Abortions are especially difficult to pin down unless there are several, allowing multiple diagnostic workups on each fetus.

Stillbirths are often not what they seem. Most may appear to be related to a slow birthing process, but records may reveal a disproportionate number that dictate further investigation [9]. It is this author's opinion that the normal incidence of stillbirths in pluriparous cows should be less than 5%, and that in primiparous cows less than 10%. If stillbirths appear excessive, did they occur in assisted or unassisted calvings? Were they to primiparous or pluriparous cows?

Etiology of reproductive inefficiency

Key management issues

The herd manager often has a major impact on reproductive inefficiency. He is the captain of the ship. The manager implements the protocols for the reproductive program and must diligently maintain a system to constantly track reproductive trends. Is reproductive performance cruising, or is the ship sinking?

It is important to have protocols in place for each component of the breeding program. Heat detection is best accomplished with tail chalking, heat detection patches, pedometers, or a computer transponder system such as Heat Watch (American Breeder Service, DeForest, Wisconsin). Many herd managers have opted for breeding programs that involve follicular recruitment and timed artificial insemination. Some of these follicular recruitment programs, such as PreSynch, OvSynch and ReSynch, discussed in the article on breeding strategies for dairy by Stevenson elsewhere in this issue, take the guesswork out of heat detection. Other managers choose a combination of heat detection methods, using tail paint and one of the timed breeding programs. Regardless of the choice, it is important to follow these protocols precisely as charted; imprecision often results in reproductive failure. This author recently evaluated a reproductive program that appeared to be correctly planned and implemented. The herd manager, however, was not entering data into the computer program so that the cows could be followed up appropriately, with either a prostaglandin or gonadotropin injection and then artificial insemination. Chaos ensued as the manager realized that cows were given the same injections they had received the previous week.

Many managers of large herds use software that allows them to track the results of various technicians who breed cows in the herd. Such software can reveal which technicians are more effective at breeding cows and obtaining pregnancies, presenting good managers the opportunity to shift personnel to tasks that best suit their skills. Of course, the disparity in results is not always a question of skill. Sometimes it can be attributed to a faulty thaw box thermometer or defective nitrogen tank, which results in damaged semen.

Impact of the energy balance on reproduction

There is probably no single issue that has a greater impact on reproduction than a cow's energy balance. A cow that has a negative energy balance may have impaired or total absence of follicular genesis. Most experts believe that primordial follicles start growing at 60 to 100 days before ovulation [10]. This implication is profound: many follicles are developing during late pregnancy before calving, or immediately after calving, when the cow's body is in a negative energy crisis! The cow is producing high levels of milk, yet her dry-matter intake is limited, so she is using her fat stores to maintain milk production. Cows that are over-conditioned will also subsequently have poor breeding performance at the next lactation, because excessive body condition almost always causes a metabolic crisis.

Lameness

Although the investigator may desire to focus on reproductive issues, he should not overlook lameness, which can cause reproductive inefficiency. Cows also affected by rumen acidosis, metabolic diseases at freshening, or laminitis, which leads to lameness, will surely be at risk for low reproductive performance, because these issues cause severe loss of body condition. The negative energy balance causes the ovaries to cease to function, and they become palpably smaller. Rumen acidosis caused by low effective fiber rations is not the only reason for lameness in cows. Lameness also may occur because of micronutrient deficiencies, poor environmental conditions, or a lack of routine foot health care, such as trimming and foot baths.

SANDERS

Recently, locomotion scoring [11] has given diagnosticians the criteria for measuring the degree of lameness. This scoring system has heightened attentiveness to lame cows, even when the condition is subtle.

Cows must have solid footing to exhibit normal estrous behavior. Slippery concrete flooring prevents cows from exhibiting normal signs of estrus. Failure to select for conformation may cause many cows in the herd to have badly shaped feet and legs. These issues are primarily a result of maternal sires in the genetic selection program.

Other factors to be considered include posterior digital dermatitis (hair warts), sole abscesses, heel cracks, and foot rot. All can have a profoundly negative effect on a herd's reproductive performance.

Dry cow transition diets

Years of research have shown that cows encountering metabolic diseases peripartum may be at higher risk for subsequent reproductive problems. For instance, cows that have milk fever, retained placenta, ketosis, or displaced abomasum are likely to become pregnant later in their production cycle.

The dry cow transition diet is one management practice that may virtually eliminate the risk associated with metabolic disease peripartum [12,13]. These rations, containing anionic salts, shift the cow's metabolic system toward acidosis. They change the dietary cation-anion difference (DCAD) to mobilize calcium from the bone reserves. The article by Melendez and Risco elsewhere in this issue addresses the specifics of these DCAD diets.

Another nutritional tool for preventing reproductive problems is Biochlor (Arm & Hammer Animal Nutrition, Princeton, New Jersey) a product that contains isonitrogenous protein and chlorine. The protein, which increases microbial synthesis in the rumen, combined with the natural occurring negative DCAD, often increases cows' dry-matter intake. Increased dry-matter intake and a negative DCAD prevent metabolic crises such as milk fever, retained placenta, ketosis, and displaced abomasum in cows at freshening. Cows on a transition diet with a minus DCAD component have a lower incidence of retained placenta, reduced days to first service, fewer services per conception, higher conception rates, shorter calving interval, and 7% to 10% increased milk production for the entire lactation (D.K. Beede, personal communication, 2004).

Impact of protein and mineral nutrition on reproduction

The article by Ferguson elsewhere in this issue addresses a number of nutritional issues that affect reproductive performance. It is important to note that excessive dietary protein or a deficit in starch may raise levels of blood urea nitrogen (BUN) and subsequently milk urea nitrogen (MUN). High BUN levels (>20 mg/dl) [14] indicate excessive dietary protein that is degraded but not recaptured and used. This raises ruminal ammonia, which the liver conjugates to urea. The urea circulates in the blood and is excreted by the kidneys, or enters the milk, as MUN. Occasionally the ammonia level rises higher than can be conjugated completely by the liver into urea. In this instance, ammonia may circulate and collect in tissue. Either condition—high BUN or tissue ammonia—is spermicidal and embryocidal; thus fertility will suffer when these diets are fed.

It is therefore important to formulate rations so that adequate energy is available for using the dietary protein and preventing high BUN.

Dietary energy has an important impact on reproduction. When a cow is in a negative energy balance, follicular development may be impaired. Cows naturally experience negative energy immediately after calving, a result of low dry-matter intake early in lactation and a large demand for energy in milk production. To summarize, every scenario that lowers a cow's dry-matter intake, ranging from metabolic diseases to poor foot health, causes a negative energy balance and puts the cows' reproductive health at risk.

Phosphorus

Phosphorus is essential for normal reproductive performance. Phosphorus deficiency is rare, because many nutritionists believe that "if a little is good, more is better," but excessive supplementation can be bad for the environment, just as phosphorus deficiency may be a problem for the cows. A deficiency problem is usually manifested in cows that are also protein or energy deficient. It is difficult to determine whether the cows are phosphorus deficient or suffering from malnutrition. They may not cycle, or may cycle but not show an outward expression of estrus. A deficiency should be suspected by evaluating body condition and analyzing the diet in conjunction with the symptoms. When a specific evaluation for phosphorus is required to eliminate confounding issues of dietary protein and energy, a small section of rib should be surgically removed and analyzed for phosphorus [15]. In some instances, phosphorus may be unavailable when high levels of heavy metals interfere with phosphorus absorption [15].

Copper

Although not as common as in years past, copper deficiency can have a major impact on many aspects of herd health and performance, including a profound influence on reproduction. Copper deficiency can be caused by a significant shortage of dietary copper, or as a result of other minerals binding to it and making it unavailable. Two minerals that can create a critical shortage of copper are molybdenum and sulfur. Soil pH and the accumulation of molybdenum by legumes are major players in copper use. Symptoms of copper deficiency include anemia, neonatal ataxia, diarrhea, anestrus, infertility, cystic ovaries, abortions, changes in hair pigmentation, reduced defense mechanism, heel cracks, spontaneous long bone fractures, myocardial fibrosis, and spontaneous rupture of the great vessels, such as the aorta [16].

Diagnosis is often an enigma. Diagnosis should be based on feed analyses, liver biopsies, serum copper or ceruloplasmin, and observation of symptoms. Hair analysis is unreliable [16]. Other tests, such as Cu, Zn superoxide dismutase, are useful, but have not been readily available.

Manganese

It is believed by the experts that manganese may cause reproductive dysfunction. In spite of this, no documented studies have demonstrated that manganese causes clinical infertility. It is known that manganese deficiency can cause testicular degeneration and defects in long-bone growth.

It is this author's opinion that supplementation to provide 40 to 60 parts per parts per million (ppm) of manganese is important in the bovine diet.

Selenium

Selenium can have a significant impact on reproduction. Selenium deficiency was such a critical issue in the past that probably more has been written about it and its effect on animal health and performance than any other mineral. Many areas around the world are considered selenium deficient [17]. It is well-documented that selenium deficiency compromises the bovine defense mechanism and causes retained placenta, cystic ovaries, infertility, and white muscle disease. It has also been shown to be closely integrated with vitamin E in its impact on bovine health.

Selenium-dependent glutathione peroxidase (Se-GPx) is a critical component in the reduction of free oxygen radicals, the defense mechanism, and the immune response. Diagnosis of deficiency is commonly done with either serum or whole blood selenium. Se-GPx can be used for diagnosis, and is especially helpful to retrospectively evaluate selenium status 60 to 90 days before the evaluation. Liver biopsies also are used for diagnosis.

Zinc

Zinc deficiency may cause reproductive inefficiency. It may cause skin lesions, lameness related to the integrity of the hoof, reduced conception rates, and decreased sperm maturation. Diagnosis is made with serum zinc analysis. One caveat is that the rubber stoppers of ordinary serum tubes are contaminated with zinc. Special vials without a residue of zinc should be used.

Implications of micronutrient deficiencies

When evaluating the status of dietary micronutrients, it is important to remember this author's observation that rarely is a single micronutrient the culprit for pervasive reproduction difficulties. One should not be complacent after identifying one deficiency, because it is common for more than one trace mineral to be lacking. It also is common for deficiencies in these minerals to be accompanied by infections such as BVDV, mycoplamosis, chlamydiosis, and other pathogens.

Impact of fat-soluble vitamins on reproduction

Vitamins A, D & E

Forages with low levels of these vitamins may adversely affect reproduction. This primarily occurs in the winter months after forages have been stored for several months [18]. Vitamin A shortages, which can result from the vitamin being tied up by excessive nitrates in the diet, may cause abortions, weak calves, and night blindness. Diagnosis is made by serum analysis. It is essential to freeze serum immediately to prevent the decay of vitamin A in the serum.

Vitamin D

Vitamin D deficiency is rarely seen in cattle because every feed company supplements vitamin and mineral packages with vitamin D_3. In addition, animals exposed to sunlight manufacture vitamin D in their skin.

Vitamin E

Vitamin E deficiency occurs in forages stored for long periods of time. This is particularly true of ensiled forages. The symptoms of deficiency include a reduced defense mechanism, cystic ovaries, high somatic cell counts (SCC), and retained placenta. It is difficult to sort out vitamin E's interactions with selenium [19]. Vitamin E is an important reducing agent in the metabolic processes to neutralize free oxygen radicals and convert them to CO_2 and water. Recent research has demonstrated the value of injected vitamin E to lower SCC and the incidence of mastitis in cows near parturition [18].

Impact of essential fatty acids on reproduction

One of the more exciting nutritional developments in food animal production is research demonstrating the benefits of feeding unsaturated and polyunsaturated fatty acids during late pregnancy and in the early postpartum period. It has been reported that the pregnancy rate can be improved as much as 19%, often with a boost in milk production of six pounds (Elliott Block, personal communication, 2004) [20].

Unsaturated and polyunsaturated fatty acids are the substrate for synthesis of the endocrine hormones used in reproduction. When these fatty acids are low, pregnancy rates tend to be lower. Indications for more unsaturated and polyunsaturated fatty acids can be determined by using CPM software (Center for Animal Health and Productivity at the University of Pennsylvania at New Bolton Center, Kennett Square, Pennsylvania) in ration formulation, with an analysis projection of fatty acids in the diet. The C:18:2 duodenal absorption of fatty acids will usually be less than 60 g/day in low unsaturated fatty acid diets. Generally, .25 lb of unsaturated and polyunsaturated fatty acids (Megalac-R, Arm & Hammer Animal Nutrition) is fed to transitional cows. This is increased to .5 lb/cow during lactation, until the cow is confirmed pregnant. Other fatty acid sources, such as fish oil, whole cottonseed, and vegetable oils, will not supply unsaturated and polyunsaturated fatty acids.

Environment and reproduction

Limited amounts of controlled research have been reported regarding environmental effects on reproduction, yet practitioners commonly observe that the environment can make a major difference on cows' reproductive performance. Slippery or defective concrete causes many injuries to dairy cows, and when cows become apprehensive on slippery concrete, they make tentative movements and little effort to demonstrate signs of estrus. Barns that have slatted floors pose a similar problem for cows, because hooves can get caught or twisted between slats.

Cows also perform poorly in hot and humid conditions. To counteract this, significant strides have been made with evaporative cooling through the use of misting systems and air movement by powerful fans located strategically over feeding areas and free stalls [21].

Free stalls that are uncomfortable for cows have an indirect impact on reproductive performance. During a quiet time of the day, nearly all of the cows should be lying in free stalls with their tails to the alley. When stalls are uncomfortable, cows tend to stand or find somewhere else to lie. If they stand for a substantial portion of the day, they tend to develop rumen acidosis. They chew their cuds less and secrete less saliva for rumen buffering, causing rumen acidosis that leads to laminitis. When cows have laminitis, they often eat less and lose weight and body condition. Low body-condition scores tend to reduce conception rates and ovarian function. This scenario is common when cows are not comfortable.

Impact of toxicities on reproduction

Mycotoxin toxicity

A number of mycotoxins affect reproduction. They range from estrogen-containing mycotoxins, such as zeralanone and deoxynivenal (DON), to mycotoxins such as T-2 toxins, other trichocethenes, and patulin, which have an indirect effect as they negatively impact the overall health of the cow. A good rule of thumb for the practitioner is that mycotoxins that are reported in ppb, with the exception of aflatoxins, are not likely to be a problem.

Although there are Food and Drug Administration (FDA) and food safety concerns with aflatoxin, the chance of having an impact on reproduction with only aflatoxin is low. Mycotoxins from the *Fusarium* spp molds, such as DON, T-2, and ochratoxins, are not likely to be a problem when fewer than five ppm. Because of their profound effect on bovine health, other toxins, such as patulin (produced by *Penicillium* spp), should never be ignored when detected.

The best method for addressing mycotoxins is to dilute or remove the offending feed; however, it is often difficult for management to do this. In these cases, mycotoxin binding agents often appear to be helpful. Unfortunately, little research on mycotoxin binding has been conducted with ruminant animals, so research data involving the control of mycotoxins in monogastric animals is often applied to ruminant rations.

Iodine toxicity

Most experts cite concerns about iodine deficiency. Although this may be a concern in countries where salt and minerals do not contain supplemental iodine, in the United States deficiency is seldom an issue. Toxicity may become an issue when cows are fed multiple sources of iodine-containing minerals. In the past, it was also common to feed kelp to dairy cows to enhance micronutrient supplementation. Kelp may contain from 100 to 1,000 ppm of iodine. This may make significant contributions to iodine toxicity [22]. Five mg/kg of iodine in the feed is toxic to dairy cows, and may cause abortions of hairless calves. Cows may also exhibit symptoms consistent with a reduced defense mechanism—unthriftiness, poor performance, and low pregnancy rates.

Milk from cows that have toxic dietary levels of iodine also poses a human health hazard. Iodine level in milk is directly correlated to dietary intake of iodine. Milk normally contains 30 to 300 ugm/ml of iodine. Levels higher than this will cause thyrotoxicosis in humans.

Vitamin D toxicity

Vitamin D toxicity, in this author's opinion, is a more significant problem than vitamin D deficiency. It occurs when dietary vitamin D levels are in excess of 40,000 international units (IU) per day in large-breed dairy cows. Occasionally this can happen when several vitamin and mineral supplements from different feed manufacturers are fed to cows. When each of these mineral sources has been laced with vitamin D, toxicity may occur. This author has determined that some diets contain vitamin D in excess of 100,000 IU/day. Vitamin D toxicity impairs ovarian function, and in some instances, can cause acute death [18,23,24]. The practitioner will have a difficult assignment making this diagnosis without carefully calculating vitamin D dietary intake and collecting blood for serum vitamin D analyses.

Poisonous plant toxicity

Numerous plants are capable of causing abortions in cattle; however, any impact poisonous plants have on reproductive performance is usually miniscule compared with the impact on the overall health of individual animals. Rarely does plant toxicity affect a whole dairy herd, but cows are more likely to die as a result of poisonous plants than from other sources of toxicity. Thus, the practitioner should check for plants such as lambs quarter, nightshade, jimson weed, fescue, and fall panicum, if any of these forages is suspected to be a major contributor to the diet.

Gossypol toxicity

Gossypol is routinely detected in whole cottonseed and cottonseed products. It has been shown that free gossypol in levels as low as 6 gm/head/day lowers fertility in bulls, and 10 gm/head/day does the same in cows. Whole cottonseed commonly contains 1.0% to 1.5% gossypol. It does not take a rocket scientist to calculate that any ration containing 4 to 5 lb/head/day of gossypol-containing whole cottonseed may contribute to herd infertility [25–27]. The important point to this discussion is that gossypol toxicity is cumulative and ultimately has a luteolytic effect on the ovaries (M.C. Calhoun, personal communication, 1996). In addition, bulls running with the herd and being fed whole cottonseed are at risk.

Inappropriate prostaglandin $F_{2\alpha}$ injection

Either because of incomplete record keeping or faulty identification, herd managers sometimes administer prostaglandin to pregnant cows, and there is probably no bovine practitioner who has not at some point in his career given an injection of prostaglandin to a cow to induce estrus, only to receive a report that the cow aborted a fetus. For cows less than 5 to 6 months pregnant, this error usually will result in an abortion.

Prevention of such incidents can be achieved only by sharpening record keeping and accurately identifying every animal. It is also important for practitioners to maintain keen pregnancy diagnosis skills to ensure no loss of pregnancies. Practitioners should consider using ultrasound examinations, particularly when herd managers are complaining of inaccuracies in pregnancy diagnosis. Herd managers should be very cautious about using pregnancy technicians in place of a veterinarian to diagnose pregnancy.

Impact of infectious diseases on reproduction

Leptospirosis, BVDV, IBR, neosporosis, and mycoplasma are considered to be in the mainstream of diseases that can affect reproductive efficiency in dairy cattle. Lesser known diseases impacting reproduction include listeriosis, salmonellosis, anaplasmosis, and babesiosis. Few dairymen are aware that every clinical case of mastitis has the potential to cause a cow to lose her pregnancy. Other articles in this issue discuss some of these diseases in more detail, including those by Grooms and Bolin, Dubey, and BonDurant.

Fixing the problem

Veterinarians and dairymen often have the "one-factor" mindset regarding the cause of a herd reproductive problem; however, it is this author's experience that one etiological diagnosis rarely is the sole cause. In many instances, after an investigation is conducted other factors not previously detected tend to crop up.

When faced with multiple factors, it helps to start by focusing on an issue that will be relatively easy to correct before taking on the more challenging ones. Chances for success also will be improved if the dairy operation stands to realize a significant financial reward by correcting the problem.

On the other hand, economic realities can delay implementation of many recommended courses of action. In such cases, managers live with the problem until they can make necessary, expensive facility and management changes. In other instances, correction of obvious problems and the rewards of doing so provide managers a comfort level at which they have no desire to pursue deeper management changes.

Prioritizing the issues to be addressed

To increase the opportunity for success, the practitioner and herd manager should select no more than a couple of factors to fix at a time. And to help raise morale, it is an excellent idea to target factors that can result in a real payoff, such as increased milk production.

Remember, it is extremely important to be able to measure the herd's performance before and after the management changes. The practitioner and management should have at least one or two barometers that can be measured weekly or monthly. This monitoring may be as simple as tracking the incidence of retained placenta, percentage of pregnancy at each herd check, interval to first service, or the pregnancy rate for the month.

Motivating key personnel

This author at times has been frustrated when working to fix a major problem, only to realize that the issues are beyond the management's scope and ability to motivate the work force. Motivating a dairy's staff can be one of the most rewarding or frustrating tasks in solving reproductive inefficiency. The key to success is getting management and employees to internalize the importance of making changes in protocols and performance. Veterinary consultants must realize, however, that many managers and key employees are set in their ways and will never change. Nonetheless, veterinarians may soften some of these seemingly un-compromising attitudes through honest, tactful communication about what the dairy operation has to gain or lose. One of the answers to getting such individuals to internalize the problem and accept the needed course of action is to make clear the profound economic impact of doing nothing.

The practitioner may find that it sometimes takes word pictures and other creative communication strategies to make a lasting, and changing, impression upon a manager. Here are a couple of examples used by this author:

Example 1

Joe was a client who often chose to exert the least effort in the management of his cows. Problems that chronically needed to be addressed in his herd were low milk production and low dry-matter intake. In addition to several other concerns, it was suspected by this author that the cows were not consuming enough water. Evaluation of the water supply indicated that additional watering locations were needed, and that the existing watering stations were extremely filthy. Joe agreed to an additional water tank, but it was soon as filthy as the other sources. Each of the tanks had a foot of black, sulfur-containing debris on the bottom, with about a foot of water on the surface. After hearing Joe's incessant excuses about not having time to clean the tanks in several discussions, this author used a camera to take Joe's photo standing beside them, explaining that the pictures would be used in a presentation on water consumption at a statewide meeting in another region of the country. This author promised to protect his identity. Joe did not say much, but it was apparent he had been reached. On subsequent visits, his tanks were clean and filled with clear water. The postscript is that Joe is no longer in the dairy business, for reasons other than the cleanliness of his water tanks.

Example 2

Tom's dairy herd had a chronic SCC problem. His sons, Terry and John, milked the cows. Frequent visits to the farm by this author revealed that they always took shortcuts in the milking preparation of each cow, in spite of promising to follow the recommended protocol. Especially galling was their refusal to wear rubber gloves during milking. After it was apparent that any further discussion about milking preparation was falling on deaf ears, this author spent a few minutes reiterating how easily their hands spread mastitis pathogens from cow to cow. A culture obtained from each of the son's hands was later brought to the dairy farm to demonstrate the pathogen load they were spreading. It was apparent that neither of them was totally ready to accept the results. So, this author asked them, "Why take a chance? Maybe you think you don't have to wear gloves to milk your cows, but you might consider slipping on a pair of gloves to protect yourselves from what's on your hands when you need to urinate!" They both had shocked looks on their faces, and they now wear gloves during milking.

Developing a plan

With input from management and key employees, the practitioner needs to develop written protocols and recommendations for correcting the identified issues. Next, the practitioner should train supervisors and employees on how to implement the plan. He should not assume that the plan is idiot-proof. Follow-up is essential—monitoring the performance of the key individuals, observing for the expected outcomes, and sharing the results with all parties involved.

Turnover of employees is common, so it is important to train new staff members in the recommended steps that are to be followed. Protocols should be reviewed and revised as needed with the existing staff, and the practitioner can discuss with the manager incentives to offer employees for a job well done.

References

[1] Pursley JR, Wiltbank MC, Stevenson JS, et al. Pregnancy rates in cows and heifers inseminated at a synchronized ovulation or synchronized estrus. J Dairy Sci 1997;80: 295–300.

[2] Wiltbank MC. Troubleshooting and improving reproductive management of lactating dairy cattle. Dairy Comp 305 Reference Manual. Madison (WI): Department of Dairy Science, University of Wisconsin Valley Ag Software; 2000.

[3] Burke JM, de la Sota RL, Risco CA, et al. Evaluation of timed insemination using a gonadotropin-releasing hormone agonist in lactating dairy cows. J Dairy Sci 1996;79: 1385–93.

[4] Pursley JR, Wiltbank MC, Stevenson JS, et al. Pregnancy rates per artificial insemination for cows and heifers inseminated at a synchronized ovulation or synchronized estrus. J Dairy Sci 1997;80:295–300.

[5] Humblot P, Camous S, Martal J, et al. Diagnosis of pregnancy by radioimmunoassay of a pregnancy-specific protein in the plasma of dairy cows. Theriogenology 1988;30(2):257–67.

[6] DesCôteaux L, Carrière PD. Evaluation of the early conception factor (ECF) dip stick test in dairy cows between days 11 and 15 post-breeding. The Bovine Practitioner 2000;34:87.

[7] Kelling CL, Grotelueschen DM, Smith DR, et al. Testing and management strategies for effective beef and dairy bBiosecurity programs. The Bovine Practitioner 2000;34(1):13–22.

[8] Nebel RL, Jobst SM, Dransfield MBG, et al. Use of a radiofrequency data communication system, HeatWatch®, to describe behavioral estrus in dairy cattle. J Dairy Sci 1997;80 (Suppl 1):151.

[9] Radostits OM, Blood DC, Gay CC, editors. Veterinary medicine, part one, section on congenital defects. London: Bailliere Tindall; 1994. p. 113.

[10] Ginther OJ, Kot K, Kulick LJ, et al. Relationships between FSH and ovarian follicular waves during the last six months of pregnancy in cattle. Journal of Reproduction and Fertility 1996;108:271–9.

[11] Sprecher DJ, Hostetler DE, Kaneene JB. Locomotion scoring of dairy cattle. Theriogenology 1997;47:1178–87.

[12] Beede DK, Risco CA, Donovan GA, et al. Nutritional management of the late pregnant dry cow with particular reference to dietary cation-anion difference and calcium supplementation. Proceedings of the 24th Annual Convention of the American Association of Bovine Practitioners, Orlando Florida, September 20, 1991.

[13] Block E. Manipulation of dietary cation-anion difference on nutritionally related production diseases, productivity and metabolic responses of dairy cows. J Dairy Sci 1994;77:1437–50.

[14] Ferguson JD, Galligan DT, Blanchard T, et al. Serum urea nitrogen and conception rate: the usefulness of test information. J Dairy Sci 1993;76:3742–6.

[15] Puls R. Mineral levels in animal health. 2nd edition. British Columbia, Canada: Sherpa International; 1994. p. 208.

[16] Sanders DE. Copper deficiency in food animals. An enigma. Compendium for Continuing Education for the Practicing Veterinarian 1983;5(8):S404–10.

[17] Smith KL, Hogan JS, Conrad HR. Selenium in dairy cattle: its role in disease resistance. Veterinary Medicine 1988;72–8.

[18] Nutrient requirements of dairy cattle. 7th revised edition. Washington, DC: National Academy Press; 2001. p. 162–8.

[19] Weiss WP. Requirements of fat-soluble vitamins for dairy cows: a review. J Dairy Sci 1998; 81:2493–501.

[20] Thomas MG, Bao B, Williams GL. Dietary fats varying in their fatty acid composition differentially influence follicular growth in cows fed isoenergetic diets. J Anim Sci 1997;75: 2512–9.

[21] Smith JF, Brouk MJ. Sept. 20, 2003. Managing heat stress in dairy facilities. Proceedings of American Association of Bovine Practitioners Annual Meeting, Vol. 35.

[22] Goss JP, Sept. 21, 2004. New developments in dairy cattle mineral nutrition. Proceedings American Association of Bovine Practitioners.

[23] Gregg WA. Hypervitaminosis D in cattle. Proceedings XVII Congreso Mundial De Veterinaria, vol. 1, Hannover 14–21. August 1963. p. 233.

[24] Herdt TH, Stowe HD. Fat-soluble vitamin nutrition for dairy cattle. Vet Clin North Am Food Anim Pract 1991;7:391–415.

[25] Risco CA. Understanding gossypol toxicity problems in feeding cotton by-products to ruminant livestock. Presented at the 11th Annual Florida Ruminant Nutrition Symposium Gainesville, FL, January, 13–14, 1993.

[26] Morgan SE. Gossypol as a Toxicant in Livestock. Vet Clin North Am Food Anim Pract 1989;5(2):251–62.

[27] Randel RD. Effects of gossypol on reproductive performance of domestic livestock. Overton (TX): Texas A & M University Agricultural Research and Extension Center; 2000.

ELSEVIER
SAUNDERS

Vet Clin Food Anim 21 (2005) 305–323

VETERINARY
CLINICS
Food Animal Practice

Reproductive Record Analysis

Cheyney Meadows, VMD

*Department of Veterinary Preventive Medicine, College of Veterinary Medicine,
The Ohio State University, A100W Sisson Hall, 1920 Coffey Road, Columbus,
OH 43210, USA*

Nationally, over 25,000 herds with more than 4 million cows participate in a Dairy Herd Improvement Association (DHIA) testing plan in conjunction with a Dairy Record Processing Center (DRPC) [1]. Countless other herds use on-farm record keeping systems to maintain information. Technological advances continue to enhance the ease and speed at which information can be recorded, transmitted, and processed, and have made records very accessible for analysis beyond interpretation of mailed test-day reports. A systematic approach to the analysis of reproductive records can yield quality information to enhance herd visits in promoting health and productivity of herds serviced by veterinarians. This article describes methods for interpreting DHIA reproductive performance data generated by off-farm DRPCs in the United States. Procedures described here have been used with data generated by two of five DRPCs listed by the Animal Improvement Programs Laboratory of the United States Department of Agriculture. The methods should be applicable using data generated by other DRPCs—although there are subtle differences among DRPCs in calculating some of the reproductive measures described, they are largely uniform because procedures and calculations are approved by DHIA [2].

Using records and presenting information

Before discussing any methodology, it is important to emphasize that analysis and interpretation of dairy records is a supplement to, but will never replace, the herd visit in the provision of services to clients. With reproductive record analysis, problems noted during a herd visit can be characterized with respect to the extent and severity of inefficiencies. Records are also useful in establishing baseline performance levels, setting

E-mail address: meadows.27@osu.edu

goals for improvement, and for monitoring changes over time. Thorough review of records can also be used to detect and initiate investigation of potential problems in herd health or management; however, any issues raised by records analysis need to be confirmed with observations made during a herd visit. Thus, interpretation of dairy records and the herd visit complement each other—problems detected on-farm can be described with the help of records review, and records review can highlight areas to inspect during a herd visit.

When sifting through herd data, it is beneficial to use techniques that simplify the process of reviewing records and make communication of findings with the client easy. Graphical summaries of reproductive indices over a history of test days are a useful way to organize information for review and presentation. Graphical exploration of the data offers opportunities to identify and illustrate relationships among measures used in analysis, as well as to describe the time course of any problems and to determine if situations are improving or worsening. Graphical analysis of herd data is usually straightforward, because herd data are typically available in electronic format, and DRPCs offer specialized software packages that can generate graphical reports. Herd data in electronic format can also be exported to productivity software packages, such as spreadsheet or database programs, for analysis.

Framework for analysis

An organized approach to records analysis assists in the extraction of useful information from the data. Fig. 1 presents a layout of a systematic approach to reproductive record analysis. It identifies key indices that are relatively easy to comprehend as they relate to each other and to herd health and management. The approach discussed here starts with an overall summary measure of reproductive performance, and then systematically examines measurable components related to it in two different periods of breeding. Each measurable component is then evaluated individually, and health and management factors impacting these components are considered for their potential to affect reproductive performance. For any measure used in analysis, it is important to be aware of benchmark values (which are often very difficult to achieve) and to be able to gauge the herd's potential for improvement.

Selecting an overall summary of reproductive performance

Average calving interval (CI) or the closely related measure average days open (DO) have been used extensively to summarize the reproductive performance of dairy herds. Cows in herds with fewer DO or shorter CI produce more milk per day of herd life [3] and yield more replacement animals [4], so lower values of DO and CI are usually preferable in terms of

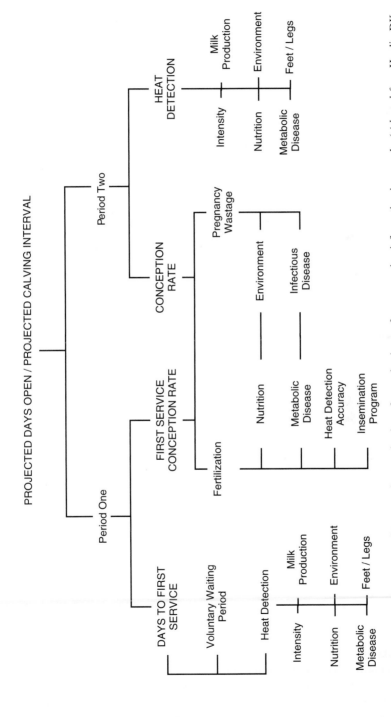

Fig. 1. Flow chart outlining a systematic approach to evaluation of reproductive performance using information in records. (*Adapted from* Hardin DK. Fertility and infertility assessment by review of records. Vet Clin North Am Food Anim Pract 1993;9(2):393; with permission.)

herd profitability [5,6]. Although longer calving intervals may be acceptable in some circumstances for high-producing (primiparous cows averaging 11,232 kg and multiparous cows averaging 12,767 kg 305-day mature equivalent milk) cows [7], it is generally agreed that a 13-month calving interval is the economically optimal target [6,8]. Using a 280-day gestation for Holstein cows, the 13-month CI corresponds to approximately 115 DO.

It is important to understand how DO and CI are calculated and reported. Typically, DRPCs report two versions of CI: (1) historical CI (HCI), which is the average time between successive calvings for the same cow; and (2) projected CI (PCI), which is based on a calculated measure known as projected DO (PDO). There are considerable limitations in using HCI to monitor herd reproductive performance. In order for a cow to have HCI measured, she must have calved at least twice, which means that the HCI only summarizes reproductive performance of multiparous cows. Also, the HCI measurement has a lot of lag, meaning that a herd with problems getting cows pregnant today will not show increased HCI until these cows finally settle and then recalve at least 9 months in the future. Likewise, if a herd makes positive changes in its reproductive program today and achieves earlier pregnancies, a shorter HCI will not be noticed for at least 9 months.

The PDO and PCI are better alternatives for monitoring overall herd reproductive efficiency, because they overcome limitations described for HCI. Projected CI is a standard gestation (usually 280 days) added to PDO, which is the weighted average of PDO for three populations of cows defined by the American Association of Bovine Practitioners (AABP) [9]:

1. For cows diagnosed pregnant, PDO is the days from calving to conception.
2. For bred cows without a pregnancy diagnosis, it is assumed that they are pregnant, and PDO is the days from calving to most recent breeding.
3. For cows beyond the voluntary waiting period (VWP) and not yet bred, and for previously bred cows that are known to be open, it is assumed that they will be inseminated and become pregnant in 10 days.

Each of the two DRPCs used by this author follow slightly different definitions for the third population of cows—one uses the greater of current days in milk (DIM) plus 10 or average days to first service for the entire herd [10]; the other uses current DIM, but only for cows more than 30 days beyond VWP [11]. The differences in PDO between the AABP methodology and that of the DRPCs are small; however, it should be noted that because the calculations for PDO assume that all bred cows of unknown status (population 2) are pregnant and that all open cows eligible to be bred (population 3) will become pregnant in a short period of time, these methods of calculation represent a minimum estimate of DO. Therefore PCI is a best-case minimum estimate of the CI that will be realized in the future [9,12].

Although PDO and PCI represent a best-case estimate of reproductive efficiency, they are still very useful measures because they are calculated using current information from as many herd members as possible [9]. Coupled with their relationship to milk and calf yield and overall herd profitability, PDO and PCI are good summary measures to begin evaluation of dairy reproductive records. Because PCI is based on PDO, the remainder of this article focuses on PDO as the overall summary measure from which to begin records analysis.

The effect of culling on projected days open

Before discussion of measurable components of efficiency in dairy records, reproductive culling needs attention. It is known to distort PDO, because open cows with extended DO are often removed from the herd and may be omitted from DRPC calculations. Reproductive failure is the most common reason for removal from the herd, with an average of 20% and a range of 0% to 45% of culling attributable to reproductive failure [13]. High reproductive culling rates will cause the PDO and PCI measures to be low [12,14]. Fig. 2 shows the relationship between PDO and reproductive culling rate for herds with different levels of reproductive efficiency. In Fig. 2, it can be seen that an inefficient herd (represented by lower heat detection rate) with high reproductive culling rate may have PDO similar to a more efficient herd (represented by higher heat detection rate) with low reproductive culling rate. This presents a challenge in record interpretation—changes in culling rate may mask some changes in PDO. It is important to be aware of this effect, particularly when herds are monitored

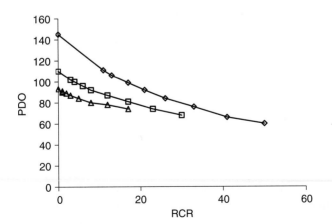

Fig. 2. Graph illustrating the relationship between predicted days open (PDO) and annual reproductive culling rate (RCR) for herds with different levels of reproductive efficiency, assuming a 50-day voluntary waiting period. Levels of reproductive efficiency are: (◇) 40% HDR, 50% CR; (□) 60% HDR, 50% CR; (△) 80% HDR, 50% CR. (*Data from* Esslemont RJ. Relationship between herd calving to conception interval and culling rate for failure to conceive. Vet Rec 1993;133:163–4.)

over time—PDO may change little in the face of improving or worsening reproduction because of changes in culling. Processing centers do report on the herd's annual culling rate and reasons for removal. The utility of reproductive indices, particularly PDO, is questionable in herds that exhibit high annual reproductive culling (over 15%) or high overall annual culling (over 45%). Also, analysts should be cautious in comparing data from different points in time if culling changes more than 10% between the points in time.

Estrus detection and conception and projected days open

Fig. 1 indicates that PDO is only a starting point for analyzing reproductive records—an understanding of measurable components of reproductive performance that are related to PDO is important. Estrus or heat detection rate (HDR) and conception rate (CR) have been identified as the two most important determinants of PDO [15], and it follows that HDR and CR should be monitored with respect to PDO.

Estrus detection and conception can be monitored in DHIA reproductive records during distinct periods of dairy cow breeding. Bailey et al [16] described record analysis during the preservice period, representing the time from calving to first insemination; and the postservice period, the time from first insemination until pregnancy diagnosis. A similar approach is used here to monitor estrus detection and conception in two distinct periods: period one is the time from calving until the outcome of the first insemination is known, whereas period two monitors cows requiring more than one service. Partitioning records analysis into periods helps to identify and characterize strengths and weaknesses of reproductive performance in relation to early (period one) or later (period two) lactation. Graphical exploration of relationships between PDO and measures of estrus detection and conception in each period are emphasized. When focusing on a single reproductive measure, it is important to be aware that changes in other measures may act to modify the effect.

Monitoring efficiency in period one

As mentioned previously, period one covers the time from calving to the outcome of the first breeding. Efficiency in this period can be monitored in DHIA records using the herd's average days to first service (DFS), and the first service conception rate (FSCR). The DFS for the herd is the average DIM when cows are inseminated for the first time, and FSCR is the proportion of cows that settle to first service [10,11]. Herds should try to have low DFS and high FSCR; however, herds must find a balance between DFS and FSCR, because there is evidence that earlier DFS is associated with a lower FSCR [17–19].

Monitoring days to first service

Herds with lower DFS have shorter HCI [20], and a recent study [15] observed that a 1-day decrease in DIM at first estrus (which was highly correlated with DFS) was associated with a 0.6-day decrease in PDO. To achieve a goal of 115 PDO, a reasonable target for DFS is VWP + 18 days [21]. A 60-day VWP is typically assumed in DRPC calculations and is appropriate for most farms [10], so a target value for DFS is between 75 and 80 days. A graphical analysis is an easy way to explore relationships between DFS and PDO.

Fig. 3 presents DHIA data from a dairy herd that demonstrates the association between DFS and PDO—generally, during periods of earlier DFS, this herd's PDO tends to decrease. Fig. 3 emphasizes the strengths of graphical exploration of records—although not perfect, a relationship between DFS and PDO has clearly presented itself and would be easy to communicate to the producer. The next step is to work with the producer to try to determine why DFS has changed over time and what can be done to ensure that cows are consistently inseminated in a timely fashion in order to reduce DFS and capture benefits of reduced PDO.

Days to first service is affected by the herd's VWP and heat detection (see Fig. 1). A shorter VWP is associated with earlier DFS [22], and herds with higher HDR have lower DFS [23]. It is worthy to mention also that calculation of PDO is affected by the herd's reported VWP, in that changing the VWP setting in DRPC calculations will change the PDO (by changing population 3 in the AABP calculation listed earlier). Producers looking to reduce DFS should consider their breeding policy with respect to VWP, but make sure that values reported to DRPCs match actual practice in the herd

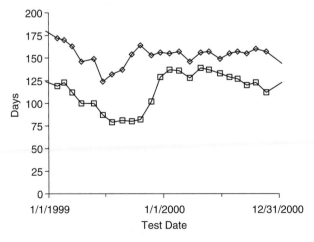

Fig. 3. Graph illustrating a relationship over time between predicted days open (◇) and days to first service (□) for a dairy herd.

[10]. Also, changing VWP from a management perspective only means that cows will be considered eligible for breeding earlier in lactation. Execution of this still requires that cows be detected in estrus and inseminated; thus estrus detection is a critical determinant of DFS, and it requires that cows are cycling, express estrus, and are observed by management. Failure to detect estrus in early lactation cows can be related to any of these factors (cycling cows, expression of estrus, detection of estrus), reflecting overlapping concerns of cow health and herd management (see Fig. 1).

Intensity of estrus detection is strictly management-related—devoting more time and effort or using multiple estrus detection aids should increase heat detection [24], and thus reduce DFS. The importance of educating herd personnel about the signs of estrus, of watching cows for estrus, and of maintaining a reliable system for recording which cows are standing cannot be overemphasized during the herd visit. Herd managers who wish to reduce DFS should consider increasing the frequency or time spent watching cows, the use of estrus detection aids, or even ovulation synchronization (OvSynch) protocols coupled with timed artificial insemination (TAI).

The effect of high milk production on overall reproductive performance has been examined numerous times, often focusing on conception in high-yielding cows. A recent study [25] used a radiotelemetry system to record frequency and duration of standing estrus behavior, and found that higher milk yield was associated with decreased duration and intensity of estrus, possibly due to increased hepatic blood flow and increased metabolic clearance of circulating estradiol. Herds with high milk yield in early lactation may present challenges in detecting estrus, and thus have delayed DFS. Again, OvSynch protocols and TAI may be of use in herds with delayed DFS associated with high milk production in early lactation.

It has been suggested that nutritional factors, such as excessive loss of body condition due to energy demands of lactation exceeding nutritional supply, can affect ovarian physiology and delay the time from calving to resumption of ovarian cyclicity [26]. High-producing cows are at risk of being in negative energy balance, but so too are average and even low producers that do not get adequate nutrition. During the herd visit, body condition of pre-fresh cows should be compared with cows in early lactation near the end of the VWP. Evidence of excessive condition loss may be a reason for delayed DFS, and producers in this situation should consider if their nutritional program can improve their reproductive performance.

Environmental conditions such as summer heat can impair ovarian function and cyclicity [27], and thus affect estrus expression and delay DFS. Producers are limited in their ability to control the weather, but efforts can be made in barn design and layout to ameliorate summer heat stress. Other environmental conditions, such as poor footing, can limit mounting activity and impair estrus expression and delay DFS. The herd visit should include an assessment of ventilation and floor surfaces of the barn if extended DFS is a problem in the herd.

Diseases in transition cows, such as milk fever, retained fetal membranes, metritis, ketosis, and displaced abomasum, have been shown to be associated with delays in time to pregnancy [28]. A possible mechanism may be that cows "start slowly," have poor feed intake, and lose body condition, which can affect heat detection and DFS. Assessment of the incidence of these diseases as well as of management actions that may increase risk of occurrence is an important aspect of the herd visit. Cow health during the time around calving can have impacts on reproductive efficiency months later.

A final important cow health factor affecting estrus expression and DFS is feet and leg health—lameness can delay DFS [29]. The herd visit should assess locomotive abilities of cows as a potential cause for delayed DFS due to impaired estrus expression; however, identification of lameness represents only a sign of an underlying problem. Potential causes of lameness are numerous, and may include management, diet, environmental conditions, or infectious disease. Again, the herd visit is very important to assess the presence, potential impact, and possible causes of lameness in relation to DFS and reproductive performance.

Monitoring first service conception rate

The second important component of PDO measured during the period one is the FSCR. In DHIA records, DRPCs report overall and service-specific CR (including FSCR) as the proportion of bred cows that are diagnosed pregnant [10,11]. It has been suggested that a normal FSCR is 45%, but that 60% FSCR is attainable [30]. Although there is an association with reduced FSCR at earlier DFS, herds should be able to achieve FSCR of 50% by 75 to 80 DFS [31].

Fig. 4 shows data from a herd that displays an association between FSCR and PDO. During the 2-year period shown, FSCR declined and PDO increased; however, the records analysis only illustrates a relationship between two measures—the critical role of the veterinarian is to consider factors that can cause a decline in FSCR and a resultant increase in PDO. The herd visit would allow exploration of potential reasons for the drop in FSCR, and allow the management team to try to correct the problem.

Because pregnancy diagnosis occurs about 5 to 6 weeks after breeding, FSCR (and overall CR) reported in records is a function of successful fertilization of the oocyte as well as implantation and maintenance of the conceptus to pregnancy diagnosis. In healthy cows, it has been suggested that successful fertilization occurs in as many as 90% of inseminations [32], but that 20% of embryos fail to survive beyond 18 days of gestation, around the time of maternal recognition of pregnancy [33]. Furthermore, pregnancy rates at day 32 of gestation can be as high as 60%, with a further loss of 15% between day 32 and day 74 [34]. Therefore, if records analysis identifies unacceptable FSCR, the herd should consider factors in period one that

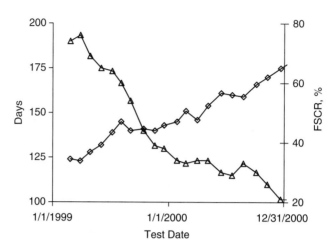

Fig. 4. Graph illustrating a relationship over time between predicted days open (◊) and first service conception rate (△), plotted on the right axis, for a dairy herd.

affect success of fertilization, as well as factors that affect pregnancy wastage. Successful fertilization can be affected by multiple factors, including the insemination program, accuracy of heat detection, nutrition, environment, metabolic disease, and infectious disease. Factors that affect pregnancy wastage are similar, and it is often difficult to differentiate problems with fertilization from problems with pregnancy maintenance.

Producers with herds that experience problems with FSCR should consider their insemination program, including semen storage, handling, thawing, and placement in the cow. Although not common, problems in the insemination program can severely affect herd reproductive performance by limiting fertilization success [16]. It is important that all personnel performing insemination are aware of and follow proper techniques to maximize the chance of fertilization when cows are submitted for insemination.

Accuracy of heat detection refers to the status of cows that are submitted for insemination, and can affect FSCR—if cows that are not in estrus are submitted for insemination, herd CR will decline [35]. In a multiherd study [19], it was found that 5% of cows submitted for insemination had high (≥1 ng/mL) milk progesterone concentration; but for individual herds, inaccuracy ranged from 0% to 60%. Increased reliance on secondary signs of estrus (such as roughened tail head, rubbed-off paint or chalk, triggered heat-mount detectors, mucus on vulva) can increase estrus detection (and reduce DFS), but may reduce CR (and FSCR) [19,36]. Kinsel and Etherington [15] observed that herds with increased HDR had shorter DFS but lower CR, perhaps due to increased reliance on secondary signs of estrus. This presents a dilemma to the producer—weighing the benefits of increased HDR (and lower DFS) against potential reductions in CR (and FSCR). Usually, it is better to favor insemination of cows (higher HDR). Barring major inaccuracies in estrus detection, it has been found that improvements in estrus detection lead to economic benefits [37]. Additional information (interestrus intervals) in the records can be used to help shed light on accuracy of estrus detection, and are discussed later.

In addition to playing a role with respect to estrus expression, nutritional factors can impact FSCR. Relating to energy balance, recent studies have suggested that loss of body condition was associated with decreased FSCR [38]. With respect to dietary protein, high milk urea nitrogen concentration, a marker of protein-to-energy balance in the diet, has been associated with decreased CR [39]. Thus, managers of herds with depressed FSCR should consider the potential for the nutritional program to impact the re-productive program.

The environment can also affect FSCR in dairy herds. Heat stress with high ambient temperature is a notable cause of depressed fertility in dairy cattle [40]. When reviewing reproductive records, one may anticipate declines in FSCR during periods of high heat. During the herd visit, facilities should be evaluated for their potential to exacerbate heat stress.

Diseases such as milk fever, retained fetal membranes, metritis, cystic ovarian disease, and even mastitis and lameness have been associated with reduced risk for pregnancy at first insemination [28]. It is difficult to differentiate an impact on fertilization from pregnancy maintenance, but a complete work-up for herds with reduced FSCR should consider high incidence of any disease condition that can delay normal uterine involution or affect reproductive tract health, as well as disease conditions that affect overall health, as potential contributors to reduced conception efficiency.

Another very important factor that can impact FSCR and overall CR in dairy herds is the presence of infectious diseases. A variety of infectious diseases can affect conception rate, either by reducing fertilization success or increasing early embryonic death (EED). Infectious agents such as bovine viral diarrhea virus (BVD), *Leptospira borgpetersenii* serovar hardjo (type hardjo-bovis), *Neospora caninum*, and bovine herpes virus type 1 (infectious bovine rhinotracheitis, IBR) are capable of causing EED, fetal loss, and abortions in dairy cattle [31]. Mangers of herds with problems in FSCR (or CR) should consider infectious disease as a potential cause for declines in DRPC reported measures. To this end, it is important to evaluate the herd's current and historical biosecurity and vaccination programs. Furthermore, any apparent abortions should be worked up through a diagnostic lab service. It is critical to do this even in the face of inconclusive results. Laboratory work-ups of abortions do not always yield definitive etiological results; a study in California found that a definitive etiology was determined in just 43% of submissions to state diagnostic laboratories [41].

The effect of ovulation synchronization protocols in period one

In the 1990s, reliable programs for synchronization of ovulation using gonadotropin hormone-releasing hormone (GnRH) and prostaglandins were developed [42]. When used, these programs effectively eliminate the need for detection of estrus and allow cows to receive TAI. In DHIA records, use of these protocols and TAI increases estrus detection to 100% in cows enrolled in the protocol. These programs are quite effective in period one at reducing DFS to a consistent uniform value [43]. Synchronization protocols and TAI can also be used in period two to ensure that cows are being inseminated. Depending on the extent of use at the herd level, DHIA records will likely show decreased DFS and increased HDR as more cows are submitted for insemination.

An important consideration when using OvSynch protocols and TAI is that CR assessed by ultrasound at 5 weeks is about 40% [43,44], which means that 60% of cows will continue to cycle and should be watched for estrus. Therefore, estrus detection is still critical for more than half of all synchronized cows. Thus, it is important to evaluate estrus detection efficiency in light of any synchronization and TAI; the records may indicate low DFS and high HDR (because of many cows being submitted for insemination), but efficiency of detection in cows following TAI may be low. Evaluation of interestrus intervals, discussed below, may help to shed light on estrus detection efficiency in herds with a high proportion of cows under OvSynch and TAI.

Monitoring efficiency in period two

Period two concerns the reproductive performance of the herd for all cows requiring multiple services to become pregnant. This period can be monitored in DHIA records using the herd's HDR, and either the services per conception (SPC) or CR. The herd HDR is the percentage of possible estruses detected (all recorded breedings are assumed to be estruses) in eligible cows during a test period [9]. The term SPC is calculated separately for all cows and pregnant cows, but this article focuses on all cows. SPC for all cows is the total number of services recorded for all cows (pregnant, open, and even cows designated as culls) divided by the number of pregnancies; CR is the inverse of SPC. Herds should strive to have high HDR and high CR (low SPC) although a balance must be struck between HDR and CR—Kinsel and Etherington [15] found a small but significant reduction in CR as HDR increased.

Monitoring heat detection rate in period two

Efficient and accurate estrus detection is the cornerstone of a successful dairy herd reproductive management program [35], and increased HDR is associated with lower PDO [45]. Heat detection of 70% or greater is considered good, and HDR less than 60% may be considered suboptimal [16]. The calculation of HDR is complex and does vary between DRPCs [10,46], but it is important to realize that calculated HDR reflects the recorded number of cows submitted for insemination, and that it does not reflect the accuracy of effort. Heat detection rate in records can be low if all breedings are not recorded; also, as mentioned earlier, HDR will be higher in herds using synchronization protocols and TAI.

Fig. 5 illustrates a relationship between HDR and PDO for a dairy herd. During most of 2000, HDR was lower and PDO higher than in most of 1999. Of particular interest is the period in late 1999 when HDR dropped and PDO increased. The herd visit should investigate how management or health conditions may have changed, and triggered a change in HDR that affected PDO.

Managers of herds with suboptimal HDR should consider that multiple factors related to management and cow health may affect success in this area (see Fig. 1). Factors that affect HDR, such as intensity of detection, milk production, nutrition, environment, metabolic disease, and feet and leg health, have been discussed with respect to DFS, and apply to problems with HDR. In many situations, herds with suboptimal HDR will also have extended DFS.

Monitoring conception in period two

The herd's CR is an important component of PDO [47], reported as the proportion of bred cows that are diagnosed pregnant [10,11]. The inverse of CR is SPC, so it is possible to calculate the SPC first and then the CR. If this

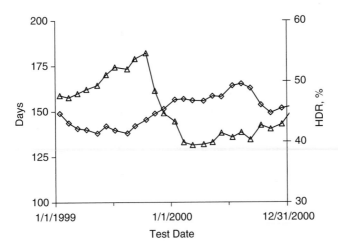

Fig. 5. Graph illustrating a relationship over time between predicted days open (◇) and heat detection rate (△), plotted on the right axis, for a dairy herd.

is done, it is important to use the SPC for all cows (which represents all breedings in the herd) rather than SPC for pregnant cows (which just uses breedings for pregnant cows). Using SPC for pregnant cows overestimates CR, because SPC for pregnant cows is less than SPC for all cows. Some have suggested a target CR of 50% [48], whereas others have suggested that SPC should be less than 2.25 (CR greater than 40%) [30].

Fig. 6 illustrates a relationship between CR and PDO for an example herd. In 2002, there was a higher CR and lower PDO, but in 2003 a drop in CR is associated with an increase in PDO. It is important to realize that the relationship does not mean that changes in CR are responsible for changes in PDO, only that the herd visit should investigate potential causes of reduced CR, and assess the potential of CR to affect PDO.

It was mentioned that when monitoring FSCR, conception is a function of successful fertilization of the oocyte as well as implantation and maintenance of the conceptus to pregnancy diagnosis. The same is true for CR, and the herd management should consider factors that affect success of fertilization as well as factors that affect pregnancy wastage, although it is difficult to differentiate failure of fertilization from pregnancy wastage. The same factors discussed when analyzing FSCR are applicable to evaluation of problems with low CR (or high SPC).

Monitoring interestrus intervals

Earlier it was mentioned that accuracy of heat detection can affect conception rate and overall reproductive performance. For cows that are bred multiple times, DRPCs calculate the days between reported breedings as the interestrus interval. The herd-level distribution of intervals into

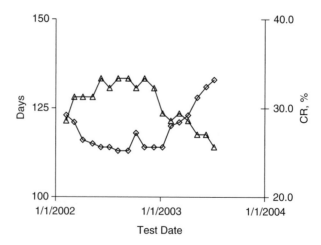

Fig. 6. Graph illustrating a relationship over time between predicted days open (◇) and conception rate (△), plotted on the right axis, for a dairy herd.

specific categories can help offer insight regarding the efficiency and accuracy of heat detection as well as provide indicators of cow health issues. Interestrus intervals are best characterized as short irregular intervals (less than 18 days between breedings), short regular intervals (18–24 days between breedings), long irregular intervals (25–35 days between breedings), long regular intervals (36–48 days between breedings), and extended intervals (49 or more days between breedings).

Short irregular intervals are suggestive of inaccurate heat detection. Assuming an estrus cycle length of 18 to 24 days, intervals of less than 18 days suggest that either of the last two breedings was to a nontrue heat. It is recommended that fewer than 15% of intervals fall in this category [30].

The short regular interval represents an ideal interval for cows bred more than once. An 18 to 24-day interval suggests that the next to last breeding was to a true heat, but did not result in a pregnancy; however, the producer successfully identified the cow open returning to another true heat at the earliest possible time. The short regular intervals should be at least 60% of intervals [30], which is consistent with an overall herd HDR of 60%; the high values suggest efficient and accurate estrus detection.

The long irregular interval may suggest both inaccuracy and inefficiency of estrus detection, problems with ovarian physiology, or EED. The 25 to 35-day interval could result from one of the last two breedings being inaccurate, coupled with a missed true heat (inefficiency). It could also arise from factors affecting follicular development and luteinization (such as heat stress, high production, or nutrition), or because a pregnancy that was appropriately recognized by the dam was lost shortly thereafter. Herds should try to keep these intervals at less than 10% of all intervals [30].

Intervals of 36 to 48 days represent late regular intervals, and are the next best to short regular intervals. Intervals of this duration represent two accurately detected heats separated by a missed heat (inefficiency). Although these suggest accuracy, the missed estrus is not ideal; intervals of this duration should represent less than 10% of all intervals [30].

Finally, intervals of 49 or more days, or extended intervals, are undesirable, and can arise due to inefficient estrus detection (two or more missed heats) or from fetal loss and abortion. These intervals should be less than 5% of all intervals [30]. In a herd considered to have efficient and accurate estrus detection, a high proportion of extended intervals may indicate unacceptable levels of fetal loss or abortion, and reasons for this, particularly infectious diseases, should be considered. Furthermore, any observed abortions should receive a full diagnostic work-up.

Interestrus intervals may also be useful in characterizing estrus detection in herds using OvSynch and TAI. In these herds, HDR may be high and DFS may be low, suggesting efficient detection of estrus (because of high numbers of cows submitted for insemination). If heat detection following TAI is inadequate, however, these herds may have low proportions of short regular interestrus intervals, and high proportions of late regular or even extended intervals. Thus, the interestrus intervals are an important adjunct to monitoring estrus detection efficiency in OvSynch herds, and it is critical to remind producers that estrus detection is very important even in bred cows—at least half of these are expected to return to estrus.

Other considerations in monitoring reproductive records

Age at first calving

Another important piece of information to examine in dairy herds with respect to reproductive performance is the average age at first calving. Before first calving, heifers do not generate revenue for the producer. Also, earlier calving ensures that replacements are ready in a timely fashion. Thus, it is good to have heifers calve by 24 months of age, but it is important that heifers be of appropriate size—at least 544 kg (1200 lbs) after first calving [49]. If a herd has delayed age at first calving, the producer and veterinarian should evaluate the heifer rearing program with respect to nutrition, housing, and health status of growing heifers.

"Slice-and-dice" analysis

Bailey et al [16] point out that the distribution of herd reproductive performance is often as important as mean values in monitoring re-productive efficiency. Therefore, they suggest "slicing" records analysis by age (lactation number) and "dicing" by stage of lactation (DIM periods). The techniques described here dice records with respect to the two periods described, but more periods can be examined. Slice-and-dice analysis is useful to help zero in on specific ages, groups, or pens to investigate during the herd visit. Too much slice and dice, however, can yield unstable performance estimates by reducing the number of cows included in each group analyzed. The technique is limited in smaller herds—it can be performed, but veterinarians should note if cow numbers in any examined group are small (fewer than 10, and certainly no fewer than 5).

Assimilating information

When analyzing dairy records and investigating relationships between various measures, it is useful to consider that multiple interactions can be occurring simultaneously. For example, PDO may not change in response to increased HDR if CR simultaneously decreases. Likewise, in many cases an increase in DFS may occur with a reduction in HDR, or FSCR and CR may decline together. Being aware of the potential for these interactions to exist improves the quality of any records analysis. Still, any hypotheses generated from records analysis should be confirmed with impressions obtained during the herd visit.

Choosing intervention strategies

Although a number of ideal performance targets have been mentioned in this article, few herds achieve these performance levels. For example, an estimate of HDR for US herds is under 50% [50], far from an ideal of 70%. Furthermore, reproductive inefficiency is often caused by a number of shortcomings related to management and cow health. Therefore, producers and veterinarians need to prioritize targets for intervention; however, it is difficult to allocate finite labor and capital resources to programs that need attention. A good rule of thumb to follow is that measures that are further from targets often present greater opportunities for improvement. Each additional DO becomes more costly to herds as CI increases [5]. Also, benefits of marginal improvement in HDR are greater for herds when HDR is low as opposed to herds in which HDR is high [37].

Summary

Review of reproductive records for dairy herds can be useful in terms of detection of potential problems, confirmation and characterization of suspected problems, and suggestion of targets for intervention in the reproductive management of the herd. An organized strategy for analysis makes it easier to identify and communicate issues to the producer, as well as to offer factors that may be undermining reproductive performance. Records review may generate hypotheses with respect to the situation in the herd, but these must be corroborated by information obtained during the herd visit. Optimal targets are difficult to achieve, but it is important to realize that the greatest potential for economic gains lies in areas that are furthest from targets.

References

[1] Wiggans GR. Dairy records processing center activity (DHI Report K-6). Animal Improvement Programs Laboratory; 2004. Available at: http://www.aipl.arsusda.gov/publish/dhi/current/drpcall.html. Accessed September 29, 2004.

[2] Uniform data collection procedures. National Dairy Herd Improvement Association, Inc; 2002. Available at: http://www.dhia.org/udcp.pdf. Accessed September 7, 2004.

[3] Louca A, Legates JE. Production losses in dairy cattle due to days open. J Dairy Sci 1968; 51(4):573–83.

[4] Britt JH. Enhanced reproduction and its economic implications. J Dairy Sci 1985;68(6): 1585–92.

[5] Plaizier JC, King GJ, Dekkers JC, et al. Estimation of economic values of indices for reproductive performance in dairy herds using computer simulation. J Dairy Sci 1997;80(11): 2775–83.

[6] Schmidt GH. Effect of length of calving interval on income over feed and variable costs. J Dairy Sci 1989;72:1605–11.

[7] Arbel R, Bigun Y, Ezra E, et al. The effect of extended calving intervals in high-yielding lactating cows on milk production and profitability. J Dairy Sci 2001;84(3):600–8.

[8] Holmann FJ, Shumway CR, Blake RW, et al. Economic value of days open for Holstein cows of alternative milk yields with varying calving intervals. J Dairy Sci 1984;67:636–43.

[9] Fetrow J, McClary D, Harman R, et al. Calculating selected reproductive indices: recommendations of the American Association of Bovine Practitioners. J Dairy Sci 1990; 73(1):78–90.

[10] DHI-202 herd summary. Fact sheet: A-1. Raleigh (NC): Dairy Records Management Systems; 1997.

[11] Herd summary description. Dairy herd improvement—Provo; 2003. Available at: www.dhiprovo.com/Pro_pgs/hs_sm02.htm. Accessed March 16, 2005.

[12] Plaizier JC, Lissemore KD, Kelton D, et al. Evaluation of overall reproductive performance of dairy herds. J Dairy Sci 1998;81(7):1848–54.

[13] Bascom SS, Young AJ. A summary of the reasons why farmers cull cows. J Dairy Sci 1998; 81(8):2299–305.

[14] Esslemont RJ. Relationship between herd calving to conception interval and culling rate for failure to conceive. Vet Rec 1993;133(7):163–4.

[15] Kinsel ML, Etherington WG. Factors affecting reproductive performance in Ontario dairy herds. Theriogenology 1998;50(8):1221–38.

[16] Bailey TL, Dascanio J, Murphy J. Analyzing reproductive records to improve dairy herd production. Vet Med (Praha) 1999;94:269–76.

[17] Tenhagen BA, Vogel C, Drillich M, et al. Influence of stage of lactation and milk production on conception rates after timed artificial insemination following OvSynch. Theriogenology 2003;60(8):1527–37.

[18] Loeffler SH, de Vries MJ, Schukken YH, et al. Use of AI technician scores for body condition, uterine tone and uterine discharge in a model with disease and milk production parameters to predict pregnancy risk at first AI in Holstein dairy cows. Theriogenology 1999; 51(7):1267–84.

[19] Reimers TJ, Smith RD, Newman SK. Management factors affecting reproductive performance of dairy cows in the northeastern United States. J Dairy Sci 1985;68(4):963–72.

[20] Slama H, Wells ME, Adams GD, et al. Factors affecting calving interval in dairy herds J Dairy Sci 1976;59:1334–9.

[21] Risco CA, Archbald LF. Dairy herd reproductive efficiency. In: Howard JL, Smith RA, editors. Food animal practice. 4th edition. Philadelphia: W.B. Saunders Company; 1999. p. 604–6.

[22] Hardin DK. Fertility and infertility assessment by review of records. Vet Clin North Am Food Anim Pract 1993;9(2):389–403.

[23] Rounsaville TR, Oltenacu PA, Milligan RA, et al. Effects of heat detection, conception rate, and culling policy on reproductive performance in dairy herds. J Dairy Sci 1979;62(9): 1435–42.

[24] Williams WF, Yver DR, Gross TS. Comparison of estrus detection techniques in dairy heifers. J Dairy Sci 1981;64(8):1738–41.

[25] Lopez H, Satter LD, Wiltbank MC. Relationship between level of milk production and estrous behavior of lactating dairy cows. Anim Reprod Sci 2004;81(3–4):209–23.

[26] Shrestha HK, Nakao T, Higaki T, et al. Resumption of postpartum ovarian cyclicity in high-producing Holstein cows. Theriogenology 2004;61(4):637–49.

[27] Wilson SJ, Marion RS, Spain JN, et al. Effects of controlled heat stress on ovarian function of dairy cattle. 1. Lactating cows. J Dairy Sci 1998;81(8):2124–31.

[28] Loeffler SH, de Vries MJ, Schukken YH. The effects of time of disease occurrence, milk yield, and body condition on fertility of dairy cows. J Dairy Sci 1999;82(12):2589–604.

[29] Barkema HW, Westrik JD, van Keulen KAS, et al. The effects of lameness on reproductive performance, milk production and culling in Dutch dairy farms. Prev Vet Med 1994; 20:249–59.

[30] Gaines JD. The role of record analyisis in evaluating subfertile dairy herds. Vet Med (Praha) 1989;84(5):532–43.

[31] Williamson NB. The interpretation of herd records and clinical findings for identifying and solving problems of infertility. Compendium Food Animal 1987;9(1):F12–24.

[32] Lucy MC. Reproductive loss in high-producing dairy cattle: where will it end? J Dairy Sci 2001;84(6):1277–93.

[33] Dunne LD, Diskin MG, Sreenan JM. Embryo and foetal loss in beef heifers between day 14 of gestation and full term. Anim Reprod Sci 2000;58(1–2):39–44.

[34] Moreira F, Orlandi C, Risco CA, et al. Effects of presynchronization and bovine somatotropin on pregnancy rates to a timed artificial insemination protocol in lactating dairy cows. J Dairy Sci 2001;84(7):1646–59.

[35] Heersche G Jr, Nebel RL. Measuring efficiency and accuracy of detection of estrus. J Dairy Sci 1994;77(9):2754–61.

[36] Gwazdauskas FC, Nebel RL, Sprecher DJ, et al. Effectiveness of rump-mounted devices and androgenized females for detection of estrus in dairy cattle. J Dairy Sci 1990;73(10):2965–70.

[37] de Vries A, Conlin BJ. Economic value of timely determination of unexpected decreases in detection of estrus using control charts. J Dairy Sci 2003;86(11):3516–26.

[38] Domecq JJ, Skidmore AL, Lloyd JW, et al. Relationship between body condition scores and conception at first artificial insemination in a large dairy herd of high yielding Holstein cows. J Dairy Sci 1997;80(1):113–20.

[39] Rajala-Schultz PJ, Saville WJA, Frazer GS, et al. Association between milk urea nitrogen and fertility in Ohio dairy cows. J Dairy Sci 2001;84(2):482–9.

[40] al-Katanani YM, Webb DW, Hansen PJ. Factors affecting seasonal variation in 90-day nonreturn rate to first service in lactating Holstein cows in a hot climate. J Dairy Sci 1999; 82(12):2611–6.

[41] Jamaluddin AA, Case JT, Hird DW, et al. Dairy cattle abortion in California: evaluation of diagnostic laboratory data. J Vet Diagn Invest 1996;8(2):210–8.

[42] Pursley JR, Mee MO, Wiltbank MC. Synchronization of ovulation in dairy cows using PGF2a and GnRH. Theriogenology 1995;44(7):915–23.

[43] Pursley JR, Kosorok MR, Wiltbank MC. Reproductive management of lactating dairy cows using synchronization of ovulation. J Dairy Sci 1997;80(2):301–6.

[44] Tenhagen BA, Drillich M, Surholt R, et al. Comparison of timed AI after synchronized ovulation to AI at estrus: reproductive and economic considerations. J Dairy Sci 2004;87(1): 85–94.

[45] Pecsok SR, McGilliard ML, Nebel RL. Conception rates. 1. Derivation and estimates for effects of estrus detection on cow profitability. J Dairy Sci 1994;77(10):3008–15.

[46] DHI-Plus for Windows [computer program]. Version 2.28.7. Provo (UT): DHI Computing Service; 2004.

[47] Pecsok SR, McGilliard ML, Nebel RL. Conception rates. 2. Economic value of unit differences in percentages of sire conception rates. J Dairy Sci 1994;77(10):3016–21.

[48] Domecq JJ, Nebel RL, McGilliard ML, et al. Expert system for evaluation of reproductive performance and management. J Dairy Sci 1991;74(10):3446–53.

[49] Gabler MT, Tozer PR, Heinrichs AJ. Development of a cost analysis spreadsheet for calculating the costs to raise a replacement dairy heifer. J Dairy Sci 2000;83(5):1104–9.

[50] Rorie RW, Bilby TR, Lester TD. Application of electronic estrus detection technologies to reproductive management of cattle. Theriogenology 2002;57(1):137–48.

ELSEVIER
SAUNDERS

Vet Clin Food Anim 21 (2005) 325–347

VETERINARY
CLINICS
Food Animal Practice

Nutrition and Reproduction in Dairy Herds

James D. Ferguson, VMD, MS

School of Veterinary Medicine, University of Pennsylvania,
New Bolton Center, 382 West Street Road, Kennett Square, PA 19348, USA

The reader is encouraged to refer to articles that deal with nutrition and reproduction and ovulation in postpartum cows [1–9].

Nutrition influences reproduction in mammals via specific nutritional deficiencies or excesses, or via toxic factors in feeds. Slight nutritional imbalances are tolerated, but moderate-to-severe nutritional imbalances progress to moderate-to-severe reduction in reproductive performance [6]. General malnutrition, or inanition, resulting in significant loss of body weight, impairs reproduction through ovulatory failure, and overnutrition and obesity also negatively impact reproduction through impaired folliculogenesis, reduced oocyte quality, and embryonic failure [10–14]. Nutrition modulates reproductive function through alteration of gonadotropin secretion, or through local effects on ovarian folliculogenesis or uterine environment. Effects appear to be mediated through metabolic hormones such as insulin, insulinlike growth factor-1 (IGF-1), growth hormone, and leptin; or through metabolic end products such as urea, glucose, and amino acids [15–21].

Because mean conception rate (CR) has declined from 66% in 1951 to 40% in 1999 [3,20,22], and estrus detection rate (HDR) has also declined to less than 50% [23], producers are concerned about relationships between nutrition and reproduction in high-producing dairy cows consuming high-quality, well-balanced rations. Genetic selection for high milk production is antagonistic for reproduction [22–25]. Because fertility in heifers has not dramatically declined, genetic selection for milk production compromises reproduction during lactation, possibly through an array of gene expression that directs nutrients to milk production and suppresses the hypothalamic-pituitary-ovarian axis. Altering specific nutrients may help reverse this trend, but increased energy intake in

E-mail address: ferguson@vet.upenn.edu

cows that were selected for higher milk production versus those that were not has not mitigated negative trends [26]. Despite the negative genetic relationship between high production and fertility [20,22,26], management can accomplish high milk production and high fertility. This is apparent, because high-producing herds tend to have better fertility than low-producing herds [27,28]. To improve reproduction, producers have been offered products that include specially designed fats, rumen protected choline, blends of rumen undegradable protein sources with and without rumen inert fat, increased vitamin supplementation, and organic complexes of trace minerals in order to try to improve reproduction. Improvement in reproduction has not been consistent across all studies investigating these products. Ultimately, the use of these products depends on whether any improvement in reproduction will be sufficient to make that use cost effective.

Good fertility is a composite of cow, bull, environmental, inseminator, and management factors. Low CR herds require a systematic approach to identify significant factors influencing performance. In addition, on many farms, 40% to 60% of cows are afflicted with a periparturient condition that reduces fertility. These conditions include dystocia, metritis, retained placenta, milk fever, ketosis, displaced abomasum, and lameness [29–33]. Often these conditions have a nutritional or management association that contributes to an increased risk of periparturient problems. Nutritional risk factors may be present in precalving or postcalving rations. The influence of nutrition on the incidence of these conditions should not be ignored when considering nutritional effects on fertility; however, this article does not specifically address these associations.

Associations of nutrition with reproduction must be examined as a continuum from precalving through pregnancy in cows with normal and abnormal parturient events, across varying age groups and season of calving. Studies of this type require large numbers of cows. Until these studies are performed, we can only describe nutritional effects on fertility in bits and pieces, and factors that confound and interact with nutritional factors on fertility can not be clearly identified.

Parturient conditions

Periparturient problems are a major factor contributing to reduced CR in dairy herds. On many farms, 40% to 60% of cows calving have one or more of the conditions outlined in Table 1 that reduce fertility [29,32,34–37]. Health problems in postpartum cows tend to occur in clusters [34,35] and have significant effects on fertility. In addition, metabolic problems have been implicated in association with cystic ovarian disease [38–40], anestrous [41], and reduced immune function [42]. Acute mastitis has been linked with development of cystic ovaries [43]. Monitoring these conditions and working

Table 1
Effects of periparturient conditions on odds ratio of conception rate and median days to diagnosis and range in incidence from a selected group of references

Condition	Fertility ratio (odds ratio)	Relative CR[a] (rmse .07) %	Median days to diagnosis	Range in incidence %
Normal cows	1.00	65		40.0 to 60.0
Metritis, chronic	.63	54	>18	1.1 to 23.0
Abnormal lochia, acute metritis	.68	56	<18	6.5 to 8.3
Systemic metritis, acute metritis	.70	57	<18	2.0 to 3.0
Retained fetal membranes	.72	57	1	4.5 to 8.6
Ketosis	.90	63	29	7.4
Lameness	.83	61	46	.3 to 3.7
Ovulatory dysfunction	.71	57	85	1.6 to 8.6
Uterine prolapse	.80	60	1	.2

Conditions not included which reduce fertility include milk fever (2%–5% incidence), displaced abomasum (3% incidence), dystocia (2% incidence), mastitis around time of insemination (24.7% prevalence during lactation, 6.9% prevalence during time of insemination [43]).
Abbreviation: CR_n, relative CR in normal cows (65%).
[a] Relative $CR = CR_n \times (OR/[CR_n \times OR + (1 - CR_n)])$.
Data from Refs. [29,32,34–37].

with management to reduce the overall incidence to less than 40% is a first step to controlling nutritional effects on reproduction. In general, these conditions influence fertility to approximately the same extent, although mechanisms of influence may be different. Metritis may act through effects on uterine involution, whereas metabolic conditions may effect the function of the hypothalamic-pituitary-ovarian axis. Importantly, many of these conditions have been linked to dry-cow nutrition and management [33].

The period from 3 weeks precalving to 3 weeks postcalving has been termed the "transition period," because during this time the cow is at risk of consuming less energy and protein than can meet requirements, and is transitioning from a nonlactating to a lactating state [44]. Feeding management in the dry period, particularly the late dry period, has significant effects on postpartum health. Prevention of periparturient disease and metabolic problems early in lactation are important components of nutrition and fertility relationships.

Minimizing metabolic problems is contingent upon management of energy and protein, not only in rations fed, but also in body tissue stores. Increasing age and body fatness are major risk factors associated with postpartum complications [45–47]. Body tissue stores have typically been estimated by assessing body condition score (BCS). The scale commonly used in the United States was developed by Wildman et al [48]. Ferguson and coauthors [49] identified principal descriptors of BCS based on Wildman's scale of 1 to 5; 1 being emaciated and 5 being obese. It is possible to separate BCS by quarter-point increments between 2.5 to 4.0

[49]. Excess body condition score at calving (BCSC) is associated with an increase risk of metritis and ketosis [46,47], milk fever [50], metritis, and cystic ovaries [47]. Low BCSC has been associated with retained placenta (RP), metritis, anestrous, and lameness [45,47]. A loss of body condition of more than .25 units of BCS during the dry period has been associated with an increase in the risk of metabolic diseases, lameness, RP, and calving problems [45,47,51].

Feeding management during the last 3 weeks before calving may be more critical in prevention of periparturient problems than any specific nutrient. This is due to typical declines in feed intake as parturition approaches, which create nutritional imbalances even with well-formulated diets. Well-managed dry-cow environments and feed delivery may encourage higher dry matter intake (DMI) and improved nutrient balance. Typically, DMI declines from 1.91% of body weight on day 21 before calving to 1.3% of body weight on day 1 before calving [44]. Over this same time period, energy requirements have increased (22.2 to 23.2 mcal/d metabolizable energy requirement [ME], day -21 versus day -1 relative to calving) and protein requirements have increased (734 g to 1051 g metabolizable protein [MP] requirement per day, day -21 versus day -1 relative to calving) [52]. Therefore, the precalving cow is at risk for negative energy and protein balance before calving. Twin pregnancies, primiparous cows, increase in BCS, and thermal stress increase the decline in DMI. In addition, higher dietary content of neutral detergent fiber (NDF), ether extract (EE), and rumen undegradable protein (RUP) is associated with decreased DMI in precalving cows [44].

In herds experiencing transition problems, the veterinarian should examine the composition of the close-up diet and ascertain the amount of time that feed is available and that cows are actually in the group before calving. With increasing herd size due to expansion, dry-cow groups are often overcrowded and calving facilities are inadequate. Rations with marginal nutrient content become limiting when DMI is further decreased because of management and environmental conditions. Areas that should be monitored include DMI per head/day for the group, NDF and nonfiber carbohydrate (NFC) content of the ration (% dry matter [DM] basis), adequate intake of metabolizable protein, dietary approaches to control milk fever (either low calcium, dry cow diets [Ca <.5% DM] or anionic salts), and adequate vitamin and trace mineral supplementation. As guidelines, DMI should be ≥ 9.5 kg/head/day (21.0 lbs), NDF should range between 36% and 45% of DM, and NFC should range between 33% and 36% of DM. Metabolizable protein should be greater than 900 g/day. A ration program needs to be used to evaluate MP supply based on diet composition and DMI. A crude monitoring tool is to examine blood or plasma urea nitrogen, which should average at least 10 mg/dl and be below 17 mg/dl for a group of at least eight cows sampled in the close-up group.

Lactating dairy cows

Energy

Reproduction effects economic returns on a dairy farm by influencing milk produced per day, calves born per year, and replacement pressure [53]. As calving interval increases, the average milk produced per day decreases, fewer calves are born per year, and the length of the dry period increases [54,55]. Most economic models support the goal that calving intervals should be less than 13 months. In seasonally calving herds using grazed pasture as forage input, more pressure is exerted on management to achieve a yearly calving cycle than in confined dairy herds that use more inputs from stored forage. To achieve at least a yearly calving interval, cows must be pregnant by 85 days postcalving. If CR is .65, HDR is .85, and insemination commences at 43 days postpartum, then 91% of cows will be pregnant by 85 days postcalving. Decreasing HDR to 65% decreases this proportion to 81%. Decreasing CR to 40% reduces the proportion pregnant by 85 days to 71%, with HDR at 85%. Because synchronization programs can force HDR to 100% through insemination on appointment at specific times postcalving, reduction in CR becomes the limiting factor in maintaining high reproductive efficiency.

Early initiation of luteal activity postcalving is conducive to improved fertility, and an increase in the number of ovulatory cycles before insemination has been associated with improvement in CR [1,20,56,57]. Cows that have normal ovulatory patterns commencing before 40 to 50 days postpartum have better reproductive performance than cows with first ovulation after 50 days postpartum, or that have extended luteal phase activity [55,58,59]. Resumption of ovarian activity extremely early postcalving was negatively associated with reproductive performance, possibly due to an increase in risk of pyometra [22,55].

Initiation of follicular waves commences by 5 days postcalving, subsequent to a surge in follicle-stimulating hormone (FSH) [1,3,19, 20,60]. Emergence of a dominant follicle usually occurs by day 10 post-calving (size >9 mm, [60]). This follicle may ovulate, regress, and a new follicular wave emerge, or it may continue to grow and develop into a cystic structure [20,60]. The proportion of cows that ovulate the first dominant follicle is variable. Savio and colleagues [61] observed that 75% of cows ovulated the first dominant follicle, whereas Beam and Butler [20] observed that 46% did so, Horan and coworkers [25] observed that 42% did so, and Darwash and associates [58] and Royal et al [22] observed that approximately 55% of cows ovulated the first dominant follicle.

Factors that influence first ovulation include age, breed, milk production, suckling, presence of the dam's calf, presence of a bull, season, periparturient health problems, and nutrition [6]. Comprehensive reviews of follicular recruitment postcalving may be found in studies by Wiltbank and coauthors [60]. As follicular waves develop postpartum, ovulation depends on the development of a dominant follicle that produces sufficient estradiol to stimulate a surge of luteinizing hormone (LH) from the pituitary. Follicular waves commence by about 5 days postpartum. These waves are preceded by a surge in FSH, and are characterized by the development of follicles from 4 to 9 mm in diameter. A dominant follicle with ovulatory potential emerges from the follicular wave, and is identifiable morphologically based on size greater than 10 mm. The dominant follicle emerges in response to an increase in plasma LH concentration and an increase in LH pulse frequency. Dominance of a follicle is associated with induction of LH receptors on thecal and granulosa cells. IGF-1 binding proteins decrease in follicular fluid, IGF-1 increases in the dominant follicle, and estradiol production increases [6,61,62]. The dominant follicle suppresses development of other contemporary follicles [63]. Ovulation of a dominant follicle depends on triggering a surge of LH by increasing estradiol in the presence of low serum progesterone [5,60]. If progesterone is high, the dominant follicle regresses, FSH surges, and another follicular wave commences [60].

Critical factors associated with the stimulation of an LH surge appear to be adequate production of estradiol by the dominant follicle and release of the hypothalamus from inhibitory effects of estradiol on LH secretion [60]. Nonovulatory follicles postcalving produce low levels of estradiol compared with follicles that ovulate [20]. Failure of ovulation is due to low estradiol production [5,20]. Metabolic factors that may link nutritional status with hypothalamic and ovarian function include insulin, IGF-1, and growth hormone (GH) [1,6,19,20,60]. Release of hypothalamus from inhibitory effects of estradiol may be dependent on energy status [60].

In lactating dairy cows, nutrient intake immediately postpartum is insufficient to meet the demands of milk production, and cows are in negative energy and protein balance [1,20,64,65]. A few cows never go into negative energy balance postcalving, but the majority of cows experience a period of weight and body condition loss that are usually maximal by 30 to 40 days postcalving. Homeorhetic controls in early lactation assure that body tissue, primarily adipose stores, will be mobilized to support milk production, despite insufficient intake of nutrients [66]. In addition, significant amounts of body protein are directed to support glucose and protein deficits in early lactation [67]. Homeorhetic controls orchestrate nutrient priorities for maintenance, growth, lactation, and reproduction. The negative energy balance and fat mobilization stimulate DMI, and cows progress to a positive energy balance by about 8 weeks postcalving (range 4–14 weeks) [20,65]. DMI typically increases at a decreasing rate from calving, and reaches a maximum around 15 weeks postpartum, whereas milk production peaks around 5 to 7 weeks postpartum and declines at a consistent rate until dry-off.

Dairy cows tolerate slight nutritional deficits and resume reproductive function by 15 to 40 days postcalving (mean 33.3 days, sem = 2.09, [68–77]). Across ten studies and 29 groups of dairy cows, time to first ovulation was negatively correlated with energy balance nadir (r = −.57, P < .008, [68–77]).

In various studies, Butler and coworkers [1,19,20,69,71,72] have correlated time to first ovulation with days to nadir of negative energy balance (NNEB). The NNEB typically occurs during the first to second week postcalving [1,65]. Beam and Butler [20] found that first ovulation occurred 19.4 + .78*NNEB (days) (r^2 = .094, P < .01), whereas de Vries and Veerkamp [65] found start of luteal activity related to nadir of energy balance (NEB) (−.125*NEB, megajoules [MJ] of net energy of lactation [NEL]/d, r^2 = .042, P < .001). De Vries and associates [64,65] observed later days to first ovulation with lower nadir of energy balance and lower total cumulative energy balance in dairy cows. Milk fat content of first test-day milk and the decrease in fat percentage could be used as indicators of negative energy balance [64,65]. They also found that resumption of luteal activity was delayed with lower nadir in energy balance [64,65]. Ten MJ of NEL/day lower NEB was associated with a delay of first ovulation by 1.25 days [64].

Emergence of a dominant follicle before the NEB is associated with reduced follicle diameter and reduction in peak estradiol plasma concentration compared with emergence of a dominant follicle after the NNEB [20]. Cows that ovulated before 21 days postpartum ovulated the first dominant follicle that emerged, and the follicle emerged after the NNEB. These cows had higher serum insulin and IGF-1 and lower GH in the first week postcalving compared with cows that did not ovulate the first dominant follicle postcalving [19,20,78]. Cows that did not ovulate the first dominant follicle postpartum averaged over 40 days to first ovulation [20]. Thus, several sequential follicular waves occurred before ovulation. Providing diets and feed management that promote increases in serum insulin and IGF-1 early postcalving and facilitate increases in DMI so that NNEB occurs before 10 days postcalving may reduce time to first ovulation and enhance fertility.

Increases in insulin and IGF-1 appear to be significant modulators of reproduction and follicular development. Feeding diets conducive to higher plasma insulin postpartum increased the proportion of cows ovulating by 50 days postpartum [15], reduced the mean interval from calving to first ovulation, and tended to reduce the interval to first service and days open (DO). Thomas and coauthors [79] found that a diet associated with elevations in serum insulin in beef cattle increased follicular growth in diets that were isoenergetic. Kendrick and colleagues [80] observed an increase in the quality of oocytes obtained from high-yielding dairy cows when corn grain was increased in the diet, and found that the improvement in quality was associated with an improvement in energy balance. Landau and coworkers [81] found that acute dietary changes that increased serum insulin (7 days prior to synchronized estrus) increased intrafollicular insulin and glucose. In general, they observed that intrafollicular insulin and glucose were higher in preovulatory follicles than in subordinate follicles. Thus, systemic changes in glucose supply may result in improved intrafollicular insulin, IGF-1, and glucose. Glucose and cholesterol are the primary metabolic fuel and steroid precursors in the ovary [82]. Diets that promote increases in insulin and IGF-1 may enhance follicular development and promote fertility; however, there is a limit to the quantity of grain that may be added to a ration for a lactating dairy cow without interfering with rumen fermentation.

In cycling heifers, dietary restriction eventually inhibits ovarian cycling when weight loss is about 19% to 25% of initial body weight [11,75,10]. Fertility also declines if reproductive function is maintained [83]. These changes are associated with declining plasma insulin, IGF-1, estradiol, and increasing GH and nonesterified fatty acids (NEFA) [10]. Plasma concentrations, pulse frequency, and amplitude of LH remained normal up to the cycle before cessation of ovulation [10]. Declines in IGF-1, insulin, and progesterone and estradiol preceded the cessation of cycling and decline in LH [10]. Plasma concentration of FSH and pulses per 8 hours increased at cessation of ovulation associated with reduced estradiol concentrations [10]. Dominant follicle and corpus luteum (CL) were smaller in the last two cycles before cessation of ovulation compared with those in control heifers [10]. Dietary restriction in cycling heifers highlights the changes in ovarian function that occur over time, concomitant with changes in metabolic hormones.

IGF-1 is a growth factor produced in the liver [84]. Over 90% of IGF-1 in blood circulates bound to insulinlike growth factor binding proteins (IGFBP), of which there are six distinct types [84]. Production of IGF-1 by the liver is stimulated by GH, and dietary supply of energy and protein are critical regulators of IGF-1 and IGFBPs. IGFs (IGF-1 and IGF-2) are important hormones linking nutrition and growth. IGF-1 is stimulatory to granulosa cells, increasing cell proliferation and steroid hormone production [85]. In cattle, IGF-1 may interact with insulin to influence cell proliferation and estradiol production, induce LH receptor induction, and contribute to selection of the dominant follicle [12]. High-energy diets fed to heifers decreased follicle IGFBP-2 and IGFBP-4, which would increase the availability of IGF-1 [12]. High-energy diets also decreased insulin resistance (increase in insulin receptors in thecal and granulosa cells) in follicles compared with low-energy diets [12]. Plasma IGF-1 decreases with nutrient restriction, and is associated with interference with normal ovarian cycling and inhibition of folliculogenesis and ovulation [62].

LH pulse frequency may be modulated by serum insulin and IGF-1 concentrations [19,20,78]. Leptin, a polypeptide produced by adipose cells, is a metabolic modifier, and may be another key component in communicating nutritional status to the hypothalamic-pituitary axis [7,86]. Leptin has been recognized as a component of the regulation of body weight and energy homeostasis, and has been linked to reproductive processes [14,86–88]. Plasmas leptin increases with body fatness. Increases in serum leptin seem to play a significant role in triggering puberty. As body fat is lost, plasma leptin decreases, which may play a role in decreasing gondadotropin secretion from the pituitary. Conversely, with extreme obesity, plasma leptin increases, and this also suppresses gonadotropin secretion. Leptin may modulate fertility in extreme states of body fatness.

As energy balance increases, ovarian follicular growth is stimulated [3,8,56,76,78]. Dominant follicles are larger and estradiol production is enhanced. Cows with more positive energy balance have larger dominant follicles, and more follicles move into follicle class 2 and class 3. The ovary appears to be stimulated by improved energy status. Following ovulation, CL are larger and progesterone production is increased [8,89]. Taken together, more positive energy balance is stimulatory to ovarian reproductive structures.

Fertility is not conferred with initiation of ovulation. Both estrus expression and conception improve with each estrous cycle through to the third estrus postcalving (Table 2) [56,57]. Repetitive estrous cycles are necessary to confer fecundity. Following calving or puberty, CR and estrus expression are influenced by sequential estrous cycle from first ovulation up to the third estrous cycle. Thus, if breeding begins at 45 to 50 days, first estrus must have occurred by 25 to 30 days to ensure adequate heat detection (and conception rate) by first insemination on the third estrus postcalving.

Progesterone may be a conditioning factor that enhances fertility on subsequent cycles. Progesterone concentrations have an influence on follicular turnover. Higher progesterone concentrations are associated with higher ovarian follicular turnover [78,89]. Higher progesterone in the cycle before breeding has been associated with improved CR at insemination at the next estrus [8,78,89]. The effect of sequential ovarian cycling may be through the conditioning of follicular growth by increasing progesterone concentration with each postpartum cycle. If progesterone concentrations do not meet a certain threshold, then oocyte quality may be reduced and

Table 2
Effect of ovulation postcalving and estrus expression

Reference	N	Percent detected estrus		
		First ovulation	Second ovulation	Third ovulation
Villa-Godoy et al [77]	32	34.4	71.9	83.3
Berghorn et al [68]	62	30.0	70.5	
Carroll et al [119]	52	23.0	27.0	43.0
Dachir et al [120]	45	13.0	56.0	65.0
Dachir et al [120] secondary signs		25.0	60.0	77.0

fertility lower. Lower progesterone is associated with larger dominant follicles, slower follicle turnover, and poorer quality ovum [89].

Progesterone concentrations rise following insemination and ovulation. Granulosa cells produce progesterone after ovulation. Progesterone is important in influencing the uterine environment for support of the developing embryo. Fertilization occurs in the oviduct, and transport of the embryo into the uterus occurs about 3 days following fertilization. Progesterone concentrations are important in preparing the uterus to receive the developing embryo. The rate of progesterone rise following insemination has been associated with pregnancy. Larson et al [90] found slower rates of rise in cows that failed to become pregnant and had extended interbreeding intervals, suggesting early embryonic death. Cows with intermediate rates of rise in progesterone following insemination failed to become pregnant, but had regular return to estrus. Progesterone concentrations may be important in influencing events before insemination (follicle development) and events following insemination (uterine environment).

Energy balance is not possible to calculate or measure on dairy farms because DMI is not known in individual cows. Several monitoring tools are available. The simplest tool to assess energy status is to estimate body condition loss (BCSL) postcalving. One unit change in BCS represents about 56 kg (120 lbs) of body weight change and about 16,742 MJ (400 Mcal) of total net energy loss, using a scale of 1 to 5, with 1 being very thin and 5 being very fat. Change in body condition correlates with cumulative negative energy balance and reflects total negative energy deficit. Typically, high-producing cows should lose about -0.5 body condition score unit by 30 days postcalving, and begin to increase in body condition score by 12 to 14 weeks postcalving.

Cows appear to tolerate modest to moderate amounts of BCSL, up to -3/4 of a condition score by 30 days postpartum. In general, one unit of BCSL has been associated with reductions in first service conception rate (FSTCR) [46,50,91–94], later days to first insemination, and later days to first ovulation [91], and with an increase in number of services [95]. Cows in lower BCS class at insemination had lower CR [91,96].

Other measures of energy balance include milk fat percentage in early lactation (day 1), change in fat percentage in early lactation, and ratio of milk fat to milk protein content on first test postcalving [65,97]. Milk protein content at second test postcalving is also correlated with NEB. Lower milk protein content is associated with lower energy balance. De Vries and coauthors [65] found the change in milk fat content from day 1 postcalving to be a better estimate of energy balance than other measures. These estimates are difficult to specifically assess, because cows usually are tested only once a month, and days postcalving on first test may vary from 3 to 45. Changes in fat and protein are rapid in the first month postcalving, thus changes in days in milk at first test may greatly bias these measures.

Because there are limits to the amount of grain that can be added to ruminant diets, and because fats are significantly higher in energy density, they have been attractive dietary supplements to increase energy density of dairy rations. Excessive inclusion of fat in dairy rations may depress rumen digestion, however, particularly if fat sources are high in polyunsaturated fatty acids (PUFA). Fat sources include high-fat byproduct feeds, high-oil seeds, oils, greases, tallow, and specialty fats processed to be inert in the rumen. To prevent negative effects of fat on rumen fermentation, specialty fats have been produced to avoid rumen degradation by complexing with calcium to form salts of long-chain fatty acids or prilling hard fat into small, low specific-gravity particles. A comprehensive review of fat in dairy diets is beyond the scope of this article, but Staples et al [8] is an excellent review of fat on fertility in dairy cows.

Supplemental dietary fat has been shown to influence ovarian processes such as follicular growth and the lifespan of induced CL, and has decreased time to first ovulation [79,19,98]. Fat feeding increased the number of large follicles, increased progesterone production, and decreased prostaglandin production from the uterus. Inclusion of fat sources high in PUFA increased serum insulin, cholesterol, and follicular concentrations of IGF-1; and decreased prostaglandin and estradiol production [8,79]. Effects may benefit fertility by stimulating ovarian function and extending the lifespan of the CL.

Effects of supplemental dietary fat on fertility have been inconsistent [8]. Using the data in Staples [8], the CR for cows fed low-fat diets was subtracted from the CR of cows fed high-fat diets. The difference in CR was regressed against the difference in milk production [8]. Part of the variation in CR response to added fat is explained by the change in milk production. If milk production increased 1.96 kg, CR was not changed. If milk production increases were higher than 1.96 kg, CR declined. If milk production increased 3 to 4 kg, CR was reduced by .12 and .27 units, respectively. If milk production increase was below 1.96 kg, CR increased. If there was no change in milk, CR was predicted to increase .14 units. The change in milk only explained 14% of the change in CR within the studies.

The proportion of cows not ovulating by 40 days postpartum, the amount of body condition loss, and the proportion of extremes in body condition at calving and 30 to 100 days postcalving are factors that should be monitored. Monitoring ovulation is problematic, because rectal palpation and infrequent ultrasound examination are not sufficient to determine timing of ovulation accurately in a sufficient proportion of cows [55,60]. Sequential milk progesterone tests can identify days to first ovulation, but must be sampled two to three times a week for identification of ovulation. Collection of milk for progesterone testing may be useful in herds with significant CR problems. Fewer than 15% of cows should have extreme BCSC: either too fat (4 or more), or too thin (less than 3). After calving, fewer than 15% of cows should be below a 2.5 in BCS.

Protein

In general, increasing levels of dietary crude protein (CP) have been associated with increases in services per pregnancy and days open [99]. More specifically, increasing rumen degraded intake protein (RDP) in excess of requirement decreases fertility [71,99–102]. Cows fed higher amounts of RDP than required experienced more irregular intervals between first and second service than cows fed diets balanced for RDP and undegradable intake protein (RUP) [90,101,102]. Elrod and coworkers [101,102] showed that a decrease in uterine pH was associated with higher degraded intake protein, and that it may be a possible cause of conception failure.

These effects in the uterine environment may be on the early embryo. Blanchard and colleagues [103] found that embryo quality was reduced in cows consuming a 16.5% CP diet that contained 70% RDP compared with cows fed a diet containing 62% RDP. The effect was not apparent in all cows, but was observed in a higher proportion of cows consuming the high RDP diet, particularly in cows in their fourth parity and older. Approximately a third of cows consuming the higher RDP diet failed to yield any fertilized embryos. Larson et al [90] found that cows with higher milk urea nitrogen (MUN) had more failed pregnancies that were associated with regular interestrus interval, based on sequential milk progesterone testing, compared with cows that became pregnant. These data suggest that higher RDP and urea concentrations are associated with fertilization failure as a cause of repeat breeding.

Sinclair and associates [104] found that higher dietary RDP increased serum ammonia and effected oocyte maturation and early blastocyst development. McEvoy et al [105] observed that plasma ammonia concentrations measured at or near insemination were negatively correlated $(r = -0.27, P < .0002)$ with pregnancy. These studies suggest that increases in serum ammonia may play a role in reducing reproductive performance in cows fed high RDP diets by influencing oocyte quality and blastocyst maturation. DeWit and coauthors [106] and Ocon and Hansen [107] found that oocytes incubated in increasing concentrations of urea had reduced proportions of fertilized oocytes that developed to blastocysts. DeWit and colleagues [106] found that increasing urea was associated with reduced fertilization and cleavage rate, but had no effect on embryos after fertilization. Ocon and Hansen [107] reported that fewer oocytes developed to blastocysts, due to decreased developmental competence. Urea reduced fertilization and cleavage rate of developing embryos. Armstrong and coworkers [12] found increased urea associated with increased nutrient supply decreased oocyte quality; however, Laven and associates [108] observed that Holstein cows fed diets high in rapidly rumen degradable nitrogen experienced no negative effects on follicular development or embryo growth, despite increases in serum urea and ammonia, suggesting that cows can adapt to short-term increases in RDP.

Few studies have examined the relationship between RUP and fertility. Westwood et al [109,110] concluded that increasing RUP in isonitrogenous diets improved feed intake, reduced serum nonesterified fatty acids post-partum, and improved reproductive performance, particularly in cows of high genetic merit. Triplett and coauthors [111] fed a basal diet to postpartum beef cows with three supplements of increasing RUP content (low RUP, 38.1%; moderate RUP, 56.3%; and high RUP, 75.6%, as a percentage of CP). Cows receiving the low RUP supplement had lower first-service CR than cows receiving the moderate and high RUP supplement (29.2% versus 57.6% and 54.6%, respectively). Overall pregnancy proportion tended to be lower for the cows receiving the low RUP supplement than those receiving the moderate and high supplements (43.2%, 61.5%, 56.4%, respectively). It is difficult to separate the effects of increasing RUP on fertility from the simultaneous reduction in RDP that occurred in these studies.

Ferguson and colleagues [100] observed that herd fertility was sensitive to elevated urea levels associated with higher RDP. Cows with serum urea nitrogen greater than 20 mg/dl had CR under 25% [100]. CR to all services declined as serum urea nitrogen increased. The data suggested that plasma urea nitrogen (PUN) concentrations above 19.8 mg/dl (3.3 mmol/l plasma urea [PU]) were detrimental to fertility. Canfield and coworkers [71] associated elevated PUN with reduced CR in an experiment with higher dietary RDP. In subsequent work [17], data from 323 cows suggested that increasing PUN was associated with reduced fertility in a stepwise fashion. Elrod and associates [101,102] observed that reduced fertility with increasing serum urea nitrogen in heifers was associated with increased interestrous interval and reduction in uterine pH early in the luteal phase. Infertility was associated with increased embryonic loss.

Several more recent studies [112–114] have found elevations in MUN to be associated with reductions in fertility. Increasing dietary CP was associated with increases in MUN [114]. The degree of negative association was lower in a study by Hojman et al [114] than in earlier studies by Melendez and coauthors [113], which only observed a negative association of higher MUN levels in summer, whereas in winter months there was no association. Cows may adapt to high urea levels and maintain fertility [109]; however, increased MUN is correlated with increased urinary urea. Urinary urea breaks down rapidly to ammonia when mixed with feces. Ammonia volatilizes rapidly from barn floors and contributes to air particulate matter and acid rain. Therefore, reducing MUN has benefits other than in reproduction.

Together, the results of various studies suggest that fertility declines in cows with PUN above 15.0 mg/dl to 16.2 mg/dl (2.5 to 2.7 mmol/l PU) [17,18,112]. Fertility appears to be further reduced when values are above 19.8 mg/dl (3.3 mmol/l PU). Cows on well-balanced diets for RDP and RUP have PUN concentrations between 10.0 to 160 mg/dl (1.7 and 2.7 mmol/l PU). Thus, high production can be supported with adequate protein and minimal urea concentrations. Table 3 presents data summarized from studies [17,18,112] for PUN and MUN category and pregnancy. In all three studies, increasing MUN is associated with a lower likelihood ratio (LR) for pregnancy or a lower risk ratio for pregnancy (see Table 3).

Veterinarians can monitor MUN as a tool to assess efficiency of protein feeding. Mean MUN between 10 to 14 mg/dl is sufficient for adequate milk production, and will ensure that there are no negative effects on repro- duction. Concentrations of MUN between 14 to 16 mg/dl should not significantly impair fertility, but do indicate that some wastage of dietary nitrogen is occurring. Increases above 16 mg/dl may not only decrease fertility, but may also increase the risk of environmental pollution from ammonia volatilization.

Phosphorus

Phosphorus is a significant environmental pollutant in water systems, increasing risk of eutrophication. Pollution is typically the result of surface soil runoff. Increasing dietary P increases fecal phosphorus, particularly water-soluble forms, which are a high risk for surface runoff. Supplementing appropriate amounts of dietary P is important to prevent environmental pollution.

A summary of studies that have examined P and fertility in dairy cows is presented in Table 4. Across all studies there is no benefit to supplement diets with more than .36% dietary P. Veterinarians should make every effort to encourage producers to reduce dietary supplementation in order to reduce environmental risks. An extensive review of P and N effects on fertility is presented in Ferguson and Sklan [115].

Vitamin E and selenium

Normal cellular metabolism is a process of controlled electron flow that produces energy (ATP) and reducing equivalence to be used for cell synthetic processes (NADH and NADPH). Metabolic processes also

Table 3
Likelihood ratio and risk ratio for multiple categories of plasma urea nitrogen or milk urea nitrogen

Ferguson et al [17]		Butler et al [18]		Rajala-Schultz et al [112][a]		
PUN, mg/dL	LR	PUN, mg/dL	LR	MUN, mg/dL	RR	LR
<10	1.43	<16	2.65	<10	2.4	2.50
10.0–14.9	1.01	16.0–18.9	1.61	10.0–12.7	1.4	.90
15.0–19.9	.90	19.0–21.9	.81	12.7–15.4	1.2	.71
20.0–24.9	.92	22.0–24.9	.80	>15.4	1.0	.56
>25.0	.53	>25.0	.73			

Abbreviations: LR, likelihood ratio; RR, risk ratio.
[a] LR calculated in Rajala-Schultz based on the RR and a pretest CR of 37.5%.

Table 4

Controlled studies in dairy cows reporting phosphorus content of diet and measures of reproductive performance

N, cows	Dietary P % of DM	CR[a]	% estrus detection	DFI[b]	Pregnant %	Reference
10	0.34	0.769	45		100	Lindsay and Archibald [121]
10	0.54	0.769	38		100	
8	0.16	0.600	79	105	86	Eckles et al [122]
16	0.37	0.385	43		100	Steevens et al [123]
16	0.55	0.476	36		100	
16	0.56	0.385	37		100	
16	0.37	0.227	32		100	
16	0.55	0.526	37		100	
16	0.56	0.357	39		100	
12	0.50	0.391	25		75	Carstairs et al [124]
12	0.40	0.538	25		58	
12	0.50	0.410	29		75	
12	0.40	0.375	29		100	
13	0.24	0.769	45	77	92	Call et al [125]
8	0.32	0.526	66	91	87	
13	0.42	0.667	50	72	77	
46	0.355	0.520	36	74	87	Brodison et al [126]
37	0.425	0.590	36	74	86	
36	0.364	0.600	33	75	86	
26	0.458	0.570	44	80	77	
40	0.342	0.630	34	79	80	
32	0.435	0.630	29	83	97	
52	0.39	0.476		55	79	Brintrup et al [127]
52	0.33	0.434		47	90	
8	0.31	0.714		70	100	Wu and Satter [128]
9	0.40	0.625		92	89	
9	0.49	0.435		67	89	
21	0.38	0.400		76	95	Wu and Satter [129]
21	0.48	0.385		77	90	
26	0.38	0.625		66	96	
27	0.48	0.476		72	86	
10	0.31	0.588		90	75	Wu et al [130]
14	0.39	0.625		77	80	
13	0.47	0.833		94	85	

[a] CR calculated as 1/(services per conception).
[b] Days to first insemination.

produce free electrons (free radicals), which result in uncontrolled electron flow and may disrupt cell membranes, protein function, DNA structure, and energy production [116]. Part of the cellular defense system of macrophages and neutrophils against foreign bacteria is to engulf and destroy these invaders through formation of free radicals within cell organelles. Antioxidants protect normal cells from damage by scavenging free radicals. Protection from free radical damage is extended by metalloenzymes, such as glutathione peroxidase, which contains selenium and vitamins A, E, and C. Vitamin E and Se have received considerable attention in ruminant diets, because E tends to be low in preserved, ensiled forages, and Se is deficient in specific regions.

Vitamin E and Se have been reported to benefit the immune status of an animal, to prevent or lower the incidence of, retained placenta, to reduce the incidence of cystic ovarian disease, to improve CR, and to prevent white muscle disease [116,117]. Benefits of vitamin E and Se in reducing the incidence of retained placenta and eliminating white muscle disease are well-established. Reports on the benefits of vitamin E and Se on immune status and reduction in the incidence of mastitis have been more recent. Effects of Se and vitamin E on reduction of cystic ovarian disease and improvement in conception rate tend to be anecdotal.

Both E and Se are important in the diet. The National Research Council (NRC) [52] recommended that vitamin E should be supplemented at 15.9 mg/kg dry matter and Se at 0.3 ppm dry matter, which recently has been reduced to 0.1 ppm because of environmental concerns. Researchers have examined the effects of feeding vitamin E at 1000 international units (IU) per head per day in the dry period on the incidence of retained fetal membranes and mastitis. These higher levels of vitamin E have been shown to reduce the incidence of mastitis postcalving [116]; however, lower levels of vitamin E have not been compared with no supplemental vitamin E. Therefore, it would be prudent to supplement at least at NRC levels, and to compare herd performance with that before no supplementation before adopting higher levels.

Blood analysis may be useful to assess Se status [118]. Plasma or serum Se reflects current supplementation and should be 0.08 to 0.12 ppm with adequate dietary supplementation. Whole blood may lag changes in plasma because of the influence of red blood cells on Se concentration. Se is contained in red blood cells in glutathione peroxidase (GSH-Px). Because red blood cells have a life span of 100 days or more, GSH-Px may not necessarily reflect current Se dietary status. When dietary Se is low, GSH-Px activity is correlated with whole blood Se. Under adequate to high conditions of Se supplementation, GSH-Px activity is not well correlated with Se level [118]. Because of the variation in the GSH-Px assay between laboratories, standards within laboratories have to be established to assess adequate blood levels within a population of cows.

Supplementation of Se and vitamin E in deficient animals has been shown to reduce the incidence of retained placenta. Increased supplementation above recommendations has shown no additional benefit on further reducing retained fetal membranes.

Summary

Selection for higher milk production has reduced fertility in dairy herds; however, management can mitigate the decline. Maintaining high rates of fertility require management of rations from the precalving through pregnancy to postcalving. Feed management that encourages high consumption is as important as provision of well-balanced rations. Body condition and body condition loss, incidence of periparturient problems, proportion of cows ovulating before 40 days postcalving, and MUN are all important considerations in monitoring nutritional effects on reproduction.

References

[1] Butler WR. Nutritional interactions with reproductive performance in dairy cattle. Anim Reprod Sci 2000;60–61:449–57.

[2] Butler WR. Review: effect of protein nutrition on ovarian and uterine physiology in dairy cattle. J Dairy Sci 1998;81:2533–9.

[3] Lucy MC. Reproductive loss in high-producing dairy cattle: where will it end? J Dairy Sci 2001;84:1277–93.

[4] Roche JF, Mackey D, Diskin MD. Reproductive management of postpartum cows. Anim Reprod Sci 2000;60–61:703–12.

[5] Rhodes FM, McDougall S, Burke CR, et al. Invited review: treatment of cows with an extended postpartum anestrous interval. J Dairy Sci 2003;86:1876–94.

[6] Jolly PD, McDougall S, Fitzpatrick LA, et al. Physiological effects of undernutrition on postpartum anoestrus in cows. J Reprod Fertil 1995;49(Suppl):477–92.

[7] Smith GD, Jackson LM, Foster DL. Leptin regulation of reproductive function and fertility. Theriogenology 2002;57:73–86.

[8] Staples CR, Burke JM, Thatcher WW. Influence of supplemental fats on reproductive tissues and performance of lactating cows. J Dairy Sci 1998;81:856–71.

[9] Montiel F, Ahuja C. Body condition and suckling as factors influencing the duration of postpartum anestrus in cattle: a review. Anim Reprod Sci 2005;85:1–26.

[10] Bossis I, Wettemann RP, Welty SD, et al. Nutritionally induced anolulation in beef heifers: ovarian and endocrine function preceding cessation of ovulation. J Anim Sci 1999;77: 1536–46.

[11] Imakawa K, Day ML, Zalesky DD, et al. Effects of 17 beta-estradiol and diets varying in energy on secretion of luteinizing hormone in beef heifers. J Anim Sci 1987;64:805–14.

[12] Armstrong DG, McEvoy TG, Baxter G, et al. Effect of dietary energy and protein on bovine follicular dynamics and embryo production in vitro: associations with the ovarian insulin-like growth factor system. Biol Reprod 2001;64:1624–32.

[13] Baptiste QS, Knights M, Lewis PE. Fertility response of yearling beef heifers after prebreeding energy manipulation, estrous synchronization and timed artifical insemination. Anim Reprod Sci 2005;85:209–21.

[14] Kendall NR, Gutierrez CG, Scaramuzzi RJ, et al. Direct in vivo effects of leptin on ovarian steroidogesesis in sheep. Reproduction 2004;128:757–65.

[15] Gong JG, Lee WJ, Garnsworthy PC, et al. Effect of dietary-induced increases in circulating insulin concentrations during the early postpartum period on reproductive function in dairy cows. Reproduction 2002;123:419–27.

[16] Kwon H, Ford SP, Bazer FW, et al. Maternal nutrient restriction reduces concentrations of amino acids and polyamines in ovine maternal and fetal plasma and fetal fluids. Biol Reprod 2004;71:901–8.

[17] Ferguson JD, Galligan DT, Blanchard T, et al. Serum urean nitrogen and conception rate: the usefulness of test information. J Dairy Sci 1993;76:3742–6.

[18] Butler WR, Calaman JJ, Beam SW. Plasma and milk urea nitrogen in relation to pregnancy rate in lactating dairy cattle. J Anim Sci 1996;74:858–65.

[19] Beam SW, Butler WR. Energy balance and ovarian follicle development prior to first ovulation postpartum in dairy cows receiving three levels of dietary fat. Biol Reprod 1997; 56:133–42.

[20] Beam SW, Butler WR. Effects of energy balance on follicular development and first ovulation in postpartum dairy cows. J Reprod Fertil 1999;54(Suppl):411–24.

[21] Tanaka T, Nagatani S, Bucholtz DC, et al. Central action of insulin regulates pulsatile luteinizing hormone secretion in the diabetic sheep model. Biol Reprod 2000;62:1256–61.

[22] Royal MD, Pryce JE, Woolliams JA, et al. The genetic relationship between commencement of luteal activity and calving interval, body condition score, production, and linear type traits in Holstein-Friesian dairy cattle. J Dairy Sci 2002;85:3071–80.

[23] Nebel RL, McGilliard ML. Interactions of high milk yield and reproductive performance in dairy cows. J Dairy Sci 1993;76:3257–68.

[24] Royal MD, Flint APF, Woolliams JA. Genetic and phenotypic relationships among endocrine and traditional fertility traits and production traits in Holstein-Friesian dairy cows. J Dairy Sci 2002;85:958–67.

[25] Horan B, Mee JF, O'Connor P, et al. The effect of strain of Holstein-Friesian cow and feeding system on postpartum ovarian function, animal production and conception rate to first service. Theriogenology 2005;63:950–71.

[26] Pryce JE, Nielsen BL, Veerkamp RF, et al. Genotype and feeding system effects and interactions for health and fertility traints in dairy cattle. Live Prod Sci 1999;57:193–201.

[27] Bagnato A, Oltenacu PA. Phenotypic evaluation of fertility traits and their association with milk production of Italian Friesian cattle. J Dairy Sci 1994;77:874–82.

[28] Windig JJ, Calus MPL, Veerkamp RF. Influence of herd environment on health and fertility and their relationship with milk production. J Dairy Sci 2005;88:335–47.

[29] Ouweltjes W, Smolders EAA, Elving L, et al. Fertility disorders and subsequent fertility in dairy cattle. Live Prod Sci 1996;46:213–20.

[30] Grohn TY, Rajala-Schultz PJ. Epidemiology of reproductive performance in dairy cows. Anim Reprod Sci 2000;60–61:605–14.

[31] McDougall S. Effects of periparturient diseases and conditions on the reproductive performance of New Zealand dairy cows. N Z Vet J 2001;49(2):60–7.

[32] Grohn YT, Erb HN, McCulloch CE, et al. Epidemiology of reproductive disorders in dairy cattle: associations among host characteristics, disease and production. Prev Vet Med 1990; 8:25–39.

[33] Curtis CR. Path analysis of dry period nutrition, postpartum metabolic and reproductive disorders, and mastitis in Holstein cows. J Dairy Sci 1985;68:2347.

[34] Lee LA, Ferguson JD, Galligan DT. Effect of disease on days open assessed by survival analysis. J Dairy Sci 1989;72:1020–6.

[35] Harman JL, Grohn YT, Erb HN, et al. Event-time analysis of the effect of season of parturition, parity, and concurrent disease on parturition-to-conception interval in dairy cows. Am J Vet Res 1996;57:640–5.

[36] Francos G, Mayer E. Analysis of fertility indices of cows with extended postpartum anestrus and other reproductive disorders compared to normal cows. Theriogenology 1988; 29:399.

[37] Francos G, Mayer E. Analysis of fertility indices of cows with reproductive disorders and of normal cows in herds with low and normal fertility. Theriogenology 1988;29:413.

[38] Oltenacu PA, Britt JH, Braun RK, et al. Effect of health status on culling and reproductive performance of Holstein cows. J Dairy Sci 1984;67:1783–92.

[39] Andersson L, Gustafsson AH, Emanuelson U. Effect of hyperketonaemia and feeding on fertility in dairy cows. Theriogenology 1991;36:521–36.

[40] Opsomer G, Wensing T, Laevens H, et al. Insulin resistance: the link between metabolic disorders and cystic ovarian disease in high yielding dairy cows? Anim Reprod Sci 1999;56: 211–22.

[41] Huszenicza G, Haraszti J, Molnar L, et al. Some metabolic characteristics of dairy cows with different post partum ovarian function. Journal of Veterinary Medicine 1988;35: 506–15.

[42] Ropstad E, Larsen HJ, Refsdal AO. Immune function in dairy cows related to energy balance and metabolic status in early lactation. Acta Vet Scand 1989;30:209–19.

[43] Schrick FN, Hockett ME, Saxton AM, et al. Influence of subclinical mastitis during early lactation on reproductive parameters. J Dairy Sci 2001;84:1407–12.

[44] Hayirli A, Grummer RR, Nordheim EV, et al. Animal and dietary factors affecting feed intake during the prefresh transition period in Holsteins. J Dairy Sci 2002;85: 3430–43.

[45] Markusfeld O, Galon N, Ezra E. Body condition score, health, yield, and fertility in dairy cows. Vet Rec 1997;141:67–72.

[46] Gillund P, Reksen O, Grohn YT, et al. Body condition related to ketosis and reproductive performance in Norwegian dairy cows. J Dairy Sci 2001;84:1390–6.

[47] Gearhart MA, Curtis CR, Erb HN, et al. Relationship of changes in condition score to cow health in Holsteins. J Dairy Sci 1990;73:3132.

[48] Wildman EE, Jones GM, Wagner PE, et al. A dairy cow body condition scoring system and its relationship to selected production characteristics. J Dairy Sci 1982;65:495–501.

[49] Ferguson JD, Galligan DT, Thomsen N. Principal descriptors of body condition in Holstein dairy cattle. J Dairy Sci 1994;77:2695–703.

[50] Heur C, Schukken YH, Dobbleaar P. Postpartum body condition score and results from the first test day milk as predictors of disease, fertility, yield, and culling in commercial dairy herds. J Dairy Sci 1999;82:295–304.

[51] Ruegg PL, Goodger WJ, Holmberg CA, et al. Relation among body condition score, milk production, and serum urea nitrogen and cholesterol concentrations in high-producing Holstein dairy cows in early lactation. Am J Vet Res 1992;53:5.

[52] National Research Council. Nutritional requirements of dairy cattle. Washington (DC): National Academy Press; 2001.

[53] Dijkhuizen AA, Stelwagen J, Renkema JA. A stochastic model for the simulation of management decisions in dairy herds, with special reference to production, reproduction, culling, and income. Prev Vet Med 1986;4:273–89.

[54] Esslemont RJ, Ellis PR. Components of herd calving interval. Vet Rec 1974;95:319–20.

[55] Opsomer G, Grohn YT, Hertl J, et al. Risk factors for postpartum ovarian dysfunction in high producing dairy cows in Belgium: a field study. Theriogenology 2000;53:841–57.

[56] Lucy MC, Staples CR, Thatcher WW, et al. Influence of diet composition, dry matter intake, milk production, and energy balance on time of postpartum ovulation and fertility in dairy cows. Anim Prod 1992;54:323–31.

[57] Thatcher WW, Wilcox CJ. Postpartum estrus as indicator of reproductive status in the dairy cow. J Dairy Sci 1973;56:608.

[58] Darwash AO, Lamming GE, Wolliams JA. The phenotypic association between the interval to post-partum ovulation and traditional measures of fertility in dairy cattle. Anim Sci 1997;65:9–16.

[59] Lamming GE, Darwash AO. The use of milk progesterone profiles to characterize components of subfertility in milked dairy cows. Anim Reprod Sci 1998;52:175–90.

[60] Wiltbank MC, Gumen A, Sartori R. Physiological classification of anovulatory conditions in cattle. Theriogenology 2002;57:21–52.

[61] Savio JD, Boland MP, Hynes N, et al. Resumption of follicular activity in the early postpartum period of dairy cows. J Reprod Fertil 1990;88:569–79.

[62] Muñoz-Gutiérrez M, Blache D, Martin GB, et al. Ovarian follicular expression of mRNA encoding the type I IGF receptor and IGF-binding protein-2 in sheep following five days of nutritional supplementation with glucose, glucosamine or lupins. Reproduction 2004;128: 747–56.

[63] Gonzalez-Bulnes A, Souza CJH, Campbell BK, et al. Systemic and intraovarian effects of dominant follicles on ovine follicular growth. Anim Reprod Sci 2004;84: 107–19.

[64] DeVries MJ, Van Der Beek S, Kaal-Lansbergen LMTE, et al. Modeling of energy balance in early lactation and the effect of energy deficits in early lactation on first detected estrus postpartum in dairy cows. J Dairy Sci 1999;82:1927–34.

[65] De Vries MJ, Veerkamp RF. Energy balance of dairy cattle in relation to milk production variables and fertility. J Dairy Sci 2000;83:62–9.

[66] Bauman DE, Currie WB. Partitioning of nutrients during pregnancy and lactation: a review of mechanisms involving homeostasis and homeorhesis. J Dairy Sci 1514;1980:63.

[67] Bell A. Regulation of organic nutrient metabolism during the transition from late pregnancy to early lactation. J Anim Sci 1995;73:2804–19.

[68] Berghorn KA, Allrich RD, Noller CH. Influence of energy balance on postpartum reproduction. Presented at Purdue University Dairy Day. August 31, 1988.

[69] Butler WR, Smith RD. Interrelationships between energy balance and postpartum reproductive function in dairy cattle. J Dairy Sci 1989;72:767.

[70] Britt JH. Nutrition, weight loss affect reproduction, embryonic death. Feedstuffs. September 21, 1992;17:12–3.

[71] Canfield RW, Sniffen CJ, Butler WR. Effects of excess degradable protein on postpartum reproduction and energy balance in dairy cattle. J Dairy Sci 1990;73:2342–9.

[72] Canfield RW, Butler WR. Energy balance, first ovulation and the effects of naloxone on LH secretion in early lactation dairy cows. J Anim Sci 1991;69:740–6.

[73] Harrison RO, Ford SP, Young JW, et al. Increased milk production versus reproductive and energy status of high producing dairy cows. J Dairy Sci 1990;73:2749–58.

[74] Jerred MJ, Carroll DJ, Combs DK, et al. Effects of fat supplementation and immature alfalfa to concentrate ratio on lactation performance of dairy cattle. J Dairy Sci 1990;73: 2842–54.

[75] Perkins B. Production, reproduction, health and liver function following overconditioning in dairy cattle [PhD thesis]. Ithaca (NY): Cornell University; 1985.

[76] Staples CR, Thatcher WW, Clark JH. Relationship between ovarian activity and energy status during the early postpartum period of high producing dairy cows. J Dairy Sci 1990; 73:938–47.

[77] Villa-Godoy A, Hughes TL, Emery RS, et al. Association between energy balance and luteal function in lactating dairy cows. J Dairy Sci 1988;71:1063–72.

[78] Thatcher WW, De la Sota RL, Shmitt EJ-P, et al. Control and management of ovarian follicles in cattle to optimize fertility. Reprod Fertil Dev 1996;8:203–17.

[79] Thomas MG, Bao B, Williams GL. Dietary fats varying in their fatty acid composition differentially influence follicular growth in cows fed isoenergetic diets. J Anim Sci 1997;75: 2512–9.

[80] Kendrick KW, Bailey TL, Garst AS, et al. Effects of energy balance on hormones, ovarian activity, and recovered oocytes in lactating Holstein cows using transvaginal follicular aspiration. J Dairy Sci 1999;82:1731–40.

[81] Landau S, Braw-Tal R, Kaim M, et al. Preovulatory follicular status and diet affect the insulin and glucose content of follicles in high yielding dairy cows. Anim Reprod Sci 2000; 64:181–97.

[82] Rabiee AR, Lean IJ. Uptake of glucose and cholesterol by the ovary of sheep and cattle and the influence of arterial LH concentrations. Anim Reprod Sci 2000;64:199–209.

[83] Heinonen M. Effect of postpartum live weight loss on reproductive functions in dairy cows. Acta Vet Scand 1988;29:249.

[84] Thissen JP, Ketelslegers JM, Underwood LE. Nutritional regulation of the insulin-like growth factors. Endocr Rev 1994;15:80.

[85] Bao B, Thomas MG, Williams GL. Regulatory roles of high-density and low-density lipoproteins in cellular proliferation and secretion of progesterone and insulin-like growth

factor I by enriched cultures of bovine small and large luteal cells. J Anim Sci 1997;75: 3235–45.

[86] Henson MC, Castracane VD. Leptin in pregnancy. Biol Reprod 2000;63:1219–28.

[87] Maciel MN, Zieba DA, Amstalden M, et al. Leptin prevents fasting-mediated reductions in pulsatile secretion of luteinizing hormone and enhances its gonadotropin-releasing hormone-mediated release in heifers. Biol Reprod 2004;70:229–35.

[88] Amstalden M, Harms PG, Welsh TH Jr, et al. Effects of leptin on gonadotropin-releasing hormone release from hypothalamic-infundibular explants and gonadotropin release from adenohypophyseal primary cell cultures: further evidence that fully nourished cattle are resistant to leptin. Anim Reprod Sci 2005;85:41–52.

[89] Burke JM, Staples CR, Risco CA, et al. Effect of ruminant grade menhaden fish meal on reproductive and productive performance of lactating dairy cows. J Dairy Sci 1997;80: 3386–98.

[90] Larson SF, Butler WR, Currie WB. Reduced fertility associated with low progesterone postbreeding and increased milk urea nitrogen in lactating cows. J Dairy Sci 1997;80: 1288–95.

[91] Pryce JE, Coffey MP, Simm G. The relationship between body condition score and reproductive performance. J Dairy Sci 2001;84:1508–15.

[92] Waltner SS, McNamara JP, Hillers JK. Relationships of body condition score to production variables in high producing Holstein cows. J Dairy Sci 1993;76:3410–9.

[93] Domecq JJ, Skidmore AL, Lloyd JW, et al. Relationship between body condition scores and conception at first artificial insemination in a large dairy herd of high yielding Holstein cows. J Dairy Sci 1997;80:113–20.

[94] Domecq JJ, Skidmore AL, Lloyd JW, et al. Relationship between body condition scores and milk yield in a large dairy herd of high yielding Holstein cows. J Dairy Sci 1997;80: 101–12.

[95] Ruegg PL, Milton RL. Body condition scores of Holstein cows on Prince Edward Island, Canada: relationships with yield, reproductive performance, and disease. J Dairy Sci 1995; 78:552–64.

[96] Syriyasathaporn W, Nielen M, Dieleman SJ, et al. A Cox proportional-hazards model with time-dependent covariates to evaluate the relationship between body-condition score and the risks of first insemination and pregnancy in a high producing dairy herd. Prev Vet Med 1998;37:159–72.

[97] Loeffler SH, de Vries MJ, Schukken YH, et al. Use of AI technician scores for body condition, uterine tone and uterine discharge in a model with disease and milk production parameters to predict pregnancy risk at first AI in Holstein dairy cows. Theriogenology 1999;51:1267–84.

[98] Lucy MC, Staples CR, Michel FM, et al. Energy balance and size and number of ovarian follicles detected by ultrasonography in early postpartum dairy cows. J Dairy Sci 1991;74: 473–82.

[99] Ferguson JD, Chalupa W. Impact of protein nutrition on reproduction in dairy cows. J Dairy Sci 1989;72:746–66.

[100] Ferguson JD, Blanchard T, Galligan DT, et al. Infertility in dairy cattle fed a high percentage of protein degradable in the rumen. J Am Vet Med Assoc 1988;192:659.

[101] Elrod CC, Butler WR. Reduction of fertility and alteration of uterine pH in heifers fed excess ruminally degradable protein. J Anim Sci 1993;71:694–701.

[102] Elrod CC, Van Amburgh M, Butler WR. Alterations of pH in response to increased dietary protein in cattle are unique to the uterus. J Anim Sci 1993;71:702–6.

[103] Blanchard T, Ferguson J, Love L, et al. Effect of dietary crude-protein type on fertilization and embryo quality in dairy cattle. Am J Vet Res 1990;51:905–8.

[104] Sinclair KD, Kuran M, Gebbie FE, et al. Nitrogen metabolism and fertility in cattle: II. Development of oocytes recovered from heifers offered diets differing in their rate of nitrogen release in the rumen. J Anim Sci 2000;78:2670–80.

[105] McEvoy TG, Robinson JJ, Aitken RP, et al. Dietary excesses of urea influence the viability and metabolism of preimplantation sheep embryos and may affect fetal growth among survivors. Anim Reprod Sci 1997;47:71–90.

[106] DeWit AAC, Cesar MLF, Kruip TAM. Effect of urea during in vitro maturation on nuclear maturation and embryo development of bovine cumulus-oocyte complexes. J Dairy Sci 2001;84:1800–4.

[107] Ocon OM, Hansen PJ. Disruption of bovine oocytes and preimplantation embryos by urea and acidic pH. J Dairy Sci 2003;86:1194–200.

[108] Laven RA, Dawuda PM, Scaramuzzi RJ, et al. The effect of feeding diets high in quickly degradable nitrogen on follicular development and embryo growth in lactating Holstein dairy cows. Anim Reprod Sci 2004;84:41–52.

[109] Westwood CT, Lean IJ, Garvin JK. Factors influencing fertility of Holstein dairy cows: a multivariate description. J Dairy Sci 2002;85:3225–37.

[110] Westwood CT, Lean IJ, Garvin JK, et al. Effects of genetic merit and varying dietary protein degradability on lactating dairy cows. J Dairy Sci 2000;83:2926–40.

[111] Triplett BL, Neuendorff DA, Randel RD. Influence of undegraded intake protein supplementation on milk production, weight gain, and reproductive performance in postpartum Brahman cows. J Anim Sci 1995;73:3223–9.

[112] Rajala-Schultz PJ, Saville WJA, Frazer GS, et al. Association between milk urea nitrogen and fertility in Ohio dairy cows. J Dairy Sci 2000;84:482–9.

[113] Melendez P, Donovan A, Hernandez J. Milk urea nitrogen and infertility in Florida Holstein Cows. J Dairy Sci 2000;83:459–63.

[114] Hojman D, Kroll O, Adin G, et al. Relationships between milk urea and production nutrition and fertility traits in Israeli dairy herds. J Dairy Sci 2004;87:1001–11.

[115] Ferguson JD, Sklan D. Effects of dietary phosphorus and nitrogen on cattle reproduction. In: Hristov AN, Pfeffer E, editors. Nitrogen and phosphorus nutrition in cattle. United Kingdom: CABI International; 2005. p. 233–53.

[116] Hurley WL, Doane RM. Recent developments in the roles of vitamins and minerals in reproduction. J Dairy Sci 1989;72:784–804.

[117] Trinder N, Hall RJ, Renton CP. The relationship between the intake of selenium and vitamin E on the incidence of retained placenta in dairy cows. Vet Rec 1973;93:641–4.

[118] Ullrey DE. Biochemical and physiological indicators of selenium status in animals. J Anim Sci 1987;65:1712–26.

[119] Carroll DJ, Jerred MJ, Grummer RR, et al. Effects of fat supplementation and immature alfalfa to concentrate ratio on plasma progesterone, energy balance, and reproductive traits of dairy cattle. J Dairy Sci 1990;73:2855–63.

[120] Dachir S, Blake RW, Harms PG. Ovarian activity of Holstein and Jersey cows of diverse transmitting abilities for milk. J Dairy Sci 1984;67:1776–82.

[121] Lindsey JB, Archibald JG. Mineral supplements for dairy cows. J Dairy Sci 1929;12: 102–16.

[122] Eckles CH, Palmer LS, Gullickson TW, et al. Effect of uncomplicated phosphorus deficiency on estrous cycle, reproduction, and composition of tissues on mature dry cows. Cornell Vet 1935;25:22–43.

[123] Steevens BJ, Bush LJ, Stout JD, et al. Effect of varying amounts of calcium and phosphorus in rations for dairy cows. J Dairy Sci 1971;54:655–61.

[124] Carstairs JA, Morrow DA, Emery RS. Postpartum reproductive function of dairy cows as influenced by energy and phosphorus status. J Anim Sci 1980;51:1122–30.

[125] Call JW, Butcher JE, Shupe JL, et al. Clinical effects of low dietary phosphorus concentrations in feed given to lactating dairy cows. Am J Vet Res 1987;48:133–6.

[126] Brodison JA, Goodall EA, Armstrong JD, et al. Influence of dietary phosphorus on the performance of lactating dairy cattle. J Agri Sci (Cambridge) 1989;112:303–11.

[127] Brintrup R, Mooren T, Meyer U, et al. Effects of two levels of phosphorus intake on performance and fecal phosphorus excretion of dairy cows. J Anim Physiol Anim Nutr (Berl) 1993;69:29–36.

[128] Wu Z, Satter LD. Milk production and reproductive performance of dairy cows fed two concentrations of phosphorus for two years. J Dairy Sci 2000;83:1052–63.

[129] Wu Z, Satter LD. Milk production during the complete lactation of dairy cows fed diets containing different amounts of protein. J Dairy Sci 2000;83:1042–51.

[130] Wu Z, Satter LD, Blohowiak AJ, et al. Milk production, estimated phosphorus excretion, and bone characteristics of dairy cows fed different amounts of phosphorus for two or three years. J Dairy Sci 2001;84:1738–48.

ELSEVIER
SAUNDERS

VETERINARY
CLINICS
Food Animal Practice

Vet Clin Food Anim 21 (2005) 349–365

Breeding Strategies to Optimize Reproductive Efficiency in Dairy Herds

Jeffrey S. Stevenson, PhD

Department of Animal Sciences and Industry, 254 Weber Hall,
Kansas State University, Manhattan, KS 66506-0201, USA

Reproductive inefficiency of dairy cattle causes great frustration and potential lost income for dairy producers [1]. Even under optimal conditions, the reproductive process is less than perfect because of the multiple factors involved in producing a live calf. To manage the complexities of the estrous cycle and the annual reproductive cycle, understanding of many interrelated physiological functions is critical. Further, reproductive efficiency involves successful management of not only the cows, but also the people who milk, feed, house, inseminate, and care for them.

Conception rates of lactating dairy cows in the United States have declined since the 1950s [2], whereas annual milk yield per cow has increased 3.3 times, from 2410 to 8061 kg [3]. Based on a sample of less-productive dairy cows in the United Kingdom, fertility also declined from the period 1975 to 1982 to the period 1995 to 1998 [4]. Between those periods, pregnancy rates after first services decreased from 56% to 40%, despite similar intervals to first service, whereas calving intervals increased from 370 to 390 days. Given the inverse relationship between milk yield and fertility, it is no wonder that a genetic antagonism exists between some reproductive traits and milk yield. This antagonism is manifested particularly in primiparous cows; however, sound management practices have overcome this inverse relationship to achieve acceptable rates of reproductive efficiency.

Although the benefits of improving reproduction are apparent, specific causes of poor reproductive performance are difficult to identify and not resolved easily. To improve reproductive efficiency, the limiting factors must be identified. In general, detecting estrus is the major limitation to achieving a pregnancy [5]. To maximize the chances of a renewed pregnancy for every heifer or cow that calves into the herd, a number of important time-dependent

E-mail address: jss@ksu.edu

doi:10.1016/j.cvfa.2005.02.006   *vetfood.theclinics.com*

components of the estrous cycle must be managed. It is critical to understand each component of the estrous cycle as well as the annual reproductive cycle (calving interval), and to determine where limited time and resources might best be concentrated to reach artificial insemination (AI) breeding goals. Maximal reproductive efficiency requires management of the calving interval. This consists of three major components: (1) the voluntary waiting period (VWP), (2) the active AI breeding period, and (3) gestation (including the dry period), plus their various integral parts (Fig. 1).

Voluntary waiting period

The first component of a calving interval (see Fig. 1) is the traditional rest period or the VWP. Duration of this period is partly a management decision. This period varies from 40 to 70 days on most farms. Part of its duration is based on the physiological need for the reproductive tract of the cow to undergo a healing process, or involution. Some, but not all studies, indicate that longer rest periods improve conception rates [6], possibly because of improvement in various uterine traits. Research indicates that when cows calve without complication, this healing process requires no

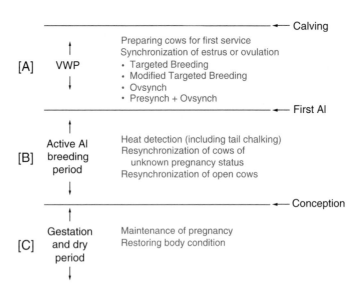

Fig. 1. The three major components of a calving interval in dairy cattle. (*A*) VWP may involve manipulation of the estrous cycle by altering follicular growth and luteal regression in preparation for insemination. (*B*) Active AI breeding period that follows first insemination if conception did not occur. It involves heat detection and resynchronization of estrus, ovulation, or both. (*C*) Gestation and the dry period follow conception. Pregnancy is maintained in the absence of embryonic or fetal loss, and the needed restoration of body condition in preparation for subsequent calving occurs.

more than 40 days [7]. Involution includes macro- and microscopic changes that prepare the reproductive tract, especially the uterus, for a renewed pregnancy.

A number of important physiological adaptations must occur during the VWP. The cow must adapt to the increased demand for nutrients by the mammary gland because of lactogenesis. During late gestation, the feto-placental unit is a major nutrient consumer, and orchestrates a homeorhetic priority of nutrient use. Once parturition occurs, the mammary gland becomes the major nutrient user. As a result, an energy prioritization is manifested that places greater priorities on use of nutrients for maintenance and growth (younger cows) of the cow and for milk secretion than for the onset of estrous cycles and the initiation of a new pregnancy. Cows that consume less dry matter than their contemporaries have delayed first ovulation and first estrus after parturition, produce less milk, and are less fertile [8].

Programmed breeding

Programmed breeding is a method to schedule and control the insemination program of lactating cows in the herd. The advantages for programming estrous cycles include: (1) convenience of scheduling labor and tasks; (2) controlling the occurrence of estrus, ovulation, or both; and (3) knowing the stage of the estrous cycle and reproductive status of groups of cows in the herd. These reproductive statuses include: (1) open cows scheduled for first services, (2) open cows scheduled for reinsemination, (3) open cows designated as culls, and (4) cows confirmed pregnant. Therefore, programmed breeding can be applied to at least two distinct groups of cows: (1) those that are scheduled for their first postpartum inseminations; and (2) those that are open at pregnancy diagnosis, but are reprogrammed to be inseminated in a new breeding cluster.

Breeding clusters

The breeding cluster is one method that can be used to organize groups of cows for programmed breeding. For example, if the VWP is 50 days, then a breeding cluster of cows can be organized to fall within a certain range of days in milk to fit the targeted first-breeding date. These cows can be identified easily using Dairy Herd Improvement Association (DHIA) software, computer records, or spreadsheet programs, or simply by keeping a chronological list of calving dates. In smaller herds (<200 cows), a cluster that calves during a 3-week period can be organized so that the freshest cow in the cluster meets the minimum acceptable VWP at the time of AI. When the VWP is 50 days, a cluster would consist of cows that are 50 to 70 days in milk during the targeted breeding week, and the average interval to first insemination for that cluster would be 60 days.

In larger herds (>200 cows), grouping cows into 1- or 2-week clusters is recommended. These clusters simplify AI breeding of cows that meet the breeding criteria on a weekly or biweekly basis. Therefore, during the period before the cows reach their targeted breeding date (based on days in milk and the VWP), estrus or ovulation is synchronized to occur during each breeding week. Usually, the synchronization period is set so that estrus or fixed-time AI (TAI) occurs during the Monday to Friday workweek or at the convenience of scheduled labor.

Once a system is in place to identify cows and heifers that satisfy those criteria for inclusion in an AI breeding cluster, then the specific programmed breeding system can be fit into a weekly management sequence. At least four programs are used for lactating dairy cows on US dairy farms: (1) Targeted Breeding, (2) Modified Targeted Breeding, (3) Ovsynch, and (4) Presynch + Ovsynch.

Targeted Breeding program

This program was promoted to synchronize the AI breeding of lactating cows in a herd [9]. Injections of prostaglandin ($PGF_{2\alpha}$) are administered 14 days apart (Fig. 2). This interval is based simply on the fact that sufficient time must pass after the first injection so that those females responding to the first injection (their corpus luteum [CL] regresses and they come into

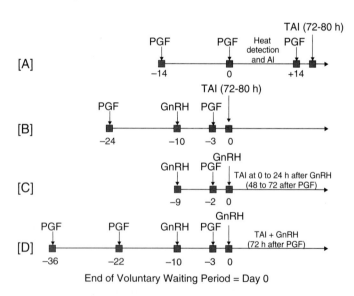

Fig. 2. Four programmed breeding systems: (*A*) Targeted Breeding; (*B*) Modified Target Breeding; (*C*) Ovsynch—the GnRH injection causes ovulation in over 50% of the cows in preparation for $PGF_{2\alpha}$-induced luteal regression; (*D*) Presynch + Ovsynch—administration of two injections of $PGF_{2\alpha}$ causes 70% of the cows to be in the early- to midluteal phase of the estrous cycle at the onset of the Ovsynch protocol.

estrus) have a new CL that is mature enough to respond to a second injection (at least on day 6 of the estrous cycle). In addition, those females that were not in a stage of the estrous cycle and who had a CL that could regress after the first $PGF_{2\alpha}$ injection should be responsive 14 days later [10]. Targeted Breeding requires that the first injection (so-called "setup injection") be given 14 days before the VWP ends. No cows are inseminated after the first injection, although up to 50% may show estrus in response to it. The second injection (first breeding injection) then is given just at the end of the VWP, so that first services can occur when cows are eligible for AI breeding. The targeted breeding program then recommends that when no estrus is detected after the second injection, a third injection (second breeding injection) be given 14 days after the second injection. If no standing estrus is detected after this third injection, then one TAI can be given at 72 to 80 hours after this third injection of $PGF_{2\alpha}$ (see Fig. 2).

Modified Targeted Breeding program

The Modified Targeted Breeding program also is another protocol to synchronize the AI breeding of lactating cows in a herd (see Fig. 2). This program was designed to force the majority of cows into the early luteal phase of the estrous cycle with a presynchronizing injection of $PGF_{2\alpha}$ before administering gonadotropin hormone-releasing hormone (GnRH). Then a 100-μg injection of GnRH is given 7 days before a second $PGF_{2\alpha}$ injection. The GnRH injection alters follicular growth by inducing ovulation of the largest follicle (dominant follicle) in the ovaries to form a new or additional CL [11]. Based on random distribution of cows throughout the estrous cycle, about 64% will be at a stage of the cycle in which a dominant follicle will ovulate in response to the GnRH-induced luteinizing hormone (LH) release from the pituitary gland [12]. Thus, estrus usually does not occur until after a $PGF_{2\alpha}$ injection regresses the natural CL, the GnRH-induced CL (formed from the follicle induced to ovulate by the first GnRH injection), or both. Therefore, a new group of follicles emerges from the ovaries (as shown by transrectal ultrasonography) within 1 to 2 days after the first injection of GnRH [11,12]. From that new group of follicles, a newly developed dominant follicle emerges, matures, and ovulates after estrus is induced by $PGF_{2\alpha}$. Following the $PGF_{2\alpha}$ injection, cows are inseminated based on detected estrus; or in the absence of estrus, one TAI can be administered at 72 to 80 hours after $PGF_{2\alpha}$.

Ovsynch

This program is similar to the previous program, except it requires no detection of estrus (see Fig. 2), and is probably the most popular protocol employed. In fact, it is described more accurately as an ovulation synchronization program; hence the name Ovsynch. A 100-μg injection of

GnRH is given 7 days before a $PGF_{2\alpha}$ injection, then a second 100-μg injection of GnRH is administered 48 hours after $PGF_{2\alpha}$, with one TAI given 0 to 24 hours later. A recent study reported no difference in pregnancy rates when 50 versus 100 μg of GnRH was injected at either time. Care must be exercised to ensure all injections are made deep intramuscular (IM). It is recommended to use 1 to 1.5-inch, 20-g needles to prevent flow back from injection sites.

Following the first GnRH injection, a dominant follicle is induced to ovulate, as described previously. Following the second GnRH injection, in the absence of elevated concentrations of progesterone after CL regression is induced by $PGF_{2\alpha}$, the preovulatory LH surge is induced so that the preovulatory follicle ovulates between 24 and 34 hours later [11]. Few cows will show estrus in this program, with about 8% to 16% showing estrus around the time of the $PGF_{2\alpha}$ injection and up to 30% showing estrus by or shortly after the second GnRH injection [13]. If cows are detected in estrus at any time, they should be inseminated according to the AM-PM rule in order to maximize conception, and the injections of $PGF_{2\alpha}$, GnRH, or both should be eliminated.

Presynch + Ovsynch

Further research with the Ovsynch protocol revealed that when cows were started on this protocol (see Fig. 2) between days 5 and 12 of the estrous cycle, diameter of the ovulatory follicle was less, but conception rates tended to be greater than at other stages of the cycle [12]. Several experiments have demonstrated improved fertility in cows when estrous cycles are presynchronized before applying the Ovsynch protocol [14–16]. This may be accomplished by one $PGF_{2\alpha}$ injection given 12 days before initiating the Ovsynch protocol, or more effectively, by two injections given 14 days apart, with the second injection given 12 days before the onset of the Ovsynch protocol (see Fig. 2). In those studies, pregnancy rates of multiparous cows were increased by 13 percentage points with one injection of $PGF_{2\alpha}$ preceding the Ovsynch protocol [14], whereas pregnancies were improved by 6 to 18 percentage points in all lactating cows when two injections of $PGF_{2\alpha}$ were employed (Table 1) [15,16]. The so-called "Presynch" procedure consists of two injections of $PGF_{2\alpha}$, given 14 days apart, with the second injection given 12 to 14 days before initiating the Ovsynch protocol (see Fig. 2). The author's group recently demonstrated that the optimal time for TAI (+GnRH injection) after the Presynch + Ovsynch protocol was at 72 hours after $PGF_{2\alpha}$ [17].

Intravaginal progesterone-releasing insert

A few studies have reported the combined use of the intravaginal progesterone-releasing controlled internal drug release (CIDR) insert with

Table 1
Comparisons of Ovsynch versus Presynch + Ovsynch in combination with an intravaginal progesterone-releasing controlled interval drug release insert in lactating dairy cows

Trait	Ovsynch		Presynch + Ovsynch		
	No CIDR % (no.)	CIDR % (no.)	No CIDR % (no.)	CIDR % (no.)	Reference
PR at day 56[a]					[18]
Noncyclic + CL at $PGF_{2\alpha}$	39 (57)	37 (46)			
Noncyclic + no CL at $PGF_{2\alpha}$	18 (37)	34 (41)			
Cyclic + CL at $PGF_{2\alpha}$	41 (175)	44 (180)			
Cyclic + no CL at $PGF_{2\alpha}$	20 (47)	40 (46)			
PR at day 32[b]	36.9 (176)		54.2 (181)		[15]
PR at day 74[b]	28.8 (177)		47.0 (180)		
PR at day 29[c]	36.3 (91)	59.3 (91)			[16]
PR at day 57[c]	19.8 (91)	45.1 (91)			
PR at day 29[d]	42.9 (154)	32.0 (150)	48.4 (153)	45.1 (157)	[16]
PR at days 40–45[e]			37 (415)	43 (414)	[20]
PR at days 40–45[f]					[19]
1st lactation	20.1	38.2			
2nd lactation	27.5	22.3			

Abbreviation: PR, pregnancy rate.

[a] Greater ($P < 0.05$) pregnancy rates for cows fitted with CIDR inserts having no CL before the $PGF_{2\alpha}$ injection.

[b] Greater ($P < 0.05$) pregnancy rates for Presynch cows.

[c] Greater ($P < 0.05$) pregnancy rates for cows fitted with CIDR inserts.

[d] Greater ($P < 0.05$) pregnancy rates for Presynch cows. No effect of CIDR insert.

[e] Greater ($P < 0.05$) pregnancy rates for Presynch + Ovsynch cows treated with CIDR inserts.

[f] Greater ($P < 0.05$) pregnancy rates for CIDR-treated first-lactation cows only.

the Ovsynch or Presynch + Ovsynch protocol in lactating dairy cows [15,16,18–20]. Pregnancy rates with the CIDR insert are improved in some studies, but not consistently (see Table 1). In some cases, regardless of cycling status before applying the Ovsynch protocol, cows treated with a CIDR insert and having a CL when $PGF_{2\alpha}$ of the Ovsynch protocol is administered, have greater pregnancy rates [16]. In other cases, only first-lactation cows benefited from the CIDR insert. In some cases, the CIDR tended to reduce pregnancy rates. Intuitively, it seems that noncycling cows should have improved pregnancy rates when treated with the Ovsynch protocol in combination with the CIDR insert. Current results, however, fail to consistently confirm that hypothesis.

Advantages of various programs

Table 2 summarizes the advantages of four programmed breeding systems described above. The best program should be simple and easy to manage, perceptions that may vary with personalities and skills of personnel

Table 2
Advantages of various programmed-breeding systems

| Item | Program | | | |
	TB	Modified TB	Ovsynch	Presynch + Ovsynch
Simplicity		X	X	
Greatest conception rates[a]	X	X		
Greatest pregnancy rates[b]			X	X
Herd size	X	X	X	X
No detection of estrus			X	X
Shorter time of program administration		X	X	
Synchronizes follicle growth and CL regression		X	X	X
Timed insemination without detection of estrus			X	X

Abbreviation: TB, targeted breeding.

[a] Conception rate = number of pregnant cows divided by the number of cows inseminated.

[b] Pregnancy rate = number of pregnant cows divided by the number of cows treated. When timed AI is used and the AI-submission rate is 100%, then conception rate = pregnancy rate.

for each herd. Simplicity could be defined as handling cows fewer times during the synchrony program. Few comparisons of programmed breeding systems have been made in field trials [9,20]. Pregnancy rates achieved in several herds after the Targeted Breeding and Ovsynch programs were similar for lactating cows, but were less for replacement heifers on the latter program [21]. Both programs improved reproductive performance over traditional programs [9] and decreased days open compared with no hormonal intervention.

The important point is not the comparison of conception rates, but whether one program produces more pregnancies per unit of time (pregnancy rate) compared with another. If conception rates are similar, pregnancy rates will be greater when TAI is used, because the AI submission rates are 100%. Therefore, all programs described have a TAI component. The Targeted Breeding program requires considerably more time to administer, including the need for detection of estrus. Where skilled cow people are involved and are adept at detecting subtle as well as major symptoms of estrus, the Targeted and Modified Targeted Breeding programs may be successful. The disadvantage of any system is the rigidity of the injection schedules to which one must conform to guarantee its success.

What adds to the complexity of these systems is the overlapping nature of the cluster groups. For example, if the Presynch + Ovsynch protocol, in which a new cluster is initiated every 2 weeks, is followed, injections must be given concurrently to three different cluster groups. Further, if pregnancy is diagnosed once weekly and open cows are started in their own separate cluster group, the complexity of more cluster groups increases. In almost every case, personnel must be disciplined and detailed in their approach to making these programs work. Otherwise, the alternative is fewer pregnancies achieved and more culling of open cows. As herd size increases and more cows are confined to concrete, the efficiency of detected estrus will decline, because the number of standing events and duration of estrus are less on concrete, where footing is not as good as it is on dirt [22]. As a result of less efficient detection of estrus or the lack of expressed estrus by cows in environments with poor footing, TAI programs have become very popular because of their predictability and the likelihood of their producing a greater proportion of the total pregnancies in the herd.

Costs of programmed breeding

Few studies have evaluated the cost-effectiveness of using the systems described above. A recent study reported the value of a pregnancy on a within-herd basis [23]. One-half of each herd was inseminated only after heat detection, and the Ovsynch protocol was applied to the remaining half of the herd. In the first herd with poor heat detection, the cost of a pregnancy was reduced significantly compared with using only heat detection. In the second herd, in which heat detection was better, the cost of the pregnancy was slightly more after Ovsynch, despite the improved reproductive performance of cows. The greatest costs of a pregnancy were associated with the losses in income associated with culling and long open periods. These two factors accounted for 68% to 83% of the total costs. What was not assessed was the value of the reduced "hassle factor" involved in being able to program inseminations and exercise some control over the breeding program.

Another study modeled the potential net returns per cow by comparing using Ovsynch in winter and summer periods in Florida versus inseminations made after detected estrus [24]. Ovsynch had greater impact on net returns during summer than during winter. Using a TAI system such as Ovsynch was a profitable alternative for managing large commercial dairy herds in which heat-detection rates were poor.

Detection of estrus

The second component of the calving interval is the period of time between the end of the VWP and when the first or subsequent estrus is detected, followed by AI and eventual conception (see Fig. 1). Duration of this period is a function of the estrus-detection rate and the level of individual cow and AI-sire fertility. Whether or not hormones are used to induce estrus before first and subsequent services, the percentage of cows detected in estrus depends on the efficiency of detecting estrus in all cows [25]. Level of cow fertility depends upon a number of factors, including fertility of the service sire, correct thawing and handling of semen, AI breeding technique, and timing of insemination. Level of fertility and estrus-detection rates are usually rate limiting to the establishment of pregnancy in a timely fashion.

The greatest limiting factor to successful fertilization is detection of estrus. Approximately 50% of the estrous periods go undetected on the average dairy farm in the United States [5]. Two important challenges exist for detecting estrus: accurately recognizing signs of estrus, and identifying all possible periods of estrus in breeding heifers and cows. One might be quite accurate in detecting cows in estrus, but still have a major estrus-detection problem because too many estrous periods go unobserved. Problems are caused by a lack of diagnostic accuracy (errors of commission) and a lack of efficient detection of all periods of estrus (errors of omission). Based on elevated progesterone on the day of AI, detection errors of commission ranged from 2% to 60% in some herds [25]. The value of improved estrus detection was estimated to range from $6 to $83 per cow per year when the probability for increasing estrus detection increased from 60% to 70% or from 20% to 30%, respectively [26]. The wide range of values occurred with fixed costs and prices, so that fluctuating prices would introduce further variation in the financial benefits.

Senger [27] described the ideal estrus-detection system as having the following characteristics: (1) continuous surveillance of the cow; (2) accurate and automatic identification of the cow in estrus; (3) operation for the productive lifetime of the cow; (4) minimal labor requirements; and (5) high accuracy and efficiency (95%) for identifying the appropriate physiological events that correlate with estrus, ovulation, or both. Several estrus-detection aids are available on the market to assist dairy producers in identifying estrus [25]. These include inexpensive tail paints, tail chalks, heat-mount detectors such as the Kamar (Kamar Inc., Steamboat Springs, Colorado) or Bovine Beacon (Omniglow Corp., W. Springfield, Massachusetts) and more expensive electronic gadgetry including pedometers, which measure increased physical activity (walking) associated with estrus, or pressure-sensitive and rump-mounted devices such as the HeatWatch system (Cow Chips LLC, Denver, Colorado), which detects and records standing activities by cows in estrus. When used properly to supplement visual observations, estrus-detection aids have a useful role in those cows in which estrus is more difficult to detect (ie, cows that are not yet inseminated, or are inseminated but still not pregnant (Fig. 3).

The key to proper timing of insemination and maximizing fertilization rates is to inseminate cows at such a time as to allow ovulation to occur when adequate numbers of motile sperm are present in the oviduct. Based on a twice-daily estrus-detection program, cows submitted for insemination should be inseminated about 12 hours after first detection in estrus. The exact time when estrus begins is unknown, but on the average, the female detected in estrus at either daily observation period has been in estrus for about 6 hours. So when inseminated 12 hours after first detection, the female

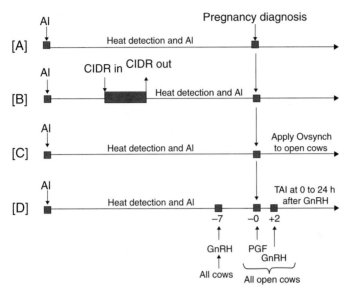

Fig. 3. Techniques used to identify cows not pregnant after first insemination and resynchronization of estrus, ovulation, or both: (*A*) standard heat detection programs; (*B*) CIDR insert is placed in cows of unknown pregnancy; (*C*) Ovsynch protocol is applied to all cows found open at pregnancy diagnosis; (*D*) Resynchronization of ovulation is initiated in cows of unknown pregnancy status. The Ovsynch protocol is then completed in all nonpregnant cows.

actually is bred about 18 hours after the onset of estrus, or approximately 6 to 12 hours before ovulation. This breeding scheme allows ample time for transport and capacitation of sperm, and a synchronized overlap of the fertile lives of both the egg and the sperm, even if the timing is off by as much as 6 hours. Studies, which were based on nonreturn rates, have shown that conception rates after once daily AI were not different from those for cows inseminated based on the AM-PM rule [28]. Results were best when inseminations were based on standing estrus and when AI occurred between 8:00 and 11:00 AM. Optimal timing of AI should occur between 4 and 12 hours after the first standing event detected by the HeatWatch system, or between 6 and 17 hours after increased pedometer readings [25].

Cows not pregnant at pregnancy diagnosis

A traditional procedure has been to give a $PGF_{2\alpha}$ injection to any cow that has a palpable CL diagnosed open at pregnancy checks. Cows were either inseminated based on subsequently detected estrus or inseminated once (80 hours) or twice (72 and 96 hours) after $PGF_{2\alpha}$. Because inseminations are based only on detected estrus, some open cows may go without reinsemination for weeks.

In addition to applying various heat-detection aids and daily monitoring of tail chalk, other techniques are available to assist in the identification of cows in estrus. Recently, the CIDR insert was introduced as a means to resynchronize estrus in nonpregnant cows [29]. It is applied to cows of unknown pregnancy status for 7 days, beginning 14 days after insemination (see Fig. 3). In response to such treatment, pregnancy rates to the initial AI were reduced slightly because of the CIDR insert; however, the CIDR increased the overall heat-detection rate after CIDR insert removal, compared with controls not given CIDR inserts. Resulting conception rates for cows after removal of the CIDR inserts were not different from those of controls.

The Ovsynch program is ideal for preparing open cows for reinsemination (see Fig. 3). It guarantees that every cow is reinseminated within at least 10 days after nonpregnant status is identified. If the open cow is detected in estrus at any time during the 10-day protocol, then the cow should be inseminated according to detected estrus, and the remaining portions of the protocol discontinued. Using this system, detection of estrus can be eliminated totally, but interinsemination intervals will approach 50 days (time to pregnancy diagnosis + 10 days for completion of the Ovsynch protocol) rather than multiples of one estrous cycle, depending on the rate of detected estrus in the herd.

A more proactive treatment [30] sets up cows on the Ovsynch protocol before their pregnancy status is known (see Fig. 3). In this treatment, all cows of unknown pregnancy status are injected with GnRH (first GnRH injection of the Ovsynch protocol) 7 days before pregnancy diagnosis. Once found not pregnant, the Ovsynch protocol is completed by injecting $PGF_{2\alpha}$, followed in 48 hours by a second GnRH injection and insemination (0 to 24 hours later). Using this scenario, in the absence of identifying the first eligible estrus after the previous insemination (20 to 24 days), all open cows were reinseminated by 2 to 3 days after diagnosed not pregnant.

Replacement heifers

Replacement heifers represent the future of the dairy herd. Herd turnover occurs about every 3 to 4 years; in other words, this rate of turnover translates into an annual culling rate of 25% to 33%, necessitating a supply of herd replacements in the form of heifers. These rather high culling rates produce a significant drain on income, because the dairy producer loses in milk income (the cull generally produces more milk than her younger replacement) and funds are expended to purchase the replacement; the producer also may lose on the value of the calf born to the replacement, depending on its genetic merit. In other words, the cost of a replacement heifer equals her purchase cost or value (if raised on the farm) plus the losses in milk yield (difference in the greater value of the milk from the cow and her replacement for what would be the remainder of the cull cow's lactation) minus the recovery value of the cull (sale price of a cull). As a result, the recovery value of the cull when sold is only about one third to one half the cost of purchasing her replacement. The time-sensitive nature of establishing pregnancy in dairy heifers dictates that excellent management inputs are required to achieve pregnancy, including the use of various hormones to manipulate the estrous cycle.

Management of heifer breeding

With tools readily available today for management of the estrous cycle, no excuse exists for failing to achieve timely pregnancies in the replacement herd. Breeding of heifers need not be wholly dependent on visually detecting estrus before AI. Various products include an orally active progestin (melengestrol acetate [MGA]), CIDR inserts, GnRH, and $PGF_{2\alpha}$. Managing the estrous cycle for the convenience of the breeder is now possible, even in large heifer-developer operations in which replacements are raised on contract for individual dairy producers or are raised for sale to other producers.

Feeding MGA (0.5 mg per heifer per day) for 14 days synchronizes estrus (long MGA; see Fig. 4). Depending on the stage of the estrous cycle in which any heifer begins the MGA feeding period, few have a functional CL after

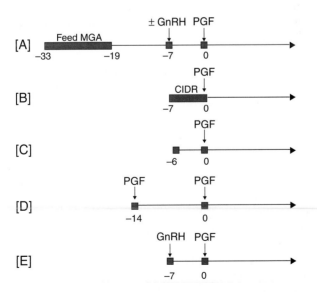

Fig. 4. Five programs for synchronization of estrus or ovulation for dairy heifer replacements: (*A*) long MGA; (*B*) CIDR insert; (*C*) visual detection of estrus; (*D*) injections of $PGF_{2\alpha}$; (*E*) Select Synch.

14 days of feeding. Most heifers show estrus within 2 to 6 days after withdrawing MGA from the feed. This estrus is quite infertile in those heifers that began MGA feeding after day 10 of their estrous cycle. Because the identity of the less fertile heifers is unknown, this first estrus is passed over, and heifers are given an injection of prostaglandin $F_{2\alpha}$ ($PGF_{2\alpha}$) 19 days after MGA withdrawal. Insemination of heifers based on detected estrus usually occurs during 5 days after $PGF_{2\alpha}$. In addition, a cleanup TAI of any noninseminated heifers at 72 to 80 hours after $PGF_{2\alpha}$ is possible, but conception rates will be approximately 60% to 75% of those achieved based on observed estrus. If GnRH is administered 7 days before $PGF_{2\alpha}$, conception rates to a single TAI at 72 hours are acceptable.

Insertion of a CIDR insert in addition to $PGF_{2\alpha}$ effectively synchronizes estrus in a short-term, 7-day period (see Fig. 4). Injection of $PGF_{2\alpha}$ 24 hours before or upon removal of the insert lyses any functional CL. Generally, inseminations occur after detected estrus during a 2 to 5-day period after insert removal. When injecting $PGF_{2\alpha}$ at the same time the insert is removed, estrus will be delayed by approximately 12 to 24 hours, and will be slightly more variable in its range of occurrence. Generally, no estrus occurs during the first 24 to 36 hours after insert removal. Insemination options include: AI based on detected estrus, AI based on detected estrus + cleanup TAI at 84 hours, or one TAI at 60 to 66 hours after $PGF_{2\alpha}$.

A more simple and less expensive method (see Fig. 4) includes detection of estrus and insemination of any heifer in estrus during 6 days. On the seventh day, $PGF_{2\alpha}$ is injected in any noninseminated heifer to induce luteolysis and estrus for subsequent insemination. The success of this method depends on the accuracy and efficiency of visual detection of estrus. Insemination should be based solely on detected estrus.

A more complicated method involves giving two injections of $PGF_{2\alpha}$ 14 days apart (see Fig. 4). One can inseminate estrus-detected heifers after the first or second of two injections, or inseminate after both injections and reduce the number of second injections to all noninseminated heifers. Timing of inseminations after the first injection should be based solely on detected estrus. Inseminations after the second of two injections should be based on detected estrus, detected estrus + a cleanup TAI at 72 to 80 hours after $PGF_{2\alpha}$, or one TAI at 72 to 80 hours. One single TAI after the second $PGF_{2\alpha}$ injection generally produces lower conception rates than those made after detected estrus.

Another technique (Select Synch; see Fig. 4) combines GnRH to induce release of follicle-stimulating hormone (FSH) and LH plus injection of $PGF_{2\alpha}$ 7 days later, before visually detected estrus. The GnRH injection in some heifers better controls follicular development and synchronizes it with luteolysis that follows $PGF_{2\alpha}$. About 10% of heifers show estrus ±24 hours of $PGF_{2\alpha}$, and therefore, for optimal results detection of estrus should begin 24 to 48 hours before $PGF_{2\alpha}$. Insemination should be based solely on detected estrus.

An alternative (Ovsynch; see Fig. 2) to the previous protocol allows for a single TAI after the injection of $PGF_{2\alpha}$. A second injection of GnRH is given to all heifers at about 48 hours after $PGF_{2\alpha}$, and then insemination occurs 0 to 24 hours later. Of course, if estrus is observed before $PGF_{2\alpha}$ or the second GnRH injection, one inseminates the heifer based on visual signs and discontinues the remainder of the injections.

This program works in replacement heifers, but better pregnancy rates can be achieved with other programs [31]. It generally is not recommended unless detection of estrus during 40 hours after $PGF_{2\alpha}$ and subsequent AI are combined with TAI (0 to 24 hours after the second GnRH injection) for all heifers not previously detected in estrus. For some unexplained reason, the first GnRH injection fails to result in ovulation of a follicle as often in heifers as it does in lactating cows [11].

All of these programs only synchronize estrus for the first AI; however, subsequent periods of estrus are quite well-synchronized in those heifers that fail to conceive to the first AI. Tail chalk or tail paint, heat-mount detectors, or more sophisticated electronic devices can be used to detect estrus before any subsequent insemination. Because heifers tend to display very pronounced signs of estrus, they are easily detected if consistent twice-daily periods of visual observation are performed. Methods described earlier for resynchronizing estrus in lactating cows are options to employ with dairy heifers (see Fig. 3).

Summary

The three components of the calving interval and their parts, outlined in Fig. 1, illustrate the key management steps in maintaining reproductive efficiency in the dairy herd. Use of the Presynch + Ovsynch program is likely to be the most efficient and least costly way to prepare clusters of cows for their best chance to conceive at first AI service. Using tail chalk or sophisticated electronic detection aids to identify normal returns to estrus at 18 to 24 days after TAI will ensure greater return rates of cows not pregnant to the first TAI. For those open cows not detected in estrus, weekly pregnancy diagnosis by ultrasonography or palpation is critical to resynchronize open cows by applying a TAI program such as the Ovsynch protocol. Once diagnosed pregnant twice, these cows should be safely pregnant, with few further fetal losses after 98 days. Many reproductive technologies used today, including programmed breeding, will be refined and incorporated into the management of cows on fewer dairy farms with more cows per farm. Despite trends for longer lactations associated with bovine somatotropin (bST) and lesser pregnancy rates, renewed lactations following parturition will continue to be essential for herd longevity of cows.

Because replacement heifers represent the future genetic investment of any dairy herd, their management is critical to herd survival and longevity. Associated costs and investments in replacements are significant at 15% to

20% of all farm costs. Timeliness of establishing pregnancy is significantly improved when using various hormonal schemes to program the estrous cycle in order to facilitate the use of AI, and to ensure that a greater proportion of heifers calve by 24 months of age. Sire selection should emphasize production traits and calving ease in order to maintain high production, but ensure fewer problems at first parturition. Because heifers are more fertile than their lactating counterparts, the best sires can be used with a much greater cost-benefit ratio.

References

[1] Call EP, Stevenson JS. Current challenges in reproductive management. J Dairy Sci 1985; 68(10):2799–805.

[2] Butler WR, Smith RD. Interrelationships between energy balance and postpartum reproductive function in dairy cattle. J Dairy Sci 1989;72(3):767–83.

[3] Lucy MC. Reproductive loss in high-producing dairy cattle: where will it end? J Dairy Sci 2001;84(6):1277–93.

[4] Royal MD, Darwash AO, Flint APF, et al. Declining fertility in dairy cattle: changes in traditional and endocrine parameters of fertility. Anim Sci 2000;70(3):487–501.

[5] Barr HL. Influence of estrus detection on days open in dairy herds. J Dairy Sci 1975;58(2): 246–7.

[6] Britt JH. Early postpartum breeding in dairy cows. A review. J Dairy Sci 1975;58(2): 266–71.

[7] Kiracofe GH. Uterine involution: its role in regulating postpartum intervals. J Anim Sci 1980;51(Suppl 2):16–28.

[8] Staples CR, Thatcher WW, Clark JH. Relationship between ovarian activity and energy status during the early postpartum period of high producing dairy cows. J Dairy Sci 1990; 73(4):938–47.

[9] Nebel RL, Jobst SM. Evaluation of systematic breeding programs for lactating dairy cows: a review. J Dairy Sci 1998;81(4):1169–74.

[10] Beal WE. Current estrus synchronization and artificial insemination programs for cattle. J Anim Sci 1998;76(Suppl 3):30–8.

[11] Pursley JR, Mee MO, Wiltbank MC. Synchronization of ovulation in dairy cows using PGF_{2a}, and GnRH. Theriogenology 1995;44(4):915–23.

[12] Vasconcelos JLM, Silcox RW, Rosa GJ, et al. Synchronization rate, size of the ovulatory follicle, and pregnancy rate after synchronization of ovulation beginning on different days of the estrous cycle in lactating dairy cows. Theriogenology 1999;52(6):1067–78.

[13] Stevenson JS, Tiffany SM, Lucy MC. Use of estradiol cypionate as a substitute for GnRH in protocols for synchronizing ovulation in dairy cattle. J Dairy Sci 2004;87(10): 3298–305.

[14] Cartmill JA, El-Zarkouny SZ, Hensley BA, et al. Stage of cycle, incidence and timing of ovulation, and pregnancy rates in dairy cattle after three timed breeding protocols. J Dairy Sci 2001;84(5):1051–9.

[15] Moreira F, Risco CA, Pires MFA, et al. Use of bovine somatotropin in lactating dairy cows receiving timed artificial insemination. J Dairy Sci 2000;83(6):1237–47.

[16] El-Zarkouny SZ, Cartmill JA, Hensley BA, et al. Pregnancy in dairy cows after synchronized ovulation regimens with or without presynchronization and progesterone. J Dairy Sci 2004; 83(4):1024–37.

[17] Portaluppi MA, Stevenson JS. Pregnancy rates in lactating dairy cows after presynchronization of estrous cycles and variations in the Ovsynch protocol. J Dairy Sci 2005;88: 914–21.

[18] Pursley JR, Fricke PM, Garverick HA, et al. Improved fertility in noncycling lactating dairy cows treated with exogenous progeserone during Ovsynch [abstract 251]. In: Abstracts of Midwest ADSA-ASAS meeting; 2001. p. 63.

[19] Moreira F, Flores R, Boucher J. Use of CIDR with a timed insemination protocol in lactating dairy cows during summer in Mexico [abstract W238]. In: Joint annual meeting abstracts of ADSA-ASAS-PSA; 2004. p. 373.

[20] Moreira F, Flores R, Boucher J, et al. Effects of CIDR inserts on first service pregnancy rates of lactating dairy cows submitted to a presynch program and on re-resynchronization of second service in Mexico [abstract 419]. In: Joint annual meeting abstracts of ADSA-ASAS-PSA; 2004. p. 256.

[21] Pursley JR, Wiltbank MC, Stevenson JS, et al. Pregnancy rates per artificial insemination for cows and heifers inseminated at a synchronized ovulation or synchronized estrus. J Dairy Sci 1997;80(2):295–300.

[22] Vailes LD, Britt JH. Influence of footing surface on mounting and other sexual behaviors of estrual Holstein cows. J Anim Sci 1990;68(1):2333–9.

[23] Tenhagen BA, Drillich M, Surholt R, et al. Comparison of timed AI after synchronized ovulation to AI at estrus: reproductive and economic considerations. J Dairy Sci 2004;87(1): 85–94.

[24] Risco CA, Moreira F, DeLorenzo M, et al. Timed artificial insemination in dairy cattle—Part II. Compend Contin Educ Pract Vet 1998;20(11):1284–90.

[25] Stevenson JS. Reproductive management of dairy cows in high milk-producing herds. J Dairy Sci 2001;84(Suppl E):E128–43.

[26] Pecsok SR, McGilliard ML, Nebel RL. Conception rates. 1. Derivation and estimates for effects of estrus detection on cow profitability. J Dairy Sci 1994;77(10):3008–15.

[27] Senger PL. The estrus detection problem: new concepts, technologies, and possibilities. J Dairy Sci 1994;77(9):2745–53.

[28] Nebel RL, Walker WL, McGilliard ML, et al. Timing of artificial insemination of dairy cows: fixed time once daily versus morning and afternoon. J Dairy Sci 1994;77:3185–91.

[29] Chenault JR, Boucher JF, Dame KJ, et al. Intravaginal progesterone insert to synchronize return to estrus of previously inseminated dairy cows. J Dairy Sci 2003;86(6):2039–49.

[30] Fricke PM, Caraviello DZ, Weigel KA, et al. Fertility of dairy cows after resynchronization of ovulation at three intervals following first timed insemination. J Dairy Sci 2003;86(12): 3941–50.

[31] Stevenson JS, Smith JF, Hawkins DE. Reproductive outcomes of dairy heifers treated with combinations of prostaglandin $F_{2\alpha}$, norgestomet, and gonadotropin-releasing hormone. J Dairy Sci 2000;83(1):1–8.

VETERINARY
CLINICS
Food Animal Practice

ELSEVIER
SAUNDERS

Vet Clin Food Anim 21 (2005) 367–381

Breeding Strategies to Optimize Reproductive Efficiency in Beef Herds

Michael L. Day, MS, PhD*, David E. Grum, MS, PhD

Department of Animal Sciences, The Ohio State University, 2027 Coffey Road, Columbus, OH 43210, USA

Our ability to synchronize estrus in beef cattle has increased substantially over the past 15 years. This advancement in success of estrous control programs has been driven by enhanced understanding of the physiology of reproduction in cattle, and the use of this knowledge toward development of new technologies and approaches. With these advances, the success rates of artificial insemination (AI) programs that use estrous control systems have been enhanced, and the number of failed AI programs has been reduced significantly. It is not uncommon to achieve pregnancy rates of 50% to 70% in timed AI programs for well-managed herds with a compact calving season; however, less than satisfactory results in terms of pregnancy rates (<50%) still occur. There are many possible reasons for poor pregnancy rates within a single herd, ranging from reproductive diseases to the use of semen of inadequate fertility. A common limitation to success of some estrous synchronization programs appears to be the incidence of anestrus in the group of females to be synchronized. Whether AI will be performed based on detected estrus or at a set time (timed AI) influences the synchronization program that is selected, and will influence the conception and pregnancy rates achieved.

Products for estrous synchronization

Several programs for estrous synchronization that involve the use of prostaglandin $F_{2\alpha}$ (PGF), progesterone or progesterone-like compounds

Research in estrous synchronization in our program has been supported by The Ohio State University, Agricultural Research and Development Center (OARDC) and Select Sires, Plain City, Ohio.
* Corresponding author.
E-mail address: day.5@osu.edu (M.L. Day).

(progestin) and gonadotropin hormone-releasing hormone (GnRH) have been developed [1–3] and are currently used in the cattle industry. These hormones are approved for use in beef cattle and are marketed under a variety of trade names and chemical forms (Table 1). Although all compounds discussed in this article are approved for use in beef cattle, several of the synchronization programs involve combination of these products in systems that are not currently approved by the Food and Drug Administration (FDA).

Estrous synchronization programs in beef heifers

Synchronization using prostaglandin $F_{2\alpha}$

The most traditional approach to estrous synchronization in the United States has been through the use of PGF. PGF regulates a female's estrous cycle by causing regression of the corpus luteum (CL), mimicking natural PGF release from the uterus. Coordinated regression of the CL in a group of females synchronizes a decline in progesterone, and results in a relatively synchronous display of estrus 2 to 5 days later. In order for PGF to be effective, females must be exhibiting normal estrous cycles (cyclic), and be in a stage of the estrous cycle when the CL is responsive to PGF. It has been established that PGF does not consistently cause luteal regression on days 1 through 5 of the estrous cycle [4], but is effective from days 6 to 17 [5]. In a summary of data (J. Chenault, unpublished data) regarding the effects of day of the estrous cycle during the "effective period" (approximately day 5 to 17 of the cycle) on luteal regression with PGF, it was determined that the response was lowest in females treated between days 5 and 9 (67%), intermediate for those treated on days 9 to 12 (77%), and greatest in females treated after day 12 (91%). After day 17 of the estrous cycle, it was difficult to determine whether regression of the CL was the result of exogenous or endogenous PGF.

Table 1
Commonly used hormones in estrous synchronization and their respective trade names

Hormone	Commercial products[a]
Gonadotropin hormone-releasing hormone (GnRH)	Cystorelin, Factrel, Fertagyl, OvaCyst
Progestins	
Progesterone	CIDR, Intravaginal progesterone-releasing insert
Synthetic progestin	Melengestrol acetate (MGA), orally-active in feed
Prostaglandin $F_{2\alpha}$ (PGF)	Lutalyse, Estrumate, ProstaMate, In Sync

[a] The commercial products often do not have the same chemical composition as the hormone produced by the animal's body. In many cases, these compounds have similar effects on the reproductive system as the native hormone.

A variety of approaches have been developed in an effort to ensure that most cyclic females have a responsive CL at the time of PGF, thereby increasing the proportion in which estrus is synchronized. A standard approach is to administer two injections of PGF 12 to 14 days apart, and AI all females during the 5 to 7 day period after the second PGF treatment. With this spacing of injections, essentially all females should possess a CL that is responsive to regression by PGF at the time of the second injection. An alteration of this approach is to administer the initial injection of PGF and inseminate those in estrus during the 3 to 7 days after PGF. Subsequently, females that do not display estrus are given a second PGF treatment 12 to 14 days after the first PGF treatment, with the presumption that these females were in the early part of the cycle at the time of the first injection, and should have a CL that is highly responsive to PGF at the time of the second injection. An alternative approach to account for cyclic females in a nonresponsive stage of the estrous cycle at the planned time of the initial PGF treatment is to detect estrus and AI heifers for 5 to 7 days preceding administration of PGF, thereby ensuring that all heifers are at least beyond day 5 to 7 of the estrous cycle at the time of PGF.

In a majority of reports in which estrus has been synchronized with PGF and AI has been performed based on detection of the PGF-induced estrus, fertility is approximately equal to that of females inseminated following detection of a spontaneous estrus. Across many experiments [6–9], which included over 1750 heifers receiving a PGF synchronization system, conception rates to the synchronized estrus ranged from 38.7% to 88%, with an average conception rate of 62.8%. In practice, perhaps the largest determinant of pregnancy rate during a synchronization period is the proportion of the females that are cyclic, because this proportion will dictate the number of females that have CL that can be regressed by PGF and lead to a synchronized estrus.

Melengestrol acetate-prostaglandin $F_{2\alpha}$ synchronization system

Currently, a system that involves the combination of the orally active progestin, melengestrol acetate (MGA), and PGF is widely used for synchronization of estrus in heifers. This approach involves feeding MGA at 0.5 mg/animal/d for 14 days, and injecting PGF 17 to 19 days after the last feeding of MGA (Fig. 1). Typically, MGA is provided as part of a daily concentrate supplement, and is carried in 4 to 5 pounds of feed. Additionally, MGA can be top-dressed on a grain/concentrate or a silage-based ration. Heifers should be allowed sufficient bunk space to ensure adequate consumption by all heifers. A short adaptation period (3–7 days) to the ration is recommended for heifers not previously receiving feed of similar composition.

In this program, feeding MGA for 14 days serves two purposes. First, this treatment synchronizes estrus in cyclic heifers in such a manner that all these

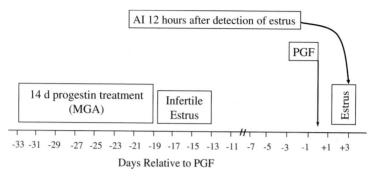

Fig. 1. The MGA-PGF synchronization program includes MGA, provided in feed for 14 days at a daily rate of 0.5 mg/animal (days −33 to −19). Conception rate at the synchronized estrus occurring immediately after cessation of MGA (day −19 to day −13) will be reduced, and animals should not be inseminated during this infertile estrus. Animals receive the recommended dose of PGF on day 0. Estrus will occur during the 5-day period after PGF, with the peak time of estrus at 48 to 72 hours after PGF. For the MGA-Select program, an injection of GnRH (100 µg) will be given on day −7, with all other treatments remaining the same.

females will be in estrus during the 7-day period following the MGA feeding period. This is accomplished through the progesterone-like actions of MGA to block estrus and ovulation in all animals during this 14-day period. Second, treatment with a progestin induces prepubertal heifers to ovulate [10,11], with the timing of the induced ovulation in prepubertal females approximately coinciding with the synchronized estrus in the cyclic females during the 7 days after MGA feeding is terminated. The synchronized estrus/ovulation that occurs during the 7 days following the last day of MGA feeding is of low fertility [12,13], however, as a result of the development of persistent ovarian follicles following extended feeding of MGA [14]. Females are not bred at this initial estrus, but an injection of PGF is given 17 to 19 days after the last feeding of MGA (approximately 10 to 16 days after the infertile estrus), when a majority of females are in the last half of their estrous cycle. By grouping all heifers at this stage of the estrous cycle, the efficacy of PGF to induce luteal regression should be great, and the resulting estrus is of normal fertility. A majority of heifers will be in estrus between the second and fourth days after PGF. Thus, an overall time frame of approximately 36 days (14 + 19 + 3) is required between the initiation of the feeding of MGA and expression of estrus with the MGA-PGF program.

In a recent experiment involving 709 heifers at four locations, the authors and associates [15] reported submission rates (estrus detection rate) of 83.4% in heifers receiving the MGA-PGF protocol during the 7 days following PGF, with the peak timing of AI occurring the third day after PGF. Conception rate in this experiment was 75.8%, resulting in a pregnancy rate of 63.2% in this group of heifers. These responses are typical of those in the published literature; in a recent review [3] the authors summarized reports that included a total of 2800 heifers and that had submission (84.8%) conception (67.2%) and pregnancy (57%) rates after receiving the MGA-PGF treatment. Investigation of the use of timed AI with the MGA-PGF system has yielded variable results. In a recent study [16] that involved over 1700 heifers, pregnancy rates were compared for heifers that were inseminated exclusively by timed AI with those inseminated following detection of estrus. Pregnancy rates were 37% for timed AI and 62% for AI based upon detection of estrus, indicating that programs which exclusively used timed AI with the MGA-PGF system are less effective. In the same report, however, the authors reported an investigation of programs that coupled a shortened period of estrus detection (3 days) with timed AI occurring at the end of 3 days in all females not detected in estrus. Pregnancy rates were similar between heifers that received the "hybrid" approach of estrus detection/timed AI and heifers in which estrus detection continued for 5 days. This approach provides a method to reduce the duration of the estrus detection period to 3 days.

Progesterone-prostaglandin $F_{2\alpha}$ program

The CIDR (Interag, Hamilton, New Zealand), which releases progesterone from an intravaginal insert, is marketed and approved in the United States to be used in combination with an injection of PGF. The CIDR is inserted for 7 days and an injection of PGF is given either 1 day before, or at the time of withdrawal of the CIDR (day 0) (Fig. 2). Females

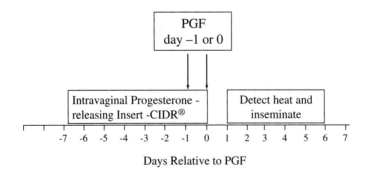

Days Relative to PGF

Fig. 2. The CIDR-PGF synchronization program includes a CIDR, inserted intravaginally on day −7 and withdrawn on day 0, and an injection of PGF at the recommended dosage given either on day −1 or day 0. Substantial differences in pregnancy rate have not been noted between the two times of PGF treatments; however, estrus will occur approximately 12 to 24 hours earlier after CIDR withdrawal if PGF is given on day −1. Estrus can occur from day 1 to 6, but a majority of females will be in estrus between days 1 and 4. In some programs, estrus detection is performed for the initial 72 hours after PGF (day 0 to 3), with AI performed based upon detection of estrus. Females not detected in estrus by hour 72 are administered 100 μg of GnRH and bred by timed AI at hour 84.

are inseminated upon detection of estrus during the 3 to 6-day period beginning on day 1. The progesterone from the CIDR suppresses heat from days 7 to 0, thus no heat detection is necessary during this time. A large experiment that included 724 yearling heifers at five locations across the United States was performed to compare the effectiveness of this approach (CIDR + PGF) with a single PGF injection (PGF) and with nonsynchronized (control) females [17]. Comparing the two synchronization treatments, the CIDR + PGF treatment increased synchronization rate by approximately 35%, and pregnancy rate by approximately 25%, during a 3-day synchronization period (day 1–3) relative to the PGF treatment. Pregnancy rates during the 3-day synchronization period were 39% for yearling heifers in the CIDR + PGF treatment. Use of the CIDR in this manner concentrated breeding, induced anestrus females to cycle, increased pregnancy rates, and did not negatively affect conception rate relative to a single PGF injection. In another report [18], use of the CIDR + PGF treatment—with AI based upon detected estrus until 84 hours, then heifers not detected in estrus bred by timed AI at hour 84 (and given an injection of GnRH)—pregnancy rate was 54.5% (n = 517) (Table 2).

Gonadotropin hormone-releasing hormone–prostaglandin $F_{2\alpha}$ programs

Several programs of estrous control in cattle that use a combination of GnRH and PGF have been developed and have been applied in heifers for estrous synchronization. The central components of all GnRH-based systems of estrous control are treatment with GnRH (or an analog), followed 6 or 7 days later with PGF (GnRH-PGF) (Fig. 3). Administration of GnRH is aimed at inducing synchronous emergence of a new wave of follicular growth in all females 1 to 2 days later, as a result of induction of ovulation of dominant follicles in the ovaries. Regression of CL 6 to 7 days later initiates

Table 2
Pregnancy rates from synchrony programs (12 locations) in heifers with breeding on either detected estrus and timed AI (hybrid approach) or exclusively with timed AI

Synchrony program[a]	Type of AI	n	Pregnancy rate (%)
CIDR-PGF	Detected estrus[b]	517	54.5
GnRH-CIDR-PGF	Detected estrus[b]	504	57.3
CIDR-PGF	60h TAI[c]	531	49.1
GnRH-CIDR-PGF	60h TAI[c]	525	53.1

[a] GnRH administered at time of CIDR insertion. CIDRs inserted for 7 days. PGF administered at time of CIDR removal.

[b] Heifers AI 12 h after observed estrus. Heifers not observed in estrus by 84 h received GnRH and were timed AI.

[c] Heifers received GnRH at time of AI.

Data from Larson JE, Lamb GC, Geary TW, et al. Synchronization of estrus in replacement beef heifers using GnRH, prostaglandin $F_{2\alpha}$ (PG) and progesterone (CIDR): a multi-locational study [abstract]. J Anim Sci 2004;82(Suppl 1):369.

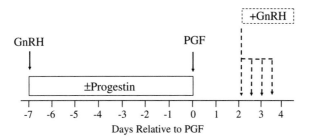

Fig. 3. All GnRH-based systems of estrous synchronization include two central components: the GnRH treatment (100 µg) given on day −7, and the recommended dosage of PGF given on day 0. The progestin treatment between GnRH and PGF is used in some programs, and most often consists of a CIDR inserted on day −7 and withdrawn on day 0, or MGA that is fed at a daily rate of 0.5 mg/animal on days −6 to −1, inclusive. For programs in which animals are bred exclusively based upon detection of estrus, detection should occur from at least day 1 to day 4. In programs that do not include a progestin, approximately 8% of animals may exhibit estrus between days −3 and 1, and may warrant detection of estrus during this time. For programs that are exclusively timed AI, the +GnRH treatment is given on day 2 or 2.5, and AI occurs either at that time, or 8 to 12 hours after GnRH. For programs that use a hybrid of estrus detection and timed AI, estrus detection is performed to day 2.5 to 3, and AI in females exhibiting estrus is performed 12 hours after detected estrus. Animals not observed in estrus during this time receive 100 µg of GnRH at hour 72 or 84, and are inseminated either at the time of GnRH or 8 to 12 hours later.

a decline in progesterone that leads to a follicular phase. If the initial GnRH injection is effective in inducing emergence of a new wave of follicles 4 to 6 days before PGF, most females will have dominant follicles of a relatively standard age and size at the time of luteal regression. Collectively, this approach should increase the precision of the timing of estrus and ovulation during the synchronization period. Moreover, this approach is designed to coordinate follicular development to the extent that a second injection of GnRH can be used 2 to 4 days after PGF (+GnRH) (see Fig. 3) to synchronize ovulation and support the use of timed AI. As indicated in Fig. 3, a progestin can also be added to the base GnRH-PGF systems.

A variety of names have arisen in the popular press and in the published literature to described the various GnRH-based programs of estrous synchronization. In the most basic system, only the GnRH and PGF (GnRH-PGF) treatments indicated in Fig. 3 are given, and females are inseminated based upon detection of estrus. The term most often used to describe this program is "Select Synch." In another program, the +GnRH treatment indicated in Fig. 3 is given to all females, usually 48 to 66 hours after PGF, and all females are given timed AI coincident with the +GnRH treatment (GnRH-PGF + GnRH).This system is usually referred to as the "CO-Synch" protocol. In some groups of animals, especially in dairy herds, an approach similar to CO-Synch is taken, with the single exception that timed AI is performed 8 to 16 hours after the +GnRH treatment, rather than coincident with this injection, requiring an additional handling of animals. This approach is commonly referred to as "Ovsynch." Some protocols use a combination of heat detection and timed AI after PGF. In these programs, estrus detection is typically performed for 72 to 84 hours after PGF, and females detected are inseminated. At 72 or 84 hours after PGF, those animals that have not exhibited estrus receive the +GnRH treatment and are bred with timed AI. The two working names in the field for this protocol are either "Hybrid-Synch" or "MSU-Synch". Finally, the option exists to add a progestin either between or preceding the GnRH and PGF treatments depicted in Fig. 3. If the progestin is applied between GnRH and PGF, and involves a CIDR, these programs are referred to as "CO-Synch + CIDR" (GnRH-CIDR-PGF + GnRH), or similar terminology, depending upon the underlying protocol (eg, Select Synch, Ovsynch, and so on). In some cases, MGA is fed for 14 days, and a GnRH program (usually Select Synch) is initiated 12 days after cessation of MGA feeding. This program is commonly referred to as "MGA-Select."

In general, use of the Select Synch program (GnRH-PGF) in heifers results in conception rates similar to those achieved with PGF or MGA-PGF programs. The authors [3] recently summarized information from four reports, in which heifers that received the Select Synch treatment and were inseminated based upon estrus detection had an average conception rate of 63.9%. The proportion of heifers detected in estrus with Select Synch is highly dependent upon the defined period of estrus detection. The occurrence of estrus outside the 3 to 5-day period after PGF is greater in heifers than cows, and is probably due to a reduced ability of the initial GnRH treatment to induce ovulation and reset follicular development in heifers [19,20]. The early occurrence of estrus (and in some cases delayed estrus) that occurs with this approach in heifers can be managed by extending the estrus detection period from 2 to 4 days before PGF, to 6 to 7 days after PGF. This relative lack of synchrony presents a greater problem when a GnRH-based, timed AI program is used in heifers. For example, when the authors' group implemented a CO-Synch program following MGA pretreatment [15], pregnancy rate to the timed AI with CO-Synch was 19% lower than when Select Synch with estrus detection was used. This agrees with other reports [3], and suggests that the CO-Synch protocol has limitations in yearling heifers. The effectiveness of the addition of a CIDR to the CO-Synch program (CO-Synch + CIDR) to overcome this limitation has been tested. The CO-Synch and CO-Synch + CIDR treatment were directly compared [21], and addition of the CIDR increased pregnancy rates to timed AI from 39% to 68%. In this report, numbers of animals were limiting; however, a recent experiment [18], which involved 12 locations and 2077 heifers, provides valuable information regarding the expectations for AI programs that involve GnRH and the CIDR. All heifers received a CIDR for 7 days, and PGF on the day of CIDR withdrawal. Two groups received GnRH at CIDR insertion (see Table 1 for detail on treatments) and treatments consisted of either timed AI at approximately 60 hours after PGF, or AI based upon detected estrus up to 84 hours, with those heifers not detected in estrus being bred by timed AI at hour 84 (hybrid approach). Statistical differences in pregnancy rates between treatments were not detected (mean pregnancy rate = 53.5%, range 49.1%–57.3); however, the GnRH-CIDR-PGF with AI on detected estrus to 84 hours and timed AI in heifers not in estrus by hour 84 (Hybrid Synch) provided the most consistent results. There appeared to be a 4% to 5% advantage of the hybrid approach over programs that relied exclusively on timed AI.

Overview

The major programs that are used to synchronize estrus in heifers are discussed in the preceding sections. For programs such as Select Synch and the PGF-based systems, fertility appears normal, and the pregnancy rates that are achieved will be determined by the proportion of females that are detected in estrus. The CO-Synch program has yielded marginal pregnancy rates in heifers in some cases. Conversely, the MGA-PGF system has been well-tested in heifers, and summarization of published reports with this system indicates a mean pregnancy rate during the synchronization period of 57%. For GnRH-based programs that include a CIDR, such as CO-Synch + CIDR and Hybrid-Synch + CIDR, pregnancy rates were 53.1% and 57.3%, respectively. Likewise, pregnancy rate was 54.5% with a CIDR-PGF program that included timed AI for heifers not detected in estrus. If only estrus detection for 3 days was used with this system, results were less desirable. In conclusion, expectations for pregnancy rates in heifers with the MGA-PGF, CO-Synch + CIDR, Hybrid Synch + CIDR, and CIDR-PGF (with hybrid approach to AI) average between 50% and 60%. Collective consideration of what is known at present suggests that there are no large differences in efficacy between these systems.

Estrous synchronization programs in beef cows

With a few exceptions, similar programs are used to synchronize estrus in postpartum beef cows as are used with yearling heifers; however, minor modifications are necessary in some cases, due to differences in physiology between cows and heifers, impacts of parturition and lactation, and time limitation of maintaining a 365-day calving interval in seasonal cattle production systems.

Synchronization using prostaglandin $F_{2\alpha}$

Programs similar to those described for heifers are used in postpartum beef cows. An extensive review of PGF-based programs in postpartum cows was published in 1990 [12]. The variability in time to estrus in programs based exclusively on the use of PGF has been assessed in cows, and estrus typically occurs 2 to 5 days after treatment. The stage of the estrous cycle at which PGF is administered influences the interval to estrus. For example, estrus was observed between 48 and 59 hours in females administered PGF between days 5 to 8 of the cycle, and between 53 and 72 hours in females treated between days 12 to 15 of the cycle [22,23]. Females in varying stages of the estrous cycle would have dominant follicles at varying stages of development at the time of treatment, and accordingly, it has been demonstrated that the time to estrus following PGF treatment on different days of the estrous cycle is a function of time required for an ovulatory follicle to develop [24,25]. This range in time to estrus is a normal physiological response in postpartum cows. Typically, this variation is accounted for in programs in which females are inseminated based upon detection of estrus, and most reports indicate that conception rate after a PGF-induced estrus is similar to that in females inseminated following a spontaneous estrus. The use of timed AI following induction of luteolysis with PGF has been investigated; however, as a result of the variability in time to estrus, conception rate to a timed AI is typically reduced as compared with insemination based upon detection of estrus [26].

The primary challenge that exists with programs based solely upon the use of PGF in postpartum cows is that at the time of the onset of the breeding season, the incidence of anestrus is approximately 50% in many herds [27]. In a program using a single injection of PGF in postpartum cows [17], only 33% of all cows treated exhibited estrus during the synchronization period, and this poor response could largely be attributed to the anestrous cows in the experiment. The incidence of anestrus in the 851 cows in this study was 53% at the time of PGF injection. A synchronized estrus of normal fertility can be achieved with PGF in cyclic females within a herd, but efficacy is limited by the incidence of anestrus when all females in a herd are treated. The precision of the synchronized estrus is acceptable for an AI program in which estrus detection is used to determine the appropriate time to AI. The synchronized estrus is not precise enough to permit timed AI in most instances.

Melengestrol acetate-prostaglandin $F_{2\alpha}$ synchronization programs

The application of the MGA-PGF system, as described for heifers (see Fig. 1), has been tested with varying degrees of success in postpartum cows [28,29]. One challenge of this program in postpartum cows is that a 15% increase in twin births has been reported [28]. The MGA-PGF system has been modified for postpartum cows [30] through the addition of an injection of GnRH given 12 days after cessation of MGA feeding (7 days before PGF), and increased twin births have not been noted. This approach, as previously described, is referred to as the MGA-Select program. The extended duration of this treatment protocol (approximately 35 days from the initiation of MGA feeding to the synchronized estrus) limits the utility of this approach in some groups of postpartum cows. For example, to maintain a consistent annual start date for the breeding season in a beef cow herd, it is necessary to initiate the breeding season approximately 80 to 85 days after the start of the preceding calving season. Thus, only cows that calved in approximately the first 40 days of the preceding calving season are eligible to be enrolled in this system. These females are the least likely to be anestrus at the onset of breeding season, and require the full range of benefits provided by the 14 days of MGA feeding. This limitation is not as great when this system is used in first-calf heifers that calved before the onset of calving in the mature cow herd. In a recent study with 609 lactating beef cows [31], an MGA-CO-Synch program resulted in a pregnancy rate of 46%.

Progesterone-prostaglandin $F_{2\alpha}$ program

The CIDR-PGF program is identical in postpartum cows and heifers (see Fig. 2). In a recent experiment [17] conducted across 6 locations with 851 postpartum beef cows (56 $\pm$ 0.6 days postpartum), 35.6% of postpartum cows that received the CIDR-PGF program became pregnant during a 3-day synchronization period in which AI was performed based upon a detected estrus. A recent experiment involving 14 locations and over 2600 cows [32] included a treatment that consisted of a CIDR-PGF system in which AI was performed 12 hours after detected estrus, and for those cows that did not exhibit estrus within 3 days, AI was performed 84 hours post-PGF with an injection of GnRH at insemination. In this experiment, 52.3% of the cows receiving the CIDR-PGF treatment with the combination of insemination on detection of estrus and timed AI became pregnant during the 84-hour period after PGF.

Gonadotropin hormone-releasing hormone–prostaglandin $F_{2\alpha}$ systems

The GnRH-based programs that are used in cows are based upon the same hormonal mechanisms of action as described for heifers, and carry identical names in the field (eg, Select Synch, CO-Synch, and so on). With the GnRH-based programs that do not include a progestin treatment, approximately 8% of cows exhibit estrus during the 2 to 3 days leading up to the time of PGF injection. These "early" heats are fertile, and cows can be inseminated 12 hours after detection. The peak estrous response will occur 2 to 3 days after PGF, with a range of 1 to 5 days. With this system, a minimum of 4 to 5 days of estrus detection after PGF and 2 days preceding PGF are required to detect estrus in most cows. A large proportion of cyclic females will be in estrus during this 7-day period. Although this protocol will initiate estrous cycles in some anestrous cows, results can be un-predictable. In programs that do not include an exogenous progestin (eg, CIDR), the action of the initial GnRH injection to induce ovulation is a critical aspect, because the necessity of progesterone pre-exposure in anestrous cows has been well-established [27]. Short-term weaning of calves preceding ovulation is also an effective means to induce onset of estrous cycles in anestrous postpartum cows [33].

The authors' group [34] recently tested the efficacy of the CO-Synch + CIDR program as compared with a CO-Synch treatment in anestrous postpartum cows. In this experiment (n = 419), anestrous cows received either the CO-Synch or CO-Synch + CIDR treatment, and all cyclic cows in the four herds received the CO-Synch program. All cows were bred by timed AI at 48 hours after PGF. Pregnancy rate to timed AI in cyclic cows was 53%, which is a typical response for this type of program in cyclic females. In anestrous cows, those receiving the CO-Synch + CIDR had a pregnancy rate of 55%, whereas in those anestrous cows not receiving the CIDR (CO-Synch only), pregnancy rate was reduced to 35%. Thus, use of the CIDR in anestrous cows in conjunction with the CO-Synch program increased pregnancy rates by 20%. Responses to CIDR treatment in anestrous cows that received the CO-Synch protocol were similar to those reported by Stevenson et al [31]. There appears to be merit in strategically using the CIDR in GnRH-based programs. The authors often recommend that producers who are using GnRH-based programs add a CIDR to a GnRH-based program in cows that are most likely to be anestrus. A typical recommendation for producers who wish to used timed AI is to use CO-Synch + CIDR in first-calf heifers (2-year-old cows), mature cows that are less than 45 days postpartum, and cows in poor body condition, and to use a CO-Synch program in all other cows (ie, those likely to be cyclic).

A recent experiment [32] was conducted to provide a comprehensive comparison of some of the most common synchronization programs used in postpartum beef cows. This experiment involved over 2600 cows across 14 locations, and compared pregnancy rates achieved with five different GnRH-based programs. Programs included CO-Synch, CO-Synch + CIDR, Hybrid Synch, Hybrid Sync + CIDR and CIDR-PGF. Cows in the two CO-Synch treatment were inseminated by timed AI in conjunction with a +GnRH treatment at approximately 60 hours after PGF. Cows in the two Hybrid Synch treatments and the CIDR-PGF treatment were inseminated based upon detection of estrus up to 84 hours after PGF, with those females not detected in estrus being bred by timed AI at 84 hours, in conjunction with a +GnRH treatment. The greatest pregnancy rate was achieved in the Hybrid Synch + CIDR treatment (57.9%), followed by the CO-Synch + CIDR (53.6%), Hybrid Synch (53.0%), CIDR-PGF (52.3%), and CO-Synch (43.4%) treatments. Pregnancy rate was greatest in the Hybrid Synch + CIDR treatment, and significantly greater than in the CIDR-PGF and CO-Synch treatments. For programs that involved a period of estrus detection and AI, Hybrid Synch + CIDR was the most effective program, whereas CO-Synch + CIDR was the most reliable timed AI program tested. This large-scale comparison provides a benchmark for expected pregnancy rates that can be achieved in postpartum cows with GnRH-based programs.

In most cases, pregnancy rates between 50% and 60% are expected, especially when a CIDR is used in conjunction with these programs [31,32].

Overview

As with heifers, a variety of programs exist for postpartum cows that will yield synchronized pregnancy rates of 50% to 60%. Variation in pregnancy rates can be associated with the program used, as well as the proportion of the cows that are anestrus at the initiation of the breeding season. There are some programs that appear to be more effective in anestrous cows than others. Thus, one variable that will influence choice of a synchronization system must be the reproductive competence of the group to be treated. In animals that are likely to be anestrus, addition of an exogenous progestin should increase the pregnancy rate achieved. Often other variables beyond efficacy will influence the choice of program for a given situation. One important consideration is the cost of the pharmaceuticals to be used for the synchronization program. At least as important as the cash costs is how an individual program meshes with the expertise of the cattle manager, the manner in which the cattle are managed, the facilities available, the value of the semen to be used, the value of a synchronized AI pregnancy relative to one that is established later in the breeding season, and the labor and expertise available for detection of estrus. Depending upon these factors, as well as other factors unique to a given situation, the most "cost-effective" program will be the system that can be successfully implemented and meet the goals of the production system.

References

[1] Day ML. Practical manipulation of the estrous cycle in beef cattle. In: Williams EI, editor. Proceedings of the 31st American Association of Bovine Practitioners. Spokane (WA): Frontier Printers, Inc.; 1998. p. 51–61.

[2] Day ML. Use of progesterone to induce and synchronize estrus: Application of the CIDR. In: Proceedings 2001 Beef Improvement Federation. San Antonio (TX): National Association of Animal Breeders; 2001. p. 13–25.

[3] Day ML, Grum DE. 2003. Estrous synchronization in heifers. In: Maxwell H, editor. Proceedings of the Annual Conference of the Society for Theriogenology. Columbus (OH): Society for Theriogenology; 2003. p. 145–154.

[4] Lauderdale JW, Seguin BE, Stellflug JN, et al. Fertility of cattle following $PGF_{2\alpha}$ injection. J Anim Sci 1974;38:964–7.

[5] Lauderdale JW. Effects of $PGF_{2\alpha}$ on pregnancy and estrous cycle of cattle [abstract]. J Anim Sci 1972;35:246.

[6] Stevenson JS, Smith JF, Hawkins DE. Reproductive outcomes for dairy heifers treated with combinations of prostaglandin $F_{2\alpha}$, norgestomet, and gonadotropin-releasing hormone. J Dairy Sci 2000;83:2008–15.

[7] Stevenson JS, Lamb GC, Cartmill JA, et al. Synchronizing estrus in replacement beef heifers using GnRH, melengestrol acetate, and $PGF_{2\alpha}$ [abstract]. J Anim Sci 1999;77(Suppl 1):225.

[8] Chenault JR, McAllister JF, Kasson CW. Synchronization of estrus with melengesterol acetate and prostaglandin $F_{2\alpha}$ in beef and dairy heifers. J Anim Sci 1990;68:296–303.

[9] Kastelic JP, McCartney DH, Olson WO, et al. Estrus synchronization in cattle using estradiol, melengestrol acetate, and PGF. Theriogenology 1996;46:1295–304.

[10] Anderson LH, McDowell CM, Day ML. Progestin-induced puberty and secretion of lutenizing hormone in heifers. Biol Reprod 1996;54:1025–31.

[11] Hall JB, Staigmiller RR, Short RE, et al. Effect of age and pattern of gain on induction of puberty with a progestin in beef heifers. J Anim Sci 1997;75:1606–11.

[12] Odde KG. A review of synchronization of estrus in postpartum cattle. J Anim Sci 1990;68: 817–30.

[13] Patterson DJ, Kiracofe GH, Stevenson JS, et al. Control of the bovine estrous cycle with melengestrol acetate (MGA): a review. J Anim Sci 1989;67:1895–906.

[14] Anderson LH, Day ML. Acute progesterone administration regresses persistent dominant follicles and improves fertility of cattle in which estrus was synchronized with melengestrol acetate. J Anim Sci 1994;72:2955–61.

[15] Johnson SK, Broweleit B, Huston JE, et al. Use of GnRH to increase the precision of estrus and augment timed insemination in heifers treated with melengesterol acetate and $PGF_{2\alpha}$. In: Kansas State University Cattlemen's Day Report. Kansas State University; 2000. p. 101–103.

[16] Johnson SK, Day ML. Methods to reduce or eliminate detection of estrus in a melengestrol acetate-$PGF_{2\alpha}$ protocol for synchronization of estrus in beef heifers. J Anim Sci 2004;82: 3071–6.

[17] Lucy MC, Billings HJ, Butler WR, et al. Efficacy of an intravaginal progesterone insert and an injection of $PGF_{2\alpha}$ for synchronizing estrus and shortening the interval to pregnancy in postpartum beef cows, peripubertal beef heifers, and dairy heifers. J Anim Sci 2001;79: 982–95.

[18] Larson JE, Lamb GC, Geary TW, et al. Synchronization of estrus in replacement beef heifers using GnRH, prostaglandin $F_{2\alpha}$ (PG), and progesterone (CIDR): a multi-location study [abstract]. J Anim Sci 2004;82(Suppl 1):369.

[19] Martinez MF, Adams GP, Kastelic JP, et al. Induction of follicle wave emergence for estrus synchronization and artificial insemination in heifers. Theriogenology 2000;54:757–69.

[20] Pursley JR, Mee MO, Wiltbank MC. Synchronization of ovulation in dairy cows using $PGF_{2\alpha}$ and GnRH. Theriogenology 1995;44:915–23.

[21] Martinez MF, Kastelic JP, Adams GP, et al. The use of progestins in regimes for fixed-time artificial insemination in beef cattle. Theriogenology 2002;57:1049–59.

[22] Stevenson JS, Schmidt MK, Call EP. Stage of estrous cycle, time of insemination, and seasonal effects and fertility of Holstein heifers after prostaglandin $F_{2\alpha}$. J Dairy Sci 1984;67: 1798.

[23] Watts TL, Fuquay JW. Response and fertility of dairy heifers following injection with prostaglandin $F_{2\alpha}$ during early, middle or late diestrus. Theriogenology 1985;23:655.

[24] Kastelic JP, Knopf L, Ginther OJ. Effect of day of prostaglandin $F_{2\alpha}$ treatment on selection and development of the ovulatory follicle in heifers. Anim Reprod Sci 1990;23:169–80.

[25] Kastelic JP, Ginther OJ. Factors affecting the origin of the ovulatory follicle in heifers with induced luteolysis. Anim Reprod Sci 1991;26:13–24.

[26] Fogwell RL, Reid WA, Thompson CK, et al. Synchronization of estrus in dairy heifers: a field demonstration. J Dairy Sci 1986;69:1665–72.

[27] Day ML. Hormonal induction of estrous cycles in anestrous, Bos taurus beef cows. Anim Reprod Sci 2004;82–83:487–94.

[28] Patterson DJ, Hall JB, Bradley NW, et al. Improved synchrony, conception rate, and fecundity in postpartum suckled beef cows fed melengestrol acetate prior to prostaglandin $F_{2\alpha}$. J Anim Sci 1995;73:954–9.

[29] Yelich JV, Mauck HS, Holland MD, et al. Synchronization of estrus in suckled postpartum beef cows with melengestrol acetate and $PGF_{2\alpha}$. Theriogenology 1995;43:389–400.

[30] Patterson DJ, Wood SL, Kojima FN, et al. Improved synchronization of estrus in postpartum suckled beef cows with a progestin-GnRH-prostaglandin $F_{2\alpha}$ protocol [abstract]. J Anim Sci 2000;78(Suppl 1):218.

[31] Stevenson JS, Lamb GC, Johnson SK, et al. Supplemental norgestomet, progesterone, or melengestrol acetate increases pregnancy rates in suckled beef cows after timed inseminations. J Anim Sci 2003;81:571–86.

[32] Larson JE, Lamb GC, Stevenson JS, et al. Synchronization of estrus in suckled beef cows using GnRH, prostaglandin $F_{2\alpha}$ (PG), and progesterone (CIDR): a multi location study [abstract]. J Anim Sci 2004;82(Suppl 1):368.

[33] Yavas Y, Walton JS. Induction of ovulation in postpartum suckled beef cows: a review. Theriogenology 2000;54:1–23.

[34] Gasser CL, Behlke EJ, Burke CR, et al. Improvement of pregnancy rate to fixed-time artificial insemination with progesterone treatment in anestrous post-partum cows [abstract]. J Anim Sci 2003;81(Suppl 2):45.

VETERINARY
CLINICS
Food Animal Practice

ELSEVIER
SAUNDERS

Vet Clin Food Anim 21 (2005) 383–408

Venereal Diseases of Cattle: Natural History, Diagnosis, and the Role of Vaccines in their Control

Robert H. BonDurant, DVM

*Department of Population Health and Reproduction, School of Veterinary Medicine,
University of California, 1 Shields Avenue, Davis, CA 95616-8230, USA*

Although the widespread use of artificial insemination has made it possible to breed cattle with minimal risk of transmitting specific venereal pathogens, sexually transmitted diseases (STDs) are still common wherever natural service is practiced. The latter includes an estimated 80% to 95% of the commercial beef cattle in North America, and as many as 40% of all dairy females in the United States (personal communication, J. Mitchell, National Association of Animal Breeders, 2005). Regional differences exist in natural service of dairy cows, but the Raleigh Dairy Records Processing Center's 2001 report is typical: In more than 10,000 Dairy Herd Improvement Association (DHIA)-supervised herds, 24% of lactating cows were bred by bulls, and in nonsupervised herds, 36% of lactating cows were naturally served (cited by Cassell et al [1]). In many parts of the country, all nulliparous heifers are bred by bulls, a custom that brings the national total percentage of females bred by natural service to about 40%.

The best-known bovine STDs are insidious, in that the etiologic agents do not cause overt disease in the male or female, but rather cause occult pregnancy loss, usually early in gestation. In commercial cow-calf operations, the result is that a significant portion of a season's calf crop is lost without anyone ever noticing something amiss; in dairy cattle, the first indication that venereal disease is operating in the herd may be that the calving-to-conception intervals are increasing, or that the interval from

Much of this work was supported by funding from the Agricultural Experiment Station (Center for Food Animal Health), University of California at Davis, and by National Research Initiative Competitive Grants Program of the US Department of Agriculture no. 98-35204-6401.

E-mail address: rhbondurant@ucdavis.edu

doi:10.1016/j.cvfa.2005.03.002
vetfood.theclinics.com

placement of cows in the "bull string" to pregnancy is widening, with the result that mature equivalent milk production is depressed by as much as 7% [2]. In either commodity, a large economic loss often occurs before the disease is recognized.

Etiologic agents

The two classic venereal agents of cattle are the gram-negative bacterium *Campylobacter fetus venerealis* and the flagellated protozoan *Tritrichomonas foetus*. As a historical note, the "o" in *T foetus* is there because nomenclature etiquette dictates that the discoverer of an organism gets to name it. This organism was discovered in Europe in the early twentieth century by Riedmüller (cited by Honigberg [3,4]), hence the British spelling; whereas *C fetus* was first described in the United States by Smith and Taylor (cited by Yabuuchi [5]). The nomenclature gets further confused when one considers that *Tritrichomonas foetus* is probably the same organism as *Tritrichomonas suis*, which was originally described in the mid-nineteenth century [6], and which, by the same etiquette, should be the rightful name of the cattle pathogen. Further nomenclature note: The bovine disease caused by *T foetus* has traditionally been called *trichomoniasis*, but recently the name *trichomonosis* has been put forward [7]. This article uses both names interchangeably.

Campylobacter fetus venerealis has had several names in the past, and to review them all is to invite confusion. It is sufficient to say that the industry still refers to the venereal disease caused by *C fetus venerealis* as "vibrio." *C fetus venerealis* is regarded by most as a subspecies of *C fetus*. Another closely related subspecies is *C fetus fetus*, which is occasionally diagnosed as a cause of sporadic abortion, but is rarely if ever transmitted venereally. Other agents are transmitted by sexual contact, but may cause different signs, or have different epidemiologic characteristics. These include *Haemophilus somnus*, *Ureaplasma*, and other mycoplasmas; and under special circumstances, *Leptospira spp* and *Brucella abortus*. Of all these pathogens, only the classic two are known to be obligate parasites of the genital tract. Among the others, *Brucella* is certainly infamous for its potential to wreak havoc on a breeding population, but the organism survives quite well outside of the reproductive tract (eg, in the supra-mammary lymph nodes) for long periods [8]. Moreover, except in cases of intrauterine artificial insemination with infected semen, venereal trans-mission of bovine brucellosis is very uncommon [9].

In spite of the fact that *C fetus* and *T foetus* are widely separated on the phylogenetic family tree, their ecology, epidemiology, and pathology are nearly identical. For this reason, this article considers the natural history of trichomoniasis and venereal campylobacteriosis together. Table 1 is a summary comparison of the two organisms and the diseases they cause.

Table 1
Summary comparison of diagnostic and prophylactic features of bovine venereal campylobacteriosis and trichomonosis

	C fetus venerealis	T foetus
Agent description	Bacterium: gram-negative curved rod 1–2 μ long (best seen in dark-field microscope). Highly motile, single polar flagellum	Protozoan: ~5 × 12 μ 3 anterior, 1 posterior flagellae. "Undulating membrane" along one side. Slowly motile (rolling, jerky)
Best sample for demonstrating organism	Preputial smegma, obtained by scraping; or vaginal mucus, obtained by aspiration.	Preputial smegma, obtained by scraping
Transport medium	Cary-Blair, Amies, Weybridge, Clark's (others)	InPouch transport/culture packet
In vitro culture	Skirrow medium; Greenbriar Plus agar; blood agar (others); microaerophilic atmosphere	InPouch transport/culture packet; Diamond's TYM medium; aerobic incubator OK
Tentative diagnosis	Positive culture and biochemical phenotyping	Positive culture based on morphology and characteristic motility
Confirm diagnosis	PCR of positive culture	PCR of positive culture
Serology—serum	Not useful (cross-reactions)	Useful in females, but not performed
Serology—vaginal mucus	Useful, but not performed	Research work only
Carrier state, female	Up to 2–6 months	1–3 months; rarely longer
Carrier state, male	The rule in bulls >3 years	The rule in bulls >3 years
Vaccine efficacy, female	Very good, with proper adjuvant	Fair to good, used as labeled
Vaccine efficacy, male	Good-very good with proper adjuvant	No data available

Abbreviations: PCR, polymerase chain reaction; TYM, trypticase yeast extract maltose.

Natural history of trichomoniasis and campylobacteriosis in cattle

Carrier state—male

The classic venereal diseases are chauvinistic; that is, the male carries the organism for long periods—probably for life—without consequence to himself, whereas the female, who typically sheds an infection after 1 to 5 months, suffers the consequences of this infection, namely early abortion and temporary infertility [10,11]. This male carrier state exists in the microenvironment of the preputial cavity, specifically on the surface of the nonkeratinized, stratified squamous epithelium of the glans penis and proximal prepuce, in the area of the fornix [12,13]. As bulls age, this epithelium becomes folded, producing deep crypts where *T foetus* or *C fetus*, or both, can apparently thrive [14,15]. *T foetus* and *C fetus*, which are facultatively anaerobic and microaerophilic organisms, respectively [16,17], are most commonly found deep within the crypts, where oxygen tension is presumably lowest.

Given equal exposure to infected females, bulls more than 3 years old (ie, those that have deeper crypts) are more likely to become infected with either of these organisms than bulls less than 3 years old [18]. Such infections may persist for the life of the bull, in spite of the presence of a measurable quantity of specific immunoglobulin in the preputial cavity [13,19,20]. These two organisms are remarkably well-adapted to the host environment, especially that of the male host.

Infection

With two notable and thankfully rare exceptions, infection with the classical agents occurs only at coitus, during natural service. The first exception reportedly occurred when an artificial inseminator, looking for secondary signs of estrus before breeding a group of cows, inserted a gloved hand into the vagina to assess the quantity and quality of cervico-vaginal mucus (CVM), and then proceeded to do the same in several more cows without changing gloves [21]. The second exception is exposure of females by artificial insemination with contaminated semen, the latter being preventable by using semen from companies following the so-called Certified Semen Services (CSS) protocol [22]. For trichomonosis, penetration of the vagina is apparently necessary, because swabbing the vulvar area with high numbers of organisms does not lead to vaginal or uterine infection [23]. Some older literature suggested that young bulls who frequently mount each other may leave an STD pathogen on the skin of the mounted bull's rump [24]. Bull studs, in an attempt to minimize opportunities for venereal infection, routinely wipe the rear quarters of the teaser animal with disinfectant. Whether such hindquarter exposure occurs in a natural mating setting is not known, but it seems unlikely. It is known that both *T foetus* and *C fetus venerealis* are susceptible to desiccation and to ultraviolet light; hence their survival time on the surface of the hair coat of a bull is probably very brief, and the opportunity for transmission between males is therefore very limited. In the case of trichomoniasis, this is borne out by personal observations of the author, who has housed large numbers of *T foetus*-infected bulls with equally large numbers of presumed uninfected bulls for as long as 16 weeks [25]. In spite of weekly cultures of preputial smegma, no new infections were identified during those 16 ensuing weeks, suggesting that bull-to-bull transmission did not occur. It may be that authors of the earlier studies saw non-*T foetus* trichomonad organisms, which we now presume to be fecal in origin [3,4,26,27]. Because bulls, particularly young bulls, tend to mount and sodomize each other [28], it is not unusual to collect feces in the preputial cavity. This fecal material may contain non-*T foetus* trichomonads, such as *Pentatrichomonas hominis* and any number of *Tetratrichomonas* species [26,29,30]. To date, none of these non-*T foetus* trichomonads has been shown to be a pathogen.

Transmission

Heterosexual STD transmission rates of 30% to 70% are reported for infected bulls breeding susceptible females [23,31]. Transmission is likely a function of the magnitude of an individual bull's infection (the number of organisms on the surface of the penis and prepuce), his libido, and his ranking in the dominance hierarchy of all breeding bulls in the herd. The female reproductive tract is at first relatively tolerant of the STD pathogens. Older literature suggests a period of trichomonad multiplication in the vagina of experimentally infected heifers, followed by a decline in numbers of parasites just before the next estrus [32]. Presumably, a similar surge and decline occurs with *C fetus*. The hormonal milieu of the reproductive tract probably influences the metabolic machinery of these parasites, as it does the host immune responses to them [33–36].

Embryo survival

STD organisms arrive in the female reproductive tract simultaneously with spermatozoa; however, in many if not most cases, fertilization occurs in spite of the presence of the pathogen. For both *T foetus* and *C fetus,* in-vitro work has shown that fertilization and early embryonic development to the hatching stage (8–10 days) are little affected by co-culture with the venereal pathogen [37,38]. Although only a few in-vivo studies of embryonic/fetal survival have been done for either of these organisms, one authoritative work [39] showed that in heifers experimentally infected with *T foetus*, conceptus deaths peaked at 50 to 70 days' gestation. So at least for trichomonosis, and probably for campylobacteriosis as well, the bulk of pregnancy loss is technically fetal (at >42 days' gestation) and not embryonic. Occasional abortions of fetuses of greater than 4 months gestational age are reported for both agents by diagnostic laboratories, but typically losses occur 2 months earlier.

Embryo death—return to cycling

A typical history of a naturally serviced, infected cow-calf herd reveals that in the first several weeks following bull exposure, estrous activity diminishes, causing the herdsman to assume that pregnancy has been established in most cows. From a physiological viewpoint, the herdsman is correct: The embryo in most cows infected with either of these organisms generally survives long enough to release sufficient interferon tau (IFNτ) to prevent the prostaglandin $F_{2\alpha}$ ($PGF_{2\alpha}$)-mediated lysis of the corpus luteum at about day 17. Then, often just before the bulls are due to be removed, an astute herdsman may notice some females returning to estrus. As noted above, fetal death among all infected females peaks at about 7 to 10 weeks.

Following death of the conceptus, estrus would be expected in 2 to 4 weeks, which, if the bulls are still available, may allow rebreeding of affected females. Because many progressive cow-calf operators try to observe as short a breeding season as possible (10–14 weeks), bulls may not be available by the time a cow aborts and clears the infection; thus venereal diseases have the potential to quietly ruin an entire year's production. Models of the economic damage that STDs can inflict predict losses of $600 to $700 per infected dairy cow [21]; in beef cattle, one model suggests up to a 35% loss in income per cow exposed to infected bulls, as the herd infection increases from one bull to two [40].

Pathology

In the male, neither of the two classical agents causes observable gross pathology. Histological changes are subtle at first, with increased accumulations of neutrophils just below the nonkeratinized, stratified squamous epithelium of the glans and prepuce, followed by an infiltrate of lymphocytes and plasma cells penetrating into the intraepithelial area, and coalescing in the subepithelium to form lymphoid nodules [13,19]. Neutrophils are occasionally seen in the crypts, but infection is not commonly manifest as grossly purulent. In the female, both of the classic organisms induce inflammation from the vaginal to the oviductal mucosae, including both the cervix and the endometrium. In the first week or 2, infiltrates are mostly superficial neutrophils [39], with a significant number of eosinophils as well [41]; but as in the bull, a moderate-to-severe mononuclear infiltrate follows, with both lymphocytes and mature plasma cells involved [41]. Subepithelial and periglandular lymphoid nodules, sometimes resembling lymphoid follicles, begin to develop after about the sixth week of infection with either pathogen [41,42]. In trichomonosis, there is also an apparent degranulation of mast cells between weeks 6 and 9 [43].

Immunity—male

Although specific immunoglobulins have been detected in small amounts in preputial secretions by some, but not all investigators [19,20,44,45], there seems to be no effective acquired immunity to these two agents in the mature male. The exact source of these immunoglobulins is not known. Note the ability of bulls to respond to systemic (ie, nonvenereal) *C fetus venerealis* antigen exposure, discussed below.

Immunity—female

In the female exposed to *T foetus*, pathogen-specific antibodies of both immunoglobulin IgA and IgG_1 isotypes are detectable in uterine and vaginal secretions by the fifth to sixth week postinfection [46]. IgA may help immobilize and agglutinate parasites, as well as prevent adhesion of the parasites to mucosal surfaces. IgG$_1$ probably mediates complement killing, and to a lesser extent, opsonization of *T foetus* or *C fetus*, both of which are extracellular pathogens [33,47]. In any case, immunity following natural infection and clearance of these STD organisms is short lived for trichomonosis, with females becoming susceptible within a year, in time for the following breeding season [48]. For *C fetus venerealis*, once the protracted vaginal carrier state is cleared (see below), a cow can be reinfected vaginally, but the uterus will remain free of infection. This uterine protection returns a cow's fertility in many cases, and lasts for up to 2 years in the absence of further antigenic stimulation [49].

As extracellular pathogens, these organisms would be expected to encounter a predominately humoral immune response from the host [47,50], and it is likely that the type of humoral response is responsible for the short duration of immunity. With both of these STD pathogens, there is a strong IgA response in the vaginal mucosa following natural infection. In contrast, when the same organism or purified antigen from that organism is administered systemically, IgG antibodies predominate [42,47,51]. Whereas the IgG antibodies are capable of opsonization (and thus enhancement of phagocytosis by extruded neutrophils or macrophages) and complement-mediated lysis of the pathogen, secretory IgA antibodies generally immobilize or agglutinate, but do not kill the organism. The moderate uterine mucosal inflammation that characterizes infection with these STD organisms may allow systemically derived IgG and complement to gain access to the lumen of the uterus, from which they would clear the organism. A relative lack of a spontaneous IgG response in the vagina, or perhaps blocking of IgG effects by vaginal IgA binding of organisms, could then explain the longer vaginal carrier state, especially for *C fetus venerealis*.

Carrier state—female

In experimental infections of nonpregnant heifers, *T foetus* infection is typically cleared from the uterus and vagina between weeks 6 and 12 following infection [39,41,42,52]. *Campylobacter* may be cleared from the uterus at about the same interval, although it is not unusual to hear of females who remain vaginally infected for several months after clearing the uterine infection. Such animals are usually only temporarily infertile—they can eventually conceive and carry a pregnancy to term—but in the meantime, they represent a threat to susceptible bulls, and indirectly, to the female herd [50,53–55]. The mechanism by which *C fetus venerealis* maintains a vaginal infection in the presence of a significant antibody response is not completely clear, but it is known that during the course of infection, the organism can undergo antigenic variation, an adaptation that may dodge the immune system, at least for a few months [56,57].

The dynamics of surface antigen profiles of *T foetus* have not been studied in as much detail, but a "carrier-cow" state has been described on multiple occasions for this organism [58–60]. In these cases, a very small proportion of cows (a fraction of 1%) in infected herds were shown to remain infected throughout pregnancy, and into the following breeding season. Because they were not intensively studied—they were not tested weekly nor even monthly—we do not know if the females were continuously infected during this period, or whether they may have actually cleared the infection and been reinfected by a bull following a mating during late pregnancy, when up to 3% of cattle may show signs of estrus [61]. Assuming that the carrier-cow phenomenon is real, it suggests that substantial efforts to rid herds of trichomonosis by attempting to provide *T foetus*-free males (see *Herd treatment for sexually-transmitted diseases*, below) can go for naught in the very next breeding season. Fortunately, such a carrier cow is a rarity.

Consequences of infection

By weeks 7 to 10, increasing inflammatory changes in the endometrium, and possibly the trophoblast, of the growing fetus apparently cause enough damage to kill the conceptus, which is typically resorbed. This conceptus death is not detectable as an expelled abortus unless it dies after the third month. In about 5% of infected cattle, a pyometra will develop, probably as a result of bacterial contamination that occurs at the time of fetal loss, when the cervix is likely to relax sufficiently to admit contamination from the outside environment. Because the pyometra occurs after a natural service, it is termed a "postcoital pyometra" to distinguish it from the more common postpartum pyometra. Venereal disease should always be suspected and ruled out when a postcoital pyometra is discovered during routine annual pregnancy examinations of beef herds, or during the examination of dairy cows housed in bull strings.

Discovery

History

Typically, there is no suspicion until the herd is examined for pregnancy. At this time, a low overall pregnancy rate is noted; in newly exposed herds it can be as low as 50% of the expected rate [62]. Gestational ages for those pregnancies that are found will be distributed over a broad range, rather than tightly bunched and attributable to an early conception date as desired. Occasionally there will be a history of the introduction of a mature bull, either voluntarily (ie, a purchased or leased bull) or involuntarily (via a weak area in the fencing, or a cotenant with an infected bull, where public lands are used for commingling breeding cattle) [63].

Physical examination findings—females

With either of these diseases, there are few abnormal findings. As mentioned above, a useful diagnostic finding is the presence of postcoital pyometra, even in a single female. This is more commonly attributed to *T foetus* than to *C fetus*. Also, depending upon the timing of pregnancy examinations relative to fetal loss, the veterinarian may detect nonpregnant uteri that have not completed involution since aborting.

Physical examination findings—males

There are almost never any overt signs or findings in bulls that can be attributed to infection by either *T foetus* or *C fetus*. Moreover, the bulls are often not available for examination by the time venereal disease is suspected, at the time of pregnancy examination. They may have been sold, or returned to the lessor, or moved to another area to breed another herd. In such cases, testing of females offers the best hope of providing a diagnosis of "trich" or "vibrio."

Differential diagnosis

A similar picture of low pregnancy rates with high variability of gestational ages can be the result of poor nutrition, especially energy deficiency, in the mid-to-late gestation period of the previous pregnancy, or in the months leading up to a heifer's first breeding [64–66]. In addition, a less likely but compatible history includes a temporary heat stress to the herd, especially the bulls, early in the breeding season. Because semen quality is still good for the first 7 to 9 days following the onset of heat stress, and recovery from such an episode does not occur until approximately 60 days after the end of the thermal insult, it would not be unusual to see a bimodal distribution of gestational ages: That is, gestational ages would be compatible with a spate of pregnancies being established early in the season by sperm that were in the epididymis during the heat stress, and therefore somewhat protected from environmental heat effects. Few cows would have midrange pregnancies, but there could be a cluster of females with early gestational pregnancies that were established more than 60 days after the offending thermal episode. The same distribution could be seen in the case of a herd that is exposed to an STD-carrying bull in the second week of a 15-week breeding season.

Ancillary testing

Serological tests in the male or female have historically been unreliable for *C fetus*, mostly because of cross-reactivity of naturally occurring host antibodies with *C fetus venerealis* [67]. A more specific assay, the vaginal mucus agglutination test, was once employed by diagnostic laboratories. This test measured the amount of specific IgA activity in the CVM. Typically, a human vaginal tampon was weighed carefully, then inserted into the vagina for several minutes, removed, and weighed again. Results were reported as agglutination activity per gram of vaginal mucus [68].

Because the local IgA response continued for up to several months following exposure, this test was useful in cases where culture of the bulls' preputial smegma was not possible. Because of relatively low sensitivity, however, the test was more useful as a herd screening tool than a diagnostic test for an individual animal. One paper describes a delayed (Type IV) hypersensitivity reaction in the skin of *Campylobacter* infected females, so cell-mediated immune responses are apparently invoked as well [69]. None of these tests of "exposure" is particularly helpful, either because they are no longer used by diagnostic laboratories, or because they cannot determine the current infection status. Fortunately, the fact that a vaginal carrier state persists for weeks or months after uterine clearance of *C fetus venerealis* suggests that CVM culture might still be rewarding, even months after exposure. Since the advent of a relatively effective vaccine (see below), there has been less demand for the development of improved diagnostic serology for genital campylobacteriosis.

The immune response to trichomonosis has been thought to remain confined within the lumen of the reproductive tract, although some early work attempted to develop delayed type hypersensitivity tests by intradermal injection of *T foetus* antigen [70,71]. More recent work has used ELISA technology to demonstrate a very weak systemic humoral response to experimental intravaginal *T foetus* infection of nonpregnant heifers [33,46,72]; however, when the more sensitive complement-mediated hemolytic assay is used, most females show a rise in circulating antibody titer beginning the third to fourth week after infection, peaking by about the seventh week [73]. No such responses have been reported in bulls. As with the vaginal mucus agglutination test for *C fetus venerealis*, the hemolytic assay for *T foetus* is more useful as a herd screening tool than for individual animal diagnostics. Unfortunately, this assay is not being offered commercially at this time. Thus, although moderately accurate serological assays that can detect herd exposure to the classic STD agents exist, they are not readily available. They are mentioned here only to emphasize that the female does mount a detectable if somewhat ineffective antibody response to *T foetus* and *C fetus venerealis*.

Definitive diagnosis

This requires demonstration of the etiologic agent. Because these two diseases need to be considered simultaneously when the history suggests an STD, appropriate samples should be taken to detect both agents.

When the bulls are not available

It is always a good idea to begin with the males: There are fewer of them, and the self-limiting nature of the infection in the female can make it difficult to isolate either *C fetus* or *T foetus* from females by the time STDs are considered. If the males are not available, CVM can be aspirated from the cranial vagina of a representative sample of cows and heifers, and submitted for laboratory culture. Specifically, a single aspirate can be divided between media specific for each of the agents. For *Campylobacter*, this will be one of several transport-enrichment media (TEM): Weybridge, Cary-Blair, Clark's, and so forth [74–77]. The organism is fastidious, and requires a complex support medium, antimicrobials to suppress growth of contaminants and commensals, and near-anaerobic atmospheric conditions [78]. It is best to contact your diagnostic laboratory before taking the samples. You may want to determine if your laboratory has had success in distinguishing *C fetus fetus* from *C fetus venerealis*. The laboratory often supplies the transport medium, along with instructions for its use. Once in the TEM, the sample is reasonably safe from modest temperature fluxes; *C fetus* can be recovered from the TEM up to 2 days after inoculation, even if shipped at room temperature. In fact, if an inoculated TEM is to be in transit more than 4 hours, it is recommended that the sample not be incubated above room temperature until it gets to the diagnostic laboratory [75].

At the laboratory, the TEM will be streaked onto selective media (eg, Skirrow medium) and incubated in a microaerophilic atmosphere (6% O_2, 7% CO_2, 7% H_2, 80% N_2) at 37°C. Following identification of typical colonies and catalase testing (both major subspecies of *C fetus* are positive), two "phenotype" tests, the glycine tolerance test and the H_2S production test, are normally run to distinguish *C fetus venerealis* from *C fetus fetus* (*C fetus venerealis* is negative in both tests [77–80]). Recently, several laboratories have produced polymerase chain reaction (PCR) assays that can distinguish *C fetus venerealis* from *C fetus fetus* [76,77,79–81]. These assays use the colonies grown from the cultured CVM or smegma, so culture is still required, but they offer the promise of more accurate classification, and a tool that can help veterinarians better estimate the prevalence of the true pathogen, *C fetus venerealis*. In some studies [81], traditional phenotyping correctly identified only 80% of *C fetus* strains, whereas PCR correctly identified 98% of *C fetus* subspecies. PCR may be combined with other molecular techniques, including restriction fragment length polymorphism (RFLP) or sequencing of the PCR-amplified product. In the RFLP procedure, the "amplicon" created by the PCR process is digested with a specific bacterial endonuclease, such as *Alu I*. Each subspecies displays its own unique pattern of DNA bands on an agarose gel after electrophoresis [76].

For *T foetus*, the remaining portion of the vaginal aspirate should be carefully inoculated into a two-chambered commercial packet (InPouch TF, Biomed Diagnostics, White City, Oregon), which should then be sealed and stored upright to prevent leakage [15]. Like *C fetus*, temporary shipment or storage (less than 24 hours) of inoculated InPouches at room temperature (20°C–25°C) will not significantly deter growth of *T foetus* [82]. Some laboratories incubate *T foetus* cultures at a slightly reduced temperature (eg, 35°C–36°C), in an effort to suppress overgrowth of gas-forming bacteria, which at best can make it difficult to identify trichomonads through the InPouch, and at worst can lead to rupture of the sealed InPouch.

Diagnosis—Male

Published work has shown that the prepuce of the bull can be sampled either by lavage or by scraping [83]. Because scraping with a plastic artificial insemination (AI) pipette is faster, easier, and less expensive, it is usually the method of choice. To minimize contamination, it is useful to cover the pipette with a plastic chemise (available from AI/embryo transfer [ET] suppliers), and to push the tip of the pipette through the end of the chemise after the pipette/chemise are in place in the proximal fornix. The scraping should be fairly vigorous, 10 to 15 strokes, sufficient to loosen epithelial cells from the penile and preputial surface. The miniscule amount of hemorrhage that sometimes results does the bull no harm. The near end of the pipette should have a 12-cc syringe attached, and the operator should keep negative pressure in the syringe while scraping. Ease up on negative pressure as the pipette is withdrawn back into the chemise, and then withdraw the pipette/chemise from the prepuce. There should be a 2- to 5-cm column of cloudy smegma in the pipette. Half of this column can be inoculated into the TEM for *C fetus*, and the other half inoculated directly into an InPouch for *T foetus*. Seal and store the InPouch as described above for CVM samples from the female.

A preliminary diagnosis of trichomoniasis is made by observing motile trichomonads directly through the InPouch at 200 to 400 magnifications. When present, the trichomonads are usually found in the corners and near the bottom of the InPouch incubation chamber. They are identifiable by their size (perhaps 10% larger than a bovine sperm head), the presence of multiple anterior flagellae, and a characteristic refractile "undulating membrane" [3,84]. Their motility is rolling, aimless, and jerky [10]. At the resolution of most clinical microscopes, the exact number of anterior flagellae (three) cannot be determined. This is why there was initially some confusion when organisms that were clearly trichomonads were isolated in InPouches from virgin bulls. The history and the culture results were seemingly incompatible; however, electron microscopy (EM) clearly showed more than three anterior flagellae in these isolates, indicating that these trichomonads were not *T foetus*. A diagnostic technique more practical than EM was needed. That need has been met by the development of polymerase chain reaction (PCR) assays of cultured trichomonads [27,29,85–88].

The sensitivity of the culture method for *T foetus* has been calculated at 80% to 90% [25,83,89–91]. The specificity of culture was for decades presumed to be 100%, but the misidentification of the so-called "virgin bull isolates" as *T foetus* has clearly shown that this estimate was too high. Thus, there undoubtedly have been false-positive results, and because there is no legal treatment for trichomoniasis in cattle, some bulls have been sent to slaughter unnecessarily. A few Western states are changing their veterinary regulatory laws regarding diagnosis of trichomoniasis. For example, in California veterinarians must be certified to take smegma samples and read the cultures, and all positive cultures must be confirmed by a positive PCR, which can be run only at a certified laboratory (see www.cdfa.ca.gov/ahfss/ah/trichomonosis_info.htm for details).

Treatment

Male

For *Campylobacter*, some of the older literature discusses the use of streptomycin for infected males and females [92]. Whether or not this is still an effective drug is probably moot, because the use of amino glycosides in food animals is generally avoided where possible, and streptomycin in particular is no longer available. Moreover, the surprising discovery that immunization of infected bulls with an appropriately adjuvanted antigen could actually clear infection from the prepuce has reduced dependence on antibiotic use [11,93,94]. Although some failures of this "immunotherapy" are reported [94,95], the general success rate appears to be high, such that treatment of valuable bulls should at least be considered. Even those bulls that "failed" to clear infection were typically culture-negative for 9 weeks or more before reverting to a positive status. This suggests that the number of organisms was greatly reduced after injection of vaccine, a finding that could be clinically useful. In other words, such bulls may be less able to transmit an infectious dose to a susceptible female for a period that represents most of a typical breeding season. Most bull vaccination protocols for *C fetus venerealis* call for inoculation of a double dose of vaccine administered on two occasions, 1 month apart. Although none of the *C fetus venerealis* vaccine preparations sold in the United States are labeled for use in bulls, the oil-adjuvanted preparations are most often used in attempts to clear a bull's genital tract of infection (see sections on treatment and prophylaxis below). One such product is Vibrin (Pfizer Animal Health, New York, New York). Injection will cause some local tissue reaction, so the primary and booster injections should be given on opposite sides of the neck.

The story is not so positive for *T foetus*, but there are suggestions that an effective therapy may be developed. As mentioned above, there is currently no legal, efficacious treatment for trichomoniasis in either the bull or the cow. Several drugs are able to kill *T foetus* in vitro, but they are either unable to affect in vivo killing or they are specifically outlawed by the Food and Drug Administration [96]. The latter include nitrofurans [97] and the substituted imidazoles (metronidazole, ipronidazole, dimetridazole) [25,98]. And, although there is a commercially available killed whole-cell *T foetus* vaccine (Trich Guard, Fort Dodge Animal Health, Overland Park, Kansas), it has no claimed efficacy in the bull. Moreover, attempts in South Africa to use *T foetus* vaccination in bulls were not successful [99]. Nevertheless, work by Clark and colleagues in Australia [100,101] showed that the majority of *T fetus* infected bulls immunized with whole-cell or membrane preparations of the parasite were able to clear the infection. The treatment was especially efficacious in bulls younger than 5 years old. There is a need for more research in this area.

Herd treatment for sexually transmitted diseases

The well-founded recommendation to abandon natural service and go to an all-AI program has plenty of scientific evidence to support it, but is hard to sell to many clients. Many commercial cow-calf operators do not have appropriate facilities for intensive procedures such as estrus detection and AI, and dairy clients who use bulls may be doing so because of difficulty they have experienced with AI programs. In either case, a veterinarian who advocates changing to an all-AI program is really advocating a change in work styles, and not every client is willing to make that change. Because one of the major objections is estrus detection, the veterinarian can make the AI program less onerous by suggesting an estrus synchronization-timed AI program. In the author's experience, it is sometimes easier to persuade the dairy client to simply try the AI program for 6 months, with or without synchronization, with the understanding that clients can return to bull breeding after that time if they still do not care for AI. This interval will allow enough time for infected cows to clear the infection. If the owner does return to a natural service breeding program after 6 months, he must replace his previous bull battery with virgin bulls exclusively. Thus, even if there are one or two carrier cows lurking in this herd, the virgin bulls are unlikely to transmit an STD from a carrier cow to a susceptible one. Table 2 is a summary comparison of methods for dealing with herds infected with *T foetus* or *C fetus*.

Prophylaxis—male

Campylobacter fetus venerealis

The same Vibrin product used to clear *Campylobacter* infection from bulls can be used prophylactically to either prevent infection or to significantly reduce the persistence of infection. Some studies [93] found that bulls inoculated once were either not infected or were only briefly infected following exposure to *C fetus venerealis*-infected females. Typically, two injections at a 1-month interval are recommended, especially if the product used does not have an oil adjuvant. In herds in which few risk factors are active (ie, no shared grazing, no fenceline contact with an infected herd, no recent introduction of mature bulls or cull cows, and so on), it is reasonable to vaccinate only the bulls, using two doses of Vibrin, with the second dose given shortly before exposure to females, and boosters given annually. Bulls thus immunized are generally unable to establish

Table 2
Summary of options for dealing with individuals or herds diagnosed with bovine venereal campylobacteriosis or trichomonosis

	C fetus venerealis	T foetus
Treatment, individual male	Antibiotics + vaccination Requires cult/sensitivity	None (slaughter)
Treatment, individual female	Antibiotics + vaccination	None (wait for natural clearance) or slaughter
Herd treatment	1. "Blitz" antibiotics + vaccination (note withdrawal times);	1. Cull all or only infected bulls, replace with virgin bulls.
	2. Cull infected bulls, replace with virgin bulls.	2. Let infection run its course in females. Separate females into pregnant >5 months, pregnant <5 months, open (cull opens)
	3. Separate females into pregnant >5 months, pregnant <5 months, open. Consider keeping open if you vaccinate them.	3. Artificial insemination
	4. Artificial insemination	

a permanent carrier state for *C fetus venerealis*. The mechanism by which a systemically administered antigen generates a protective response on what is essentially a skin surface is not known.

Tritrichomonas foetus

For trichomoniasis, the label for the available *T foetus* vaccine claims neither prophylactic nor therapeutic efficacy in the bull. This does not necessarily mean that there is no beneficial effect in the bull, but rather suggests that such efficacy has not been tested. The author is aware of anecdotal accounts of bulls being treated for trichomoniasis by multiple injections of Trich Guard, and in some of these there appeared to be clearance, as inferred from one or two negative preputial cultures following immunotherapy. But multiple cultures, spanning a period equivalent to a breeding season, need to be done to prove clearance. Such studies are often prohibitively expensive.

Prophylaxis—female

Campylobacter fetus venerealis

Initial immunization of females requires two injections of bacterin, with the second coming shortly before exposure to bulls. This will maximize antibody levels at the time when exposure is most likely. Annual boosters should follow, again given no more than 3 weeks before exposure to bulls, if possible. Immunization induces an IgG response, and probably enhances the IgA response that follows natural exposure. The protective antibodies are of the IgG_1 and IgG_2 subclasses, and protect against uterine infection, although transient vaginal infection can still occur following natural service to an infected bull. The most thorough test of efficacy of vibrio vaccines is now 25 years old, and was conducted in a guinea pig abortion model [102]. These studies indicated that oil adjuvant significantly enhanced the protection conferred by the vaccine against abortion in guinea pigs, and are the bases of our current recommendations for vaccine selection [103]. The findings are confirmed by bovine studies as well [104].

Tritrichomonas foetus

A prospective clinical trial [105] compared pregnancy and calving rates between beef heifers vaccinated with Trich Guard and control heifers. All heifers were exposed to infected bulls at estrus, and received an intravaginal challenge with a very large number of *T foetus* organisms (nearly 10 million) as well. At calving, twice as many vaccinated heifers calved as did control heifers (61% versus 31%), so it appears that the vaccine offered at least some protection. The relatively low calving rate even among the vaccinates suggests that either the vaccine induced only a partially protective response or the challenge dose was overwhelming. The lack of a nonimmunized, nonchallenged group hampered interpretation of this study, because we cannot know what the normal calving rate was for this herd in this geographic area; but it is clear that the vaccine had a positive overall effect.

Where vaccination fits in the control of these diseases

With a highly efficacious and inexpensive vaccine available for *C fetus venerealis*, it is relatively easy to incorporate vaccination into the routine management of a herd's reproductive program. Although many practitioners claim that they do not see venereal campylobacteriosis, it is still prevalent wherever natural service is practiced. Diagnostic laboratories in the Western United States still report a few cases of *C fetus venerealis* each year. This is in spite of widespread vaccination. The author believes that the extensive use of an efficacious vaccine is largely responsible for holding this disease in check, and that cessation of vaccination will invite epizootics of venereal campylobacteriosis.

The role of vaccine in the control of trichomoniasis is more complicated, partly because the efficacy of the vaccine is less than that for *C fetus venerealis*, and partly because the vaccine is considerably more expensive. To help answer the question "Should I vaccinate for trichomoniasis?," a mathematical simulation model was developed [106]. This model takes into account a variety of inputs, including such risk factors as the number and age of bulls, the known status of the disease in the local geographic area, the use of shared grazing, the failure to test bulls for trichomoniasis before the breeding season, and so on. It also takes into account the cost of vaccine, the value of the weaned calf, the cost of veterinary time and expertise, and labor costs associated with vaccinating. Using this model, the use of trich vaccine in females was warranted if shared grazing (eg, on public lands) is used, if bulls are not tested before the season begins, and if at least two thirds of bulls used are more than 3 years old. It is important to note that avoidance of all risk factors showed a better economic return than vaccinating, but when this is not feasible for a given herd the simulation indicates that vaccination will significantly decrease economic losses due to *T foetus*-induced pregnancy disruption.

Nonclassical agents that may be spread by venereal route

These are discussed only briefly, because each agent has a body of literature attached that goes beyond the scope of this article.

Haemophilus somnus

This gram-negative bacteria, better known as an agent of respiratory disease and thromboembolic meningoencephalitis (TEME), has been frequently isolated from the genitalia of cattle [107]. In bulls examined at the time of slaughter, the organism has been isolated from the preputial cavity in pure culture. In contrast to the classical venereal agents, *H somnus* was more commonly isolated from younger bulls. Whether *H somnus* is a component of the normal preputial flora and a possible source of infection for respiratory and central nervous systems diseases is not known. It is known that *H somnus* frequently infects the seminal vesicular glands of young bulls [108], an event that probably generates the anti-*H somnus* IgG, IgM, and IgA that can be demonstrated in the bull's reproductive tract fluids [109].

The organism has also been isolated frequently from cows that have vaginal discharges due to endometritis or cervicitis or vaginitis. Curiously, according to one clinical report [110], in every dairy involved in a protracted outbreak of acute *H somnus*-associated vaginitis-endometritis, all cows had been bred by natural service. Without an AI control group to compare, it is not possible to know with certainty that the *H somnus* was sexually transmitted.

As a predominately extracellular organism [111], *H somnus* is probably held in check by an antibody-mediated rather than cell-mediated immune response. There is evidence that IgG_2 is the more protective subtype of immunoglobulin against *H somnus* [112,113]; however, the organism has a complex set of immune-avoidance mechanisms, including the ability to bind immunoglobulin at sites other than the antigen recognition site, for example, the Fc region of the immunoglobulin [112,114].

Ureaplasma diversum

This urea-splitting *Mycoplasma*, formerly referred to as "T strain" *Mycoplasma*, has been associated with granular vulvo-vaginitis and infertility since 1980, when Doig first attributed the lesions to infection with *U diversum* [115–117]. The condition is painful, and affected cows resist inspection of the affected area. The granularity of the vulvar/vestibular region is caused by accumulations of leukocytes in clusters just below the epithelium. The inflammatory process can ascend to involve the cervix and endometrium, and is thought to contribute significantly to embryonic death (before day 42). According to most authors, *U diversum* is readily transmitted at coitus, although it can also exploit other means of transmission as well, including contaminated semen, direct contact, and congenital infection during passage through the birth canal. Diagnosis involves physical examination, which includes inspecting the vulva and vestibular mucosae for generalized hyperemia and small, pale, raised granules. The organism can be cultured in special media, which is inoculated via a cotton swab that is rubbed into a lesion. Recently, as for other infectious organisms, a PCR test has been developed [118]. The test is apparently more sensitive than culture.

Many parts of the *Ureaplasma* story are confusing, not the least of which is that many animals harbor the organism without showing signs. In one study [119], *U diversum* was isolated from 43% of 240 dairy cows, 27% of 118 beef cows, 47% of 91 beef heifers, and 67% of 34 beef bulls. None of these animals manifested any lesions; however, the proportion of animals having lesions that had positive cultures was significantly higher than the normal group (without lesions). An attempt to examine strain differences as a possible explanation for the presence of the organism in so many normal animals was inconclusive. In another epidemiologic study of beef replacement heifers [120], animals that had low body condition scores (≤ 5.5) immediately before breeding were more likely to harbor the organism, and later at pregnancy examination, culture-negative heifers were more likely to be pregnant. Taken together, one can conclude that *Ureaplasma diversum is* an opportunistic reproductive pathogen, that it can be venereally transmitted (although other routes are exploited), and that we still have not recognized some important risk factors that render one culture-positive heifer affected while another culture-positive herdmate remains normal.

Individual animals may benefit from antibiotic therapy. Initial reports used 1 g of tetracycline administered intrauterine in an effort to clear the uterus, although it is not obvious that this also cleared the vaginal/vulvar reservoir of organisms. Systemic antibiotics appear to have more justification, although the milk discard required for most of the drugs that are effective against ureaplasma (macrolides, tetracyclines) is an important consideration in dairy cows. Herd-level control involves minimizing exposure of the upper reproductive tract to the organism. Soon after the first descriptions of ureaplasma-associated endometritis and salpingitis, inseminators were advised to use a sheathed insemination pipette/Cassou gun, to minimize the possibility of pushing lower reproductive tract organisms, especially *Ureaplasma*, into the uterine lumen. The idea was to move the sheathed pipette quickly through the vagina to the fornix, then to "pop" the pipette through the flimsy plastic chemise and into the cervix as quickly as possible. No commercial vaccine is currently available for *U diversum*.

Leptospira

Historically, most of the concern about *Leptospira* and genital infection in cattle has been concerned with transmission via frozen semen, rather than by coitus. Because leptospires readily survive freezing and thawing, some concern was warranted. This organism was once thought to maintain its carrier state only in the kidney, but beginning in the 1980s, evidence accumulated that indicated a carrier state in the male and female reproductive tracts [121]. Moreover, there is evidence of venereal transmission, and a suggestion of infertility as a result.

The fastidious nature of the many serovars of *Leptospira interrogans* make them difficult to grow in culture, and the time-honored alternative of interpreting microscopic agglutination titers has often been confusing. Newer immune-based tests and molecular diagnostic assays [122], and combinations thereof, including an assay that separates organisms immunomagnetically before probing the genomic DNA by PCR [123], should increase the sensitivity of our diagnostic ability for Leptospira-induced pregnancy failure. For now, the gold standard diagnostic for "lepto" is still cultivation of the organism, but we are currently at the point where immuno and molecular tests are likely to surpass the standard.

Etiologic agents

The *Leptospira* species and serovars common to cattle are zoonotic agents. The hardjo serovars are the most problematic for cattle. In fact, two different species of leptospires, *L interrogans*, serovar *hardjo*, type hardjoprajitno and *L borgpetersenii* type hardjobovis have similar if not identical serological reactivity. These serovars tend to cause the majority of lepto-associated pregnancy loss, with *L borgpetersenii* predominating in the United States. Until recently, all such loss was thought to be the result of hematogenous delivery of *L interrogans* serovar hardjoprajitno spirochetes to the pregnant uterus. Recent advances in the correct identification of the actual infecting strain of Leptospira offer the prospect of better protection by vaccines. Until recently, most of the Unites States was vaccinating for the wrong leptospire (reviewed in BonDurant [124]). Proper identification of the pathogen, and now a monovalent vaccine (SpiroVac, Pfizer) that contains antigens from the appropriately identified leptospires, offer the hope of more effective prophylaxis than we have had heretofore.

Treatment

Whether the vaccine can clear the carrier state of an infected female has not been thoroughly tested. Antibiotics are probably still required for clearance. Streptomycin, the former favorite for this purpose, is not available [125], but the following have been effective: a single injection of oxytetracycline (20 mg/kg IM), tilmicosin (10 mg/kg, SC), or multiple injections of ceftiofur sodium (2.2 or 5 mg/kg, IM, once daily for 5 days, or 20 mg/kg, IM, once daily for 3 days) [126]. Appropriate withdrawal times must be honored. Vaccination of females with a monovalent bacterin is recommended before breeding age, and then annually thereafter. Interestingly, both Pfizer's *L borgpetersenii* bacterin and another manufacturer's monovalent *L interrogans* hardjoprajitno bacterin (Leptavoid, Schering Plough, Kenilworth, New Jersey) induced robust, protective Type I responses against the *borgpetersenii* strain, whereas pentavalent lepto vaccines did not generate such a response [127]. Further, the Type I response following a monovalent hardjo immunization protected against a different serovar, *L interrogans*, serovar *grippotyphosa*. The Type I response is characterized by an enhanced cell-mediated response, measured in part by detection of sustained elevated interferon gamma (IFNγ), and relatively increased antigen-specific IgG$_2$ [127–129]. The class switch to IgG$_2$ may be important, because IgG$_2$ is a more effective opsonin than IgG$_1$, and the extracellular spirochetes are presumably more readily phagocytized in the presence of specific IgG$_2$ [130]. Little is known about the efficacy of vaccinating males, although the topic can be controversial. Bulls whose semen is exported need to have minimal serological reaction to the hardjo serovars, and vaccination obviously raises the titers of those reactions. Some have argued that the microscopic agglutination titers are an indication of protection, and that stud bulls should be vaccinated, regardless of the increase in titer that vaccination will cause [121].

References

[1] Cassell BG, Jobst SM, McGilliard ML, et al. Evaluating sire selection practices using lifetime net income functions. J Dairy Sci 2002;85(12):3492–502.

[2] Akhtar S, Riemann HP, Thurmond MC, et al. The association between antibody titres against *Campylobacter fetus* and milk production efficiency in dairy cattle. Vet Res Commun 1993;17(3):183–91.

[3] Honigberg BM. Trichomonads of veterinary importance. In: Kreier J, editor. Parasitic protozoa. Boca Raton (FL): Academic Press, Inc.; 1978. p. 207–73.

[4] Honigberg BM. Structure, taxonomic status, and host list of *Tritrichomonas batachorum* (Perty). J Parasitol 1953;39(2):191–208.

[5] Yabuuchi E. Legitimacy of the names of subspecies of *Campylobacter fetus* proposed by Veron and Chatelain, 1980. Ann Microbiol (Paris) 1983;134A(1):3–8.

[6] Tachezy J, Tachezy R, Hampl V, et al. Cattle pathogen *Tritrichomonas foetus* (Riedmuller, 1928) and pig commensal Tritrichomonas suis (Gruby & Delafond, 1843) belong to the same species. J Eukaryot Microbiol 2002;49(2):154–63.

[7] Kassai T, Cordero DC, Euzeby J, et al. Standardized nomenclature of animal parasitic diseases (SNOAPAD). Vet Parasitol 1988;29(4):299–326.

[8] Wilfert CM. Brucella. In: Joklik WK, Willett HP, Amos DB, editors. Zinsser microbiology. Norwalk (CT): Appleton-Century-Crofts; 1984. p. 665–71.

[9] Roberts S. Diseases and accidents of the gestation period. In: Roberts S, editor. Veterinary obstetrics and genital diseases. Ann Arbor (MI): Edward Brothers, Inc.; 1971. p. 107–200.

[10] BonDurant RH. Diagnosis, treatment, and control of bovine trichomoniasis. Comp Cont Educ Pract Vet 1985;7:S179–88.

[11] Ball L, Dargatz DA, Cheney JM, et al. Control of venereal disease in infected herds. Vet Clin North Am Food Anim Pract 1987;3(3):561–74.

[12] BonDurant RH, Honigberg BM. Trichomonads of veterinary importance. In: Krier JP, editor. Parasitic protozoa, vol. 9. 2nd edition. San Diego (CA): Academic Press; 1994. p. 168–77.

[13] Rhyan JC, Wilson KL, Wagner B, et al. Demonstration of *Tritrichomonas foetus* in the external genitalia and of specific antibodies in preputial secretions of naturally infected bulls. Vet Pathol 1999;36(5):406–11.

[14] Hammond DM, Bartlett DE. The distribution of *Trichomonas foetus* in the preputial cavity of infected bulls. Am J Vet Res 1943;4:443–9.

[15] BonDurant RH. Pathogenesis, diagnosis, and management of trichomoniasis in cattle. Vet Clin North Am Food Anim Pract 1997;13(2):345–61.

[16] Müller M. The hydrogenosome. The eukaryotic microbial cell. Cambridge, UK: Cambridge View Press; 1980. p. 127–43.

[17] Wang CC, Wang AL, Rice A. *Tritrichomonas foetus*: partly defined cultivation medium for study of the purine and pyrimidine metabolism. Exp Parasitol 1984;57(1): 68–75.

[18] Christensen HR, Clark BL, Parsonson IM. Incidence of *Tritrichomonas foetus* in young replacement bulls following introduction into an infected herd. Aust Vet J 1977;53(3): 132–4.

[19] Campero CM, Hirst RG, Ladds PW, et al. Measurement of antibody in serum and genital fluids of bulls by ELISA after vaccination and challenge with *Tritrichomonas foetus*. Aust Vet J 1990;67(5):175–8.

[20] Flower PJ, Ladds PW, Thomas AD, et al. An immunopathologic study of the bovine prepuce. Vet Pathol 1983;20(2):189–202.

[21] Goodger WJ, Skirrow SZ. Epidemiologic and economic analyses of an unusually long epizootic of trichomoniasis in a large California dairy herd. J Am Vet Med Assoc 1986; 189(7):772–6.

[22] Howard TH, Vasquez LA, Amann R. Antibiotic control of *Campylobacter fetus* by three extenders of bovine semen. J Dairy Sci 1982;65(8):1596–600.

[23] Clark BL, Dufty JH, Parsonson IM. Studies on the transmission of *Tritrichomonas foetus*. Aust Vet J 1977;53(4):170–2.

[24] Hammond DM, Bartlett DE. Establishment of infection with *Trichomonas foetus* in bulls by experimental exposure. Am J Vet Res 1943;4:61–5.

[25] Skirrow S, BonDurant R, Farley J, et al. Efficacy of ipronidazole against trichomoniasis in beef bulls. J Am Vet Med Assoc 1985;187(4):405–7.

[26] Castella J, Muanoz E, Ferrer D, et al. Isolation of the trichomonad *Tetratrichomonas buttreyi* (Hibler et al., 1960) Honigberg, 1963 in bovine diarrhoeic faeces. Vet Parasitol 1997;70(1–3):41–5.

[27] BonDurant RH, Gajadhar A, Campero CM, et al. Preliminary characterization of a *Tritrichomonas foetus*-like protozoan isolated from preputial smegma of virgin bulls. The Bovine Practitioner 1999;33(2):124–7.

[28] Jezierski TA, Koziorowski M, Goszczynski J, et al. Homosexual and social behaviours of young bulls of different geno- and phenotypes and plasma concentrations of some hormones. Appl Anim Behav Sci 1989;24:101–13.

[29] Hayes DC, Anderson RR, Walker RL. Identification of trichomonadid protozoa from the bovine preputial cavity by polymerase chain reaction and restriction fragment length polymorphism typing. J Vet Diagn Invest 2003;15(4):390–4.

[30] Parker S, Campbell J, McIntosh K, et al. Diagnosis of trichomoniasis in 'virgin' bulls by culture and polymerase chain reaction. Can Vet J 2003;44(9):732–4.

[31] Christensen HR, Clark BL. Spread of *Tritrichomonas foetus* in beef bulls in an infected herd [letter]. Aust Vet J 1979;55(4):205.

[32] Bartlett DE, Hammond DM. Pattern of fluctuations in number of *Trichomonas foetus* occurring in the bovine vagina during initial infections. Am J Vet Res 1945; 6:91–5.

[33] Corbeil LB. Immunization and diagnosis in bovine reproductive tract infections. Adv Vet Med 1999;41:217–39.

[34] Wira CR, Fahey JV, Abrahams VM, et al. Influence of stage of the reproductive cycle and estradiol on thymus cell antigen presentation. J Steroid Biochem Mol Biol 2003;84(1): 79–87.

[35] Bondurant RH. Inflammation in the bovine female reproductive tract. J Anim Sci 1999; 77(Suppl 2):101–10.

[36] Cobb SP, Watson ED. Immunohistochemical study of immune cells in the bovine endometrium at different stages of the oestrous cycle. Res Vet Sci 1995;59(3): 238–41.

[37] Bielanski A, Ghazi DF, Phipps-Todd B. Observations on the fertilization and development of preimplantation bovine embryos in vitro in the presence of *Tritrichomonas foetus*. Theriogenology 2004;61:821–9.

[38] Bielanski A, Sampath MI, Graham JK, et al. In vitro fertilization of bovine ova in the presence of *Campylobacter fetus* subsp. *venerealis*. Reprod Domest Anim 1994;29(8): 488–93.

[39] Parsonson IM, Clark BL, Dufty JH. Early pathogenesis and pathology of *Tritrichomonas foetus* infection in virgin heifers. J Comp Pathol 1976;86(1):59–66.

[40] Rae DO. Impact of trichomoniasis on the cow-calf producer's profitability. J Am Vet Med Assoc 1989;194(6):771–5.

[41] Anderson ML, BonDurant RH, Corbeil RR, et al. Immune and inflammatory responses to reproductive tract infection with *Tritrichomonas foetus* in immunized and control heifers. J Parasitol 1996;82(4):594–600.

[42] BonDurant RH, Corbeil RR, Corbeil LB. Immunization of virgin cows with surface antigen TF1.17 of *Tritrichomonas foetus*. Infect Immun 1993;61(4):1385–94.

[43] Corbeil LB, Campero CM, Rhyan JC, et al. Mast cells and TH2 uterine immune responses during trichomoniasis. Vet Pathol 2005, in press.

[44] Soto P, Parma AE. The immune response in cattle infected with *Tritrichomonas foetus*. Vet Parasitol 1989;33(3–4):343–8.

[45] Corbel MJ. Detection of antibodies to *Campylobacter fetus* (*Vibrio fetus*) in the preputial secretions of bulls with vibriosis. Br Vet J 1974;130(3):51–3.

[46] Skirrow SZ, BonDurant RH. Immunoglobulin isotype of specific antibodies in reproductive tract secretions and sera in *Tritrichomonas foetus*-infected heifers. Am J Vet Res 1990;51(4):645–53.

[47] Corbeil LB, Anderson ML, Corbeil RR, et al. Female reproductive tract immunity in bovine trichomoniasis. Am J Reprod Immunol 1998;39(3):189–98.

[48] Dennett DP. Trichomoniasis of beef cattle in North Queensland. Vic Vet Proc 1976;34:22.

[49] Corbeil LB, Schurig GG, Duncan JR, et al. Immunity in the female bovine reproductive tract based on the response to *Campylobacter fetus*. Adv Exp Med Biol 1981; 137:729–43.

[50] Corbeil LB, Duncan JR, Schurig GD, et al. Bovine venereal vibriosis variations in immunoglobulin class of antibodies in genital secretions and serum. Infect Immun 1974; 10(5):1084–90.

[51] Corbeil LB, Schurig GD, Duncan JR, et al. Immunoglobulin classes and biological functions of Campylobacter (Vibrio) fetus antibodies in serum and cervicovaginal mucus. Infect Immun 1974;10(3):422–9.

[52] Skirrow SZ, BonDurant RH. Induced Tritrichomonas foetus infection in beef heifers. J Am Vet Med Assoc 1990;196(6):885–9.

[53] Clark BL. Venereal diseases of cattle. In: Veterinary Review, no. 1 [pamphlet]. Sydney, Australia: University of Sydney Post Graduate Foundation for Veterinary Science; 1971. p. 5–27.

[54] Clark BL, Dufty JH, Monsbourgh MJ. Observations on the isolation of Vibrio fetus (venerealis) from the vaginal mucus of experimentally infected heifers. Aust Vet J 1969; 45(5):209–11.

[55] Schurig GD, Hall CE, Burda K, et al. Infection patterns in heifers following cervicovaginal or intrauterine instillation of Campylobacter (Vibrio) fetus venerealis. Cornell Vet 1974; 64(4):533–48.

[56] Corbeil LB, Schurig GG, Bier PJ, et al. Bovine venereal vibriosis: antigenic variation of the bacterium during infection. Infect Immun 1975;11(2):240–4.

[57] Wesley IV, Bryner JH. Antigenic and restriction enzyme analysis of isolates of Campylobacter fetus subsp venerealis recovered from persistently infected cattle. Am J Vet Res 1989;50(6):807–13.

[58] Morgan BB. Studies on the trichomonad carrier-cow problems. J Anim Sci 1944;(3):437.

[59] Skirrow S. Identification of trichomonad-carrier cows. J Am Vet Med Assoc 1987;191(5): 553–4.

[60] Mancebo OA, Russo AM, Carabajal LL, et al. Persistence of Tritrichomonas foetus in naturally infected cows and heifers in Argentina. Vet Parasitol 1995;59(1):7–11.

[61] Roberts S. Examinations for pregnancy. In: Roberts S, editor. Veterinary obstetrics and genital diseases. 2nd edition. Ann Arbor (MI): Edwards Bros; 1971. p. 14–35.

[62] Dedie K, Pohl R, Romer H, et al. Distribution, survey and control of venereal campylobacteriosis in bull keeping cooperatives. Tierarztl Umsch 1982;37(2):80–96.

[63] Gay JM, Ebel ED, Kearley WP. Commingled grazing as a risk factor for trichomonosis in beef herds. J Am Vet Med Assoc 1996;209(3):643–6.

[64] Randel RD. Nutrition and postpartum rebreeding in cattle. J Anim Sci 1990;68(3):853–62.

[65] Short RE, Bellows RA, Staigmiller RB, et al. Physiological mechanisms controlling anestrus and infertility in postpartum beef cattle. J Anim Sci 1990;68(3):799–816.

[66] Maas J. Relationship between nutrition and reproduction in beef cattle. Vet Clin North Am Food Anim Pract 1987;3(3):633–46.

[67] Duncan JR, Wilkie BN, Winter AJ. Natural and immune antibodies for Vibrio fetus in serum and secretions of cattle. Infect Immun 1972;5(5):728–33.

[68] Kendrick JW. The vaginal mucus agglutination test for bovine vibriosis. J Am Vet Med Assoc 1967;150(5):495–8.

[69] Corbeil LB, Corbeil RR, Winter AJ. Bovine venereal vibriosis: activity of inflammatory cells in protective immunity. Am J Vet Res 1975;36:403–6.

[70] Kerr WR, Robertson M. Effect of ACTH, cortisone, sphingomyelin, sphingosine and phenergan (antihistamine) in inhibiting the skin reaction in cattle sensitized to Trichomonas foetus antigen. J Hyg (Lond) 1952;50(3):354–75.

[71] Kerr WR. The intradermal test in bovine trichomoniasis. Vet Rec 1944;56(34):303–5.

[72] Ikeda JS, BonDurant RH, Corbeil LB. Bovine vaginal antibody responses to immunoaffinity-purified surface antigen of Tritrichomonas foetus. J Clin Microbiol 1995; 33(5):1158–63.

[73] BonDurant RH, Van Hoosear KA, Corbeil LB, et al. Serological response to in vitro-shed antigen(s) of Tritrichomonas foetus in cattle. Clin Diagn Lab Immunol 1996;3(4):432–7.

[74] Monke HJ, Love BC, Wittum TE, et al. Effect of transport enrichment medium, transport time, and growth medium on the detection of *Campylobacter fetus* subsp *venerealis*. J Vet Diagn Invest 2002;14(1):35–9.

[75] Garcia MM, Stewart RB, Ruckerbauer GM. Quantitative evaluation of a transport-enrichment medium for *Campylobacter fetus*. Vet Rec 1984;115(17):434–6.

[76] Eaglesome MD, Sampath MI, Garcia MM. A detection assay for *Campylobacter fetus* in bovine semen by restriction analysis of PCR amplified DNA. Vet Res Comm 1995;19: 253–63.

[77] Hum S, Brunner J, McInnes A, et al. Evaluation of cultural methods and selective media for the isolation of *Campylobacter fetus* subsp *venerealis* from cattle. Aust Vet J 1994;71(6): 184–6.

[78] Bryner JH. Bovine abortion caused by *Campylobacter fetus*. In: Kirkbride CA, editor. Laboratory diagnosis of livestock abortion. Ames (IA): Iowa State University Press; 1990. p. 70–81.

[79] Wagenaar J, Van Vergen M, Newell DG, et al. Comparative study using amplified fragment length polymorphism fingerprinting, PCR genotyping, and phenotyping to differentiate *Campylobacter fetus* strains from animals. J Clin Microbiol 2001;39(6):2283–6.

[80] Salama SM, Garcia MM, Taylor DE. Differentiation of the subspecies of *Campylobacter fetus* by genomic sizing. Int J Syst Bacteriol 1992;42(3):446–50.

[81] Hum S, Quinn K, Brunner J, et al. Evaluation of a PCR assay for identification and differentiation of *Campylobacter fetus* subspecies. Aust Vet J 1997;75(11):827–31.

[82] Bryan LA, Campbell JR, Gajadhar AA. Effects of temperature on the survival of *Tritrichomonas foetus* in transport, Diamond's and InPouch TF media. Vet Rec 1999; 144(9):227–32.

[83] Schönmann MJ, BonDurant RH, Gardner IA, et al. Comparison of sampling and culture methods for the diagnosis of *Tritrichomonas foetus* infection in bulls. Vet Rec 1994;134(24): 620–2.

[84] Fitzgerald PR. Bovine trichomoniasis. Vet Clin North Am Food Anim Pract 1986;2: 277–82.

[85] Felleisen RS, Lambelet N, Bachmann P, et al. Detection of *Tritrichomonas foetus* by PCR and DNA enzyme immunoassay based on rRNA gene unit sequences. J Clin Microbiol 1998;36(2):513–9.

[86] Felleisen RS. Comparative sequence analysis of 5.8S rRNA genes and internal transcribed spacer (ITS) regions of trichomonadid protozoa. Parasitology 1997;115:111–9.

[87] Ho MS, Conrad PA, Conrad PJ, et al. Detection of bovine trichomoniasis with a specific DNA probe and PCR amplification system. J Clin Microbiol 1994;32(1):98–104.

[88] Parker S, Lun ZR, Gajadhar A. Application of a PCR assay to enhance the detection and identification of *Tritrichomonas foetus* in cultured preputial samples. J Vet Diagn Invest 2001;13:508–13.

[89] Parker S, Campbell J, Gajadhar A. Comparison of the diagnostic sensitivity of a commercially available culture kit and a diagnostic culture test using Diamond's media for diagnosing *Tritrichomonas foetus* in bulls. J Vet Diagn Invest 2003;15(5):460–5.

[90] Parker S, Campbell J, Ribble C, et al. Sample collection factors affect the sensitivity of the diagnostic test for *Tritrichomonas foetus* in bulls. Can J Vet Res 2003;67(2):138–41.

[91] Parker S, Campbell J, Ribble C, et al. Comparison of two sampling tools for diagnosis of *Tritrichomonas foetus* in bulls and clinical interpretation of culture results. J Am Vet Med Assoc 1999;215(2):231–5.

[92] Garcia MM, Ruckerbauer GM, Eaglesome MD, et al. Detection of *Campylobacter fetus* in artificial insemination bulls with a transport enrichment medium. Can J Comp Med 1983; 47(3):336–40.

[93] Bouters R, De Keyser J, Vandeplassche M, et al. Vibrio fetus infection in bulls: curative and preventive vaccination. Br Vet J 1973;129(1):52–7.

[94] Vasquez LA, Ball L, Bennett BW, et al. Bovine genital campylobacteriosis (vibriosis): vaccination of experimentally infected bulls. Am J Vet Res 1983;44(8):1553–7.

[95] Hum S, Brunner J, Gardiner B. Failure of therapeutic vaccination of a bull infected with *Campylobacter fetus*. Aust Vet J 1993;70(10):386–7.

[96] Guest GB, Solomon SM. FDA extra label use policy—1992 revisions. J Am Vet Med Assoc 1993;20:1620–3.

[97] Cole BA. Effects, in vitro, of seven nitrofurans on the survival of *Trichomonas foetus*. Am J Vet Res 1950;11(40):315–6.

[98] Kimsey PB, Darien BJ, Kendrick JW, et al. Bovine trichomoniasis: diagnosis and treatment. J Am Vet Med Assoc 1980;177(7):616–9.

[99] Herr S, Ribeiro LM, Claassen E, et al. A reduction in the duration of infection with *Tritrichomonas foetus* following vaccination in heifers and the failure to demonstrate a curative effect in infected bulls. Onderstepoort J Vet Res 1991;58(1):41–5.

[100] Clark BL, Dufty JH, Parsonson IM. Immunisation of bulls against trichomoniasis. Aust Vet J 1983;60(6):178–9.

[101] Clark BL, Emery DL, Dufty JH. Therapeutic immunisation of bulls with the membranes and glycoproteins of *Tritrichomonas foetus* var brisbane. Aust Vet J 1984;61(2):65–6.

[102] Bryner JH, Foley JW, Thompson K. Comparative efficacy of ten commercial *Campylobacter fetus* vaccines in the pregnant guinea pig: challenge with *Campylobacter fetus* serotype A. Am J Vet Res 1979;40(3):433–5.

[103] Bryner JH, Firehammer BD, Wesley IV. Vaccination of pregnant guinea pigs with *Campylobacter fetus*: effects of antigen dose, *Campylobacter* strain, and adjuvant type. Am J Vet Res 1988;49(4):449–55.

[104] Kendrick JW, Williams J, Crenshaw GL, et al. Fertility and immune reaction of heifers vaccinated with an adjuvanted *Vibrio fetus* vaccine. J Am Vet Med Assoc 1971;158(9): 1531–5.

[105] Kvasnicka WG, Hanks D, Huang JC, et al. Clinical evaluation of the efficacy of inoculating cattle with a vaccine containing *Tritrichomonas foetus*. Am J Vet Res 1992;53(11):2023–7.

[106] Villarroel A, Carpenter TE, BonDurant RH. Development of a simulation model to evaluate the effect of vaccination against *Tritrichomonas foetus* on reproductive efficiency in beef herds. Am J Vet Res 2004;65(6):770–5.

[107] Humphrey JD, Little PB, Stephens LR, et al. Prevalence and distribution of *Haemophilus somnus* in the male bovine reproductive tract. Am J Vet Res 1982;43(5):791–5.

[108] Grotelueschen DM, Mortimer RG, Ellis RP. Vesicular adenitis syndrome in beef bulls. J Am Vet Med Assoc 1994;205(6):874–7.

[109] Stefaniak T. Detection of the *Haemophilus somnus* antibodies in the bulls' reproductive tract fluids using the ELISA. I. Elaboration of the ELISA for the detection of the specific antibodies in the IgG, IgM and IgA classes. Arch Vet Pol 1993;33(1–2):79–88.

[110] Last RD, Macfarlane MD, Jarvis CJ. Isolation of *Haemophilus somnus* from dairy cattle in kwaZulu-Natal. An emerging cause of 'dirty cow syndrome' and infertility? J S Afr Vet Assoc 2001;72(2):95.

[111] Corbeil LB. Antibodies as effectors. Vet Immunol Immunopathol 2002;87(3–4):169–75.

[112] Widders PR, Dowling SC, Gogolewski RP, et al. Isotypic antibody responses in cattle infected with *Haemophilus somnus*. Res Vet Sci 1989;46(2):212–7.

[113] Stefaniak T. Detection of the *Haemophilus somnus* antibodies in the bulls' reproductive tract fluids using the ELISA. II. Occurrence of specific antibodies in bulls from three bull rearing centers. Arch Vet Pol 1993;33(1–2):89–105.

[114] Widders PR, Smith JW, Yarnall M, et al. Non-immune immunoglobulin binding by *Haemophilus somnus*. J Med Microbiol 1988;26(4):307–11.

[115] Doig PA, Ruhnke HL, Palmer NC. Experimental bovine genital ureaplasmosis. II. Granular vulvitis, endometritis and salpingitis following uterine inoculation. Can J Comp Med 1980;44(3):259–66.

[116] Doig PA, Ruhnke HL, Palmer NC. Experimental bovine genital ureaplasmosis. I. Granular vulvitis following vulvar inoculation. Can J Comp Med 1980;44(3):252–8.

[117] Doig PA, Ruhnke HL, MacKay AL, et al. Bovine granular vulvitis associated with ureaplasma infection. Can Vet J 1979;20(4):89–94.

[118] Vasconcellos CM, Blanchard A, Ferris S, et al. Detection of *Ureaplasma diversum* in cattle using a newly developed PCR-based detection assay. Vet Microbiol 2000; 72(3–4):241–50.

[119] Mulira GL, Saunders JR. Humoral and secretory antibodies to *Ureaplasma diversum* in heifers following subcutaneous vaccination and vaginal infection. Can J Vet Res 1994; 58(2):104–8.

[120] Sanderson MW, Chenoweth PJ, Yeary T, et al. Prevalence and reproductive effects of *Ureaplasma diversum* in beef replacement heifers and the relationship to blood urea nitrogen level. Theriogenology 2000;54(3):401–8.

[121] Eaglesome MD, Garcia MM. Microbial agents associated with bovine genital tract infections and semen. Part I. *Brucella abortus, Leptospira, Campylobacter fetus* and *Tritrichomonas foetus*. Vet Bull 1992;62(8):743–63.

[122] Redstone JS, Woodward MJ. The development of a ligase mediated PCR with potential for the differentiation of serovars within *Leptospira interrogans*. Vet Microbiol 1996;51(3–4): 351–62.

[123] Yan KT, Ellis WA, Montgomery JM, et al. Development of an immunomagnetic antigen capture system for detecting leptospires in bovine urine. Res Vet Sci 1998;64(2):119–24.

[124] BonDurant RH. Controlling what we can control: limiting embryonic/fetal death. In: Proceedings of the American Association of Bovine Practitioners 37th Annual Meeting. Stillwater (OK): American Association of Bovine Practioners; 2004. p. 97–112.

[125] Gerritsen MJ, Koopmans MJ, Olyhoek T. Effect of streptomycin treatment on the shedding of and the serologic responses to *Leptospira interrogans* serovar hardjo subtype hardjobovis in experimentally infected cows. Vet Microbiol 1993;38(1–2):129–35.

[126] Alt DP, Zuerner RL, Bolin CA. Evaluation of antibiotics for treatment of cattle infected with *Leptospira borgpetersenii* serovar hardjo. J Am Vet Med Assoc 2001;219(5):636–9.

[127] Brown RA, Blumerman S, Gay C, et al. Comparison of three different leptospiral vaccines for induction of a type 1 immune response to *Leptospira borgpetersenii* serovar Hardjo. Vaccine 2003;21(27–30):4448–58.

[128] Naiman BM, Blumerman S, Alt D, et al. Evaluation of type 1 immune response in naive and vaccinated animals following challenge with *Leptospira borgpetersenii* serovar Hardjo: involvement of WC1(+) gammadelta and CD4 T cells. Infect Immun 2002;70(11):6147–57.

[129] Naiman BM, Alt D, Bolin CA, et al. Protective killed *Leptospira borgpetersenii* vaccine induces potent Th1 immunity comprising responses by CD4 and gammadelta T lymphocytes. Infect Immun 2001;69(12):7550–8.

[130] McGuire TC, Musoke AJ, Kurtti T. Functional properties of bovine IgG1 and IgG2: interaction with complement, macrophages, neutrophils and skin. Immunology 1979;38(2): 249–56.

ELSEVIER
SAUNDERS

Vet Clin Food Anim 21 (2005) 409–418

VETERINARY
CLINICS
Food Animal Practice

The Effect of Semen Quality on Reproductive Efficiency

James M. DeJarnette, MS

*Reproduction Specialist, Select Sires, Inc., 11740 US 42,
Plain City, OH 43064, USA*

The effects of semen quality on reproductive efficiency in cattle are well-documented but only modestly understood. Despite 60-plus years of commercial experience in artificial insemination (AI) in the bovine, and an accompanying number of years in research and technology adaptation, our ability to use in-vitro assessments of semen quality to predict the fertility potential of a semen sample seldom explains more than 50% to 60% of the variation among males. Opportunities for enhanced accuracy of fertility predictions may reside in identification of novel semen attributes associated with male fertility; however, an equal amount of progress may reside in the appropriate use and interpretation of presently available measures of semen quality.

Principles of semen quality and fertility

The concepts of compensable and uncompensable semen quality traits and their interactions with numbers of sperm in the inseminate dose are essential to understanding the relationship of semen quality to fertility (Fig. 1) [1,2]. Compensable semen quality traits are those that respond to increasing cell numbers per dose with increased fertility, and are generally believed to be associated with measures of sperm viability (ie, motility, acrosomal, cell-membrane integrity, and the like). Uncompensable semen quality traits are those that do not respond to increased numbers of sperm per dose with increased fertility. Uncompensable traits appear to be closely associated with abnormal sperm morphology, DNA integrity, and the ability of the male to sustain normal embryonic development following fertilization [3,4]. The "threshold" is the value beyond which further

E-mail address: jmdejarnette@selectsires.com

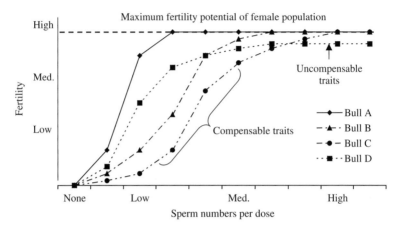

Fig. 1. Relationship of sperm numbers per dose and fertility for bulls of varying semen quality. (*Adapted from* Salisbury GW, VanDemark NL. Significance of semen quality. In: Physiology of reproduction and artificial insemination in cattle. 1st edition. San Francisco (CA): WH Freeman and Co.; 1961. p. 361; with permission.)

increases in sperm numbers per dose fail to increase fertility, and may be achieved by satisfying the semen demand of the female population (see bulls A, B, & C in Fig. 1) or when uncompensable semen quality traits become the limiting factor (see bull D in Fig. 1). Because of the heterogeneous nature of sperm populations, the rate at which individual bulls and ejaculates approach the threshold and the maximum level of fertility obtainable is a function of the severity and ratio of compensable and uncompensable sperm defects within the sample.

Assays of compensable semen quality components

Compensable semen quality attributes are those that influence accessibility of a viable sperm population to the ovum proximal to the time of ovulation. Thereby, assessment of sperm motility is a foundation measure for this component of the spermiogram. Likewise, various tests designed to measure the proportions of live sperm and those that have functional intact membranes would be expected to reflect compensable semen quality attributes. Assessment of these traits, however, is theoretically more indicative of the numbers of sperm that will be required per dose to reach maximum fertility potential than it is of the absolute level of fertility that may be achieved.

Visual, microscopic assessment of sperm motility is the classic measure of semen quality. This procedure is simple, rapid, and inexpensive; however, it is also highly subjective. Visual estimates of motility can be biased and either over- or underestimated as a function of sperm concentration within the sample. Repeatability of visual motility estimates is often marginal, both within and across technicians evaluating the same samples. Similarly, procedural, environmental, and technician variances across laboratories make it difficult to precisely define minimum standards, and it is often necessary for each laboratory to establish independent scales for assessment of sperm motility. Although the actual motility values obtained may be quite different across laboratories, a moderate to high degree of correlation across laboratories should be expected when all are performing to standards.

The computer-assisted semen analyzer (CASA) is a more objective method of sperm motility assessment. In addition to percentage of sperm motility, these systems can provide information related to patterns of sperm motion, including linearity, velocity, and frequency and amplitude of head displacement. Although these systems tend to lend precision and re-peatability to motility estimates, is it arguable as to whether or not correlations with fertility are improved [5,6]. Similar to visual motility assessments, comparison of actual measures of sperm motility across laboratories is of limited value, because of variation in procedures and parameter settings necessary to optimize individual machine performance [7]. In addition to purchasing and operating costs, application of CASA in the domestic animal andrology laboratory is further limited by the inability to distinguish between nonmotile sperm and particulate matter in the extender, which biases estimates of both concentration and motility [7,8].

Acrosomal membrane integrity is another common measure of sperm viability known to be associated with fertility. Numerous live/dead staining procedures are available to facilitate estimations of the "viable" populations of spermatozoa in a semen sample under field conditions, with relatively inexpensive brightfield-microscopy [8]; however, staining and fixation procedures can themselves represent a source of variation in the semen analysis. Use of wet-smears of unfixed bovine spermatozoa evaluated for the presence of absence of the acrosomal ridge, using differential interference contrast microscopy, is a validated alternative to fixation [9]. Similar to CASA analysis of sperm motility, flow cytometric analysis of sperm viability presents an opportunity to increase the precision and repeatability of viability analysis [10,11]; however, as with the CASA, this increased precision comes at considerable expense, with marginal, if any, gain in predictive value, which limits application in commercial andrology laboratories serving domestic livestock species.

Although it is common practice to evaluate viability of cryopreserved semen immediately after thawing, numerous studies indicate that 2 to 4 hours of incubation at 37°C before evaluation significantly improves correlations of both motility and acrosome integrity with fertility [12–14]. The pre-evaluation thermal stress induced by incubation is believed to mimic the stress that may be imposed upon deposition in the fe-male reproductive tract, and thereby facilitates detection of latent sperm damage that is otherwise undetectable immediately post-thaw. Alternatively, exposing sperm to a hypo-osmotic solution before evaluation for presence of membrane swelling is a means to induce stress for detection of latent sperm damage [15], and has demonstrated similar correlations with fertility as other measures of semen quality [16].

Assays of uncompensable semen quality components

As mentioned previously, uncompensable semen quality attributes are those believed to be closely associated with the ability of spermatozoa within a sample to sustain embryo development following fertilization. Therefore, uncompensable traits largely impact the maximum level of fertility that is obtainable from a given semen sample, more than they impact the threshold numbers of sperm required to achieve maximum fertility [2]. Normal sperm morphology is the most routinely measured semen quality attribute that is known to be associated with both embryo quality [17,18] and embryonic survival [3,4].

Assessment of normal sperm morphology is an essential component of the spermiogram, and it is generally accepted that samples should possess ≥70% morphologically normal spermatozoa. This is particularly true with respect to abnormalities associated with sperm head shape, which some laboratories justly argue should not exceed 20% of the sperm in the sample. The underlying sperm defect believed to be more directly responsible for this association between sperm morphology and fertility, however, is the DNA integrity within the condensed sperm head [19,20]. Furthermore, this influence appears to extend beyond the abnormal or misshapen population, in which otherwise normally shaped sperm possess perturbations in chromatin structure [21]. Thus, although morphological defects of the sperm tail and of the acrosomal membrane are largely believed to be compensable defects that can be overcome with sufficient sperm concentration per dose, this does not preclude the possibility that samples with significant numbers of tail and acrosomal defects may also possess abnormal chromatin structure in otherwise normal sperm. On the contrary, the significant correlation among many semen quality attributes suggests that such an association is highly probable. Seldom is the semen sample deficient in a single attribute. When quality deteriorates, as in response to heat stress, multiple viability and morphology defects occur simultaneously [22,23]. Thus, distinguishing which trait among the multitude of sperm defects within a sample is actually responsible for observed fertility responses becomes a daunting task.

Computer automation of sperm morphology analysis holds promise to enhance sensitivity for detection of uncompensable semen quality attributes [24]. Mild acid or heat denaturation before fluorescent staining can now be used to reveal heterogeneity in chromatin structure, and can be quantified using fluorescent microscopy [21] or flow cytometry [20]; however, in addition to equipment expense, these procedures appear to be quite tedious and time/environment-sensitive, which limits their implementation for use in domestic animals. Evaluation of embryo quality distributions following in-vivo [17] or in-vitro [25] fertilization are useful bioassays of sperm competency, but impractical for routine use on a large scale.

Threshold numbers of sperm per dose

Early research related extension rates for bovine semen to be used in AI supported the concept of threshold numbers of sperm per dose, as proposed by Salisbury and VanDemark [1]. These studies typically revealed that as cell numbers per dose were increased, fertility, as measured by nonreturn rates in the female population, responded in a curvilinear fashion [26–28]. These studies also indicated that individual bulls/ejaculates vary in the rate or slope of the fertility response and in the minimum numbers of sperm required to maximum fertility (see Fig. 1). It was apparent that threshold sperm numbers varied depending on semen quality, and were more closely associated with the numbers of "live" or "motile" sperm per dose than with total numbers of sperm per dose. Based on results of the above and other studies of the era, it became generally accepted that bovine AI organizations should target 8 to 10 × 10^6 motile sperm per dose for most bulls, and perhaps as high as 15 × 10^6 motile sperm per dose for bulls of below average semen quality or fertility.

Subsequent to these early studies, considerable commercial advances have been realized in almost all aspects of the AI industry, including, but not limited to, semen processing, extender formulation, freezing rates, package type, microbial control, and semen evaluation. As a result, current cryopreservation procedures not only result in increased percentages of sperm that survive the freeze-thaw process, but have also likely diminished the magnitude of latent cryopreservation injury. It is thereby likely that the inherent functional quality of a sperm that survives today's cryopreservation procedures is much greater than that of sperm surviving cryopreservation technology available 30 to 40 years ago. This concept is supported by more recent dose titration studies that indicate threshold sperm numbers on the order 2.5 to 5 × 10^6 total sperm per AI dose (ie, ~1 to 3 × 10^6 motile sperm; [29–31]). Although a recent global survey of semen-processing practices at major AI organizations [32] reports the average cryopreserved AI dose contains approximately 20 × 10^6 total spermatozoa (range 10 to 40 × 10^6), the previously cited studies imply that these numbers are 2 to 20 times greater than the minimum numbers required. These data also imply that international or veterinary standards that continue to dictate inefficiently high semen dilutions rates ($\geq$8 × 10^6 motile/dose) should be revisited to consider more recent data and technology advances.

The relationship between sperm numbers per dose and fertility is often further biased by the AI center semen-quality control program. Bulls that produce below average or marginal quality semen often achieve below average fertility levels, despite compensatory increases in cell numbers per dose. In contrast, bulls that produce above average semen quality can often maintain above average fertility, even when extended to below average cell numbers per dose. Thus, as opposed to the research setting, an artifact of the AI center quality control program is that the correlation between cell numbers per dose and fertility in the commercial setting is often negative [33,34].

The spermiogram in perspective

The complexity of the above interactions often limits the diagnostic value of a given semen evaluation procedure, particularly with respect to the positive fertility diagnosis. As implied by Amann and Hammerstedt [35], the relationships of semen quality to fertility should be investigated for degrees of "association" rather than for degrees of "correlation." Fertile sperm are those that possess sufficient levels of all known and unknown semen characteristics necessary to achieve fertilization and sustain embryo development; however, semen samples that possess sufficient levels of all known traits must still be considered of questionable fertility, because the sample could be deficient in other traits unknown or unmeasured. Therefore, the accuracy of negative or below average fertility diagnosis will likely always be more accurate than the positive or acceptable diagnosis. Greater accuracy in the positive fertility diagnosis comes by default, through identification and measurement of greater numbers of semen quality attributes that are associated with fertility. Thus researchers should abandon attempts to correlate semen attributes with fertility in lieu of more diagnostic approaches to simply identify the subfertile samples (or sires) that should be removed from the population [35].

Fortunately, many measures of semen quality known to be associated with fertility are highly correlated with each other [13,20]. Selection and screening for one trait typically enriches the retained population for multiple semen quality attributes, whereas screening and discarding collections based on multiple semen quality traits significantly reduces the probability that semen of less than acceptable fertility will be retained. Although multiple-trait regression analysis can sometimes yield quite high correlations with fertility, most of the variation is explained by the first two or three components included in the model, and little additive predictive value is provided by inclusion of additional parameters [6,14]. These correlations also imply, however, that new technologies of semen evaluation must be closely scrutinized for the "additive" predictive value imparted over existing methodologies. What does the newly identified attribute or procedure tell us over and above what we already know? Is it more predictive, or simply a different method to measure the same trait? If the latter, greater accuracy, sensitivity, or more efficient utility of implementation must be demonstrated if wide-scale application is to be expected. Otherwise, the new technology may simply represent a more tedious or expensive method to measure what was already measured, which seems to be the primary hurdle that has limited application of many validated technologies, such as flow cytometry, CASA, and numerous in-vitro fertilization assays of sperm function.

Finally, and perhaps most importantly, attempts to associate semen quality with fertility usually fail to acknowledge that the accuracy or variance of the fertility estimate is typically the limiting factor. The intense screening and culling of ejaculates, along with compensatory increases in cell numbers per dose by AI center quality control programs, tend to minimize variation in the quality of commercial semen released for sale. Additionally, sire fertility estimates are often confounded by the multitude of environmental and herd management factors that are only modestly accounted for in the evaluation model [12,35,36]. Furthermore, most estimates of sire fertility are associated with large confidence intervals as a function of small sample size and the inherent variance associated with a binomial distribution. Therefore it is not surprising that sire fertility estimates produced from the use of commercial semen tend to lack in variation, and that more than 90% of sires are determined to be within ±3% of average fertility and statistically indistinguishable from each other [37]. In reality, methods of evaluating semen quality are likely much more sensitive than our ability to accurately measure fertility within the narrow range represented in the commercial AI population. Our ability to accurately identify and measure novel semen quality attributes associated with fertility will likely reside in our ability to recognize and accept this limitation, and in turn adapt more sensitive experimental models for assessment of sire/semen fertility. To these ends, early insemination models in conjunction with fixed-time AI may magnify differences in sperm longevity that are undetectable in conventional insemination models [2,38]. Similarly, heterospermic insemination has proven to provide an extremely sensitive model to magnify minute differences in semen fertility potential [14], and should be exploited to enhance future research related to components of semen quality.

Summary

The impact of the male or inseminate on reproductive efficiency is the function of a complex series of interactions between numbers of sperm per dose and the ratio and severity of compensable and uncompensable sperm defects in the sample. Because of the correlation among many semen quality traits, screening for one trait often enriches the retained population for multiple attributes; however, these correlations also confound our ability to identify which semen quality attribute is most closely associated with the observed fertility response. Likewise, newly identified semen quality attributes or evaluation procedures must be considered in light of these potential correlations with existing methodologies to determine the additive value over prior technology. These limitations may be largely overcome if semen quality attributes are evaluated with a diagnostic approach to identify subfertile populations not identified using existing technology, rather than attempting to "correlate" results with fertility. Perhaps most importantly, researchers attempting to associate semen quality with fertility must acknowledge that the fertility estimate is typically the least accurate of all measures being considered.

References

[1] Salisbury GW, VanDemark NL. Significance of semen quality. In: Physiology of reproduction and artificial insemination in cattle. 1st edition. San Francisco (CA): WH Freeman and Co.; 1961. p. 359–79.

[2] Saacke RG. AI fertility: are we getting the job done? In: Proceedings of the 17th Technical Conference on Artificial Insemination and Reproduction. Columbia (MO): National Association of Animal Breeders; 1998. p. 6–13.

[3] Kidder HE, Black WG, Wiltbank JN, et al. Fertilization rates and embryonic death rates in cows bred to bulls of different levels of fertility. J Dairy Sci 1954;37:691–7.

[4] Bearden HJ, Hansel WM, Bratton RW. Fertilization and embryonic mortality rates of bulls with histories of either low or high fertility in artificial breeding. J Dairy Sci 1956;39: 312–8.

[5] Budworth PR, Amann RP, Chapman PL. Relationships between computerized measurements of motion of frozen-thawed bull sperm and fertility. J Androl 1988;9:41–54.

[6] Farrell PB, Presicce GA, Brockett CC, et al. Quantification of bull sperm characteristics measured by computer-assisted sperm analysis (CASA) and the relationship to fertility. Theriogenology 1998;49:871–9.

[7] Verstegen J, Iguer-Ouada M, Onclin K. Computer assisted semen analyzers in andrology research and veterinary practice. Theriogenology 2002;57:149–79.

[8] Garner DL. Ancillary test of bull semen quality. Vet Clin North Am Food Anim Practice 1997;13:313–30.

[9] Saacke RG, Marshall CE. Observation on the acrosomal cap of fixed and unfixed bovine spermatozoa. J Reprod Fertil 1968;16:511–4.

[10] Garner DL, Thomas CA, Joerg HW, et al. Fluorometric assessments of mitochondrial function and viability in cryopreserved bovine spermatozoa. Biol Reprod 1997;57: 1401–6.

[11] Thomas CA, Garner DL, DeJarnette JM, et al. Fluorometric assessments of acrosomal integrity and viability in cryopreserved bovine spermatozoa. Biol Reprod 1997; 56:991–8.

[12] Saacke RG, White JM. Semen quality tests and their relationship to fertility. In: Proceedings of the 4th Technical Conference on Artificial Insemination and Reproduction. Columbia (MO): National Association of Animal Breeders; 1972. p. 22–7.

[13] Linford E, Glover FA, Bishop C, et al. The relationship between semen evaluation methods and fertility in the bull. J Reprod Fertil 1976;47:283–91.

[14] Saacke RG, Vinson WE, O'Connor ML, et al. The relationship of semen quality and fertility. In: Proceedings 8th Technical Conference on Artificial Insemination and Reproduction. Columbia (MO): National Association of Animal Breeders; 1980. p. 71–8.

[15] Correa JR, Zavos PM. The hypoosmotic swelling test: its employment as an assay to evaluate the functional integrity of the frozen-thawed bovine sperm membrane. Theriogenology 1994; 42:351–60.

[16] Correa JR, Pace MM, Zavos PM. Relationships among frozen-thawed sperm characteristics assessed via the routine semen analysis, sperm functional tests and fertility of bulls in an artificial insemination program. Theriogenology 1997;48:721–31.

[17] DeJarnette JM, Saacke RG, Bame J, et al. Accessory sperm: their importance to fertility and embryo quality, and attempts to alter their numbers in artificially inseminated cattle. J Anim Sci 1992;70:484–91.

[18] Saacke RG, Nadir S, Dalton J, et al. Accessory sperm evaluation and bull fertility (an update). In: Proceedings of the XV Technical Conference on Artificial Insemination and Reproduction. Columbia (MO): National Association of Animal Breeders; 1994. p. 57–67.

[19] Evenson DP, Darznikiewicz Z, Melamed MR. Relation of mammalian sperm chromatin heterogeneity to fertility. Science 1980;240:1131–4.

[20] Ballachey BE, Evenson DP, Saacke RG. The sperm chromatin structure assay: relationship with alternate tests of semen quality and heterospermic performance of bulls. J Androl 1988; 9:109–15.

[21] Acevedo N, Bame J, Kuehn LA, et al. Effects of elevated testicular temperature on spermatozoal morphology and chromatin stability to acid denaturation in the bovine [abstract]. Biol Reprod 2001;64(Suppl 1):217–8.

[22] Vogler CJ, Saacke RG, Bame JH, et al. Effects of scrotal insulation on viability characteristics of cyropreserved semen. J Dairy Sci 1991;74:3827–35.

[23] Vogler CJ, Bame JH, DeJarnette JM, et al. Effects of elevated testicular temperature on morphology characteristics of ejaculated spermatozoa in the bovine. Theriogenology 1993; 40:1207–19.

[24] Parrish JJ, Ostermeier GC, Pace MM. Fourier harmonic analysis of sperm morphology. In: Proceedings of the 17th Technical Conference on Artificial Insemination and Reproduction. Columbia (MO): National Association of Animal Breeders; 1998. p. 25–31.

[25] Zhang BR, Larsson B, Lundeheim N, et al. Relationship between embryo development in vitro and 56-day nonreturn rates of cows inseminated with frozen-thawed semen from dairy bulls. Theriogenology 1997;48:221–31.

[26] Willett EL, Larson GL. Fertility of bull semen as influenced by dilution level, antibiotics, spermatozoan numbers and the interaction of these factors. J Dairy Sci 1952;35:899.

[27] Sullivan JJ, Elliott FI. Bull fertility as affected by an interaction between motile spermatozoa concentration and fertility level in artificial insemination. In: Proceedings of the VI International Congress on Animal Reproduction and Artificial Insemination. Paris: Internationl Congress on Animal Reproduction and Artificial Insemination; 1968. p. 1307.

[28] Sullivan JJ. Sperm numbers required for optimum breeding efficiency in cattle. In: Proceedings of the III Techical Conference on Artificial Insemination and Reproduction. Columbia (MO): National Association of Animal Breeders; 1970. p. 36–43.

[29] Filseth O, Komisrud K, Graffer T. Effect of dilution rate on fertility of frozen bovine semen. In: Proceedings of the XII International Congress on Reproduction and Artificial Insemination. Hague: International Congress on Animal Reproduction and Artificial Insemination; 1992. p. 1409–11.

[30] van Giessen RC, Zuidberg CA, Wilmink W, et al. Optimum use of a bull with high genetics. In: Proceedings of the XII International Congress on Animal Reproduction and Artificial Insemination. Hague: International Congress on Animal Reproduction and Artificial Insemination; 1992. p. 1493.

[31] den Daas JHG, de Jong G, Lansbergen LMTE, et al. The relationship between the number of spermatozoa inseminated and the reproductive efficiency of individual dairy bulls. J Dairy Sci 1998;81:1714–23.

[32] Vishwanath R. Artificial insemination: the state of the art. Theriogenology 2003;59: 571–84.

[33] DeJarnette JM. Interactive effects of semen quantity, semen quality and insemination techniques on conception rates of artificially inseminated cattle. In: Jordan ER, editor. Proceedings National Reproduction Symposium. Sponsored by USDA-Extension Service in cooperation with the Texas Agricultural Extension Service and the American Association of Bovine Practitioners. Pittsburg, PA, September 22–23, 1994. p. 139–50.

[34] DeJarnette JM. Industry application of technology in male reproduction. In: Funston RL, Myers TL, editors. Proceedings Applied Reproductive Strategies in Beef Cattle. North Platte, NE, September 1–2, 2004. North Central Region Bovine Reproduction Task Force. p. 201–17.

[35] Amann RP, Hammerstedt RH. In vitro evaluation of semen quality: an opinion. J Androl 1993;14:397–406.

[36] Foote RH. Fertility estimation: a review of past experience and future prospects. Anim Reprod Sci 2003;75:119–39.

[37] Clay JS, McDaniel BT. Computing mating bull fertility from DHI nonreturn data. J Dairy Sci 2001;84:1238–45.

[38] Macmillan KL, Watson JD. Fertility differences between groups of sires relative to the stage of oestrus at the time of insemination. Anim Prod 1975;21:243–9.

ELSEVIER
SAUNDERS

VETERINARY
CLINICS
Food Animal Practice

Vet Clin Food Anim 21 (2005) 419–436

Potential Applications and Pitfalls of Reproductive Ultrasonography in Bovine Practice

Paul M. Fricke, PhD[a],*, G. Cliff Lamb, PhD[b]

[a]*Department of Dairy Science, University of Wisconsin, 1675 Observatory Drive, Madison, WI 53706-1284, USA*
[b]*North Central Research and Outreach Center, University of Minnesota, 1861 Highway 169E, Grand Rapids, MN 55744, USA*

In 1986, O.J. Ginther stated that "gray-scale diagnostic ultrasonography is the most profound technological advance in the field of large animal research and clinical reproduction since the introduction of transrectal palpation and radioimmunoassay of circulating hormones" [1]. From a research standpoint, it is hard to imagine that many of the discoveries and procedures related to ovarian, uterine, and fetal function in cattle that we apply today would have been possible without the application of real-time, brightness modality (B-mode) ultrasonography to the study of reproductive function. Transition of ultrasound technology from a specialized research tool to a practical tool for managing reproduction on dairy and beef operations has already begun. Early integration of ultrasound technology to the cattle industry included applications such as transvaginal follicular aspiration and oocyte recovery [2–4], and as a complementary technology for embryo transfer procedures. These applications, however, are specialized and will not likely constitute widespread use of ultrasound technology. The purpose of this article is to examine practical applications of ultrasound to the dairy and beef industries that may cause widespread implementation of this technology in the future.

Detailed information on the principles of ultrasonography is beyond the scope of this article and has been reviewed elsewhere [4]. In general, linear-array, real-time, B-mode ultrasound scanners are best suited for veterinary applications involving dairy cattle reproduction. Most ultrasound machines

---

* Corresponding author.
E-mail address: pmfricke@wisc.edu (P.M. Fricke).

consist of a console unit that contains the electronics, controls, and a screen upon which the ultrasound image is visualized by the operator; and a transducer, which emits and receives high-frequency ultrasound waves. Linear-array transducers consist of a series of piezoelectric crystals arranged in a row. These crystals emit high-frequency sound waves on being energized. The configuration of a linear-array transducer results in a rectangular image on the field of scan (as opposed to the pie-shaped image produced by a sector transducer). Currently, a veterinary-grade ultrasound machine equipped with one rectal transducer can be purchased for $8,000 to $16,000. Image quality varies widely among veterinary-grade ultrasound machines, and generally increases with the cost of the unit. More expensive machines are available, but are not necessary for routine reproductive examinations.

Bovine reproductive organs are most commonly scanned per rectum, using a linear-array transducer specifically manufactured for transrectal use; however, specialized applications, including ovum pickup and follicle ablation, involve a transvaginal approach using a sector transducer. Linear-array transducers of 5.0 and 7.5 MHz frequency ranges are most commonly used in cattle to perform reproductive ultrasound examinations, and most veterinary ultrasound scanners are compatible with probes of different frequencies. Depth of tissue penetration of sound waves and image resolution is dependent on and inversely related to the frequency of the transducer. Thus, a 5.0 MHz transducer results in greater depth of tissue penetration and lesser image detail, whereas a 7.5 MHz transducer results in lesser depth of tissue penetration and greater image detail. An ultrasound scanner equipped with a 5.0 MHz transducer is most useful for bovine practitioners conducting routine reproductive examinations; however, small ovarian structures such as developing follicles' are best imaged with a 7.5 MHz transducer. Nonreproductive applications of ultrasound, such as evaluation of carcass traits in live cattle, employ a 3.5 MHz probe.

From a practical standpoint, many bovine practitioners have struggled with the decision to incorporate ultrasound technology into their practice. Although some have embraced ultrasound technology as a reproductive management tool, many remain skeptical about the practical implementation and economic benefits of reproductive ultrasound for their practices or their clients. Transrectal palpation is the oldest and most widespread method for assessment of the female reproductive tract in vivo and for early pregnancy diagnosis in cattle [5]. Two events must transpire before the decision to replace transrectal palpation with transrectal ultrasound as the method of choice for female reproductive ultrasound examinations is made. First, transrectal ultrasonography must be proven to exceed transrectal palpation in accuracy or in the ability to gather information with which to implement management decisions. Thus, the first section of this article reviews several practical reproductive applications for transrectal ultrasonography. Second, transrectal ultrasonography must be practically integrated into a systematic, on-farm reproductive management strategy in the beef and dairy industries, and these management schemes must empirically be demonstrated to exceed the status quo of the industry (ie, transrectal palpation) in reproductive performance and economic returns. Thus, the second section of this article reviews implementation strategies for use of transrectal ultrasonography in dairy and beef production systems.

Practical applications of ultrasonography for beef and dairy cattle

Pregnancy diagnosis

Diagnosis of nonpregnancy early post-breeding can improve reproductive performance in beef and dairy operations by decreasing the interval between successive artificial insemination (AI) services, and by coupling a non-pregnancy diagnosis with an aggressive strategy to rapidly and efficiently rebreed these animals [6]. Reports have indicated the detection of an embryonic vesicle in cattle as early as 9 [7], 10 [8], or 12 days [9] of gestation. In these situations, the exact date of insemination was known, and ultrasonography was simply used as a confirmation of pregnancy or to validate that detection of an embryo was possible within the first 2 weeks of pregnancy. By contrast, Kastelic and Ginther [10] monitored pregnancy in pregnant and nonpregnant yearling heifers that had been inseminated. Diagnosis of pregnancy in heifers on day 10 through day 16 of gestation resulted in a positive diagnosis for pregnant or nonpregnant of less than 50%. On days 18, 20, and 22 of gestation, accuracy of pregnancy diagnosis improved to 85%, 100%, and 100%, respectively. Although evidence of a pregnancy via ultrasound during days 18 to 22 of gestation yields excellent results, a technician needs to ensure that confusion between fluid accumulation in the chorioallantois during early pregnancy [10] and uterine fluid within the uterus during proestrus and estrus are not confused when making the diagnosis.

Several further reports [11–14] also indicate the presence of an embryonic vesicle as early as day 25 of gestation. Although Hanzen and Delsaux [12] used a 3.0 MHz transducer for pregnancy diagnosis, they concluded that by day 40 of gestation, a positive diagnosis of pregnancy was 100% accurate, whereas overall diagnosis of pregnancy and absence of pregnancy from day 25 of gestation proved to be correct in 94% and 90% of cases, respectively. In 148 dairy cows, pregnancy diagnosis from day 21 to day 25 was 65% accurate, whereas diagnosis of pregnancy from day 26 to day 33 was 93% accurate [13]. In their conclusions, the authors state that probable causes of misdiagnosis from day 21 to day 26 were either an accumulation of proestrus or estrus uterine fluid, or the accumulation of pathological fluid in the uterus, or cows were diagnosed pregnant but experienced early embryonic loss.

Although the authors have indicated that an embryonic vesicle is detectable by ultrasound as early as 9 days of gestation, accuracy of detection approaches 100% after day 25 of gestation. For practical purposes, the efficiency (ie, speed and accuracy) of a correct diagnosis of pregnancy should be performed in females that are at least 26 days post-breeding. This information can be used to determine the age of bovine fetuses with a high degree of accuracy [4,7,9]. Crown-rump length measurements were summarized by Hughes and Davies (Table 1) [15]. There was a significant correlation (r = 0.98) between embryo age and crown-rump length.

Identification of cows carrying twin fetuses

In dairy cattle, twinning is an unavoidable outcome of reproduction, and is undesirable because it reduces overall dairy farm profitability and reproductive efficiency [16,17]. By contrast, under certain beef cattle production systems, twinning may be considered a desirable trait that can enhance the overall profitability of the production enterprise by increasing weaned calf weight produced per cow in the herd [18,19]. In either case, it is desirable to know which females are carrying twins, so that management can be tailored to enhance survival of the calves and minimize problems during the periparturient period.

Cows carrying twin fetuses can be accurately identified using transrectal ultrasonography by 40 to 55 days post-AI [19–21]. Because the majority of twinning in dairy cattle occurs due to multiple ovulations [22,23], the presence of two or more corpus luteum (CL) on the ovaries at the time of pregnancy diagnosis is an excellent indicator of cows with an increased risk for twinning. Overall, the incidence of double ovulation in lactating dairy cows after synchronization of ovulation using the Ovsynch protocol was 14.1% [24], and the frequency of double ovulation was nearly threefold greater for cows with greater-than-average milk production near the time of AI than for cows with less-than-average milk production near the time of AI [25].

In dairy production systems, several management scenarios can be considered upon identification of a cow carrying twins, including culling,

Table 1
Fetal crown-rump length in relation to age in weeks

| Fetal age (wk) | No. of observations | Crown-rump length (mm) | | |
		Minimum	Maximum	Mean
4	25	6	11	8.9
5	35	8	19	12.8
6	50	16	26	20.2
7	47	23	36	27.7
8	41	36	52	45.5
9	48	39	71	62.4
10	43	61	101	87.4
11	39	95	118	106.5
12	32	107	137	121.8

Data from Hughes EA, Davies DAR. Practical uses of ultrasound in early pregnancy in cattle. Vet Rec 1989;124:45.

abortion and rebreeding, or continued management until parturition [26]. Continued management of the cow can be avoided either by culling the cow or by aborting the twin pregnancy, usually through administration of an luteolytic agent such as postglandin $F_{2\alpha}$ ($PGF_{2\alpha}$). Several factors argue against aborting a twin pregnancy with the intent of rebreeding the cow, however. First, although the calving interval would vary widely among cows subjected to abortion, the estimated average calving interval of cows subjected to induced abortion and rebreeding exceeds 500 days ($\sim$18 months), based on average reproductive performance and management indices for lactating cows [26]. Second, cows calving twins are at greater risk for subsequent twinning [27]. Third, establishing pregnancy in lactating dairy cows is difficult, and a pregnancy represents an inherent value to the dairy farm that is forfeited by electively aborting the pregnancy. Finally, cows carrying twins experience greater rates of early embryonic loss than cows carrying singles, and on occasion lose one fetus while maintaining the other [28]. Elective abortion of a twin pregnancy early during gestation that may result in the birth of a single calf at parturition is not a sound management practice. Based on these considerations and depending on the value of the dam and calf, culling to avoid continued management of a cow carrying twins is a better alternative to aborting the pregnancy. At present, information on twinning management in dairy cattle is inadequate, and further research is needed to make sound management decisions regarding twinning [26].

Assessment of fetal sex

Transrectal ultrasound can be used to detect the sex of bovine fetuses in utero. Sex is determined by evaluating the morphology and location of the genital tubercle using ultrasound, and is a reliable and accurate method for sex determination beginning on day 55 to 60 of gestation [29,30]. Attempts to determine fetal sex earlier can be inaccurate due to incomplete migration of the genital tubercle. Fetuses at 48 to 119 days of age have been successfully sexed [30–33]. The procedure is reliable, and accuracy has ranged from 92% to 100% [31–33]. Beal et al [33] noted that of 85 fetuses predicted to be male, 84 were confirmed correct, resulting in 99% accuracy. In addition, of 101 fetuses predicted to be female, 98 were confirmed correct, resulting in 97% accuracy. Recently, Lamb [34] determined the sex of 112 fetuses in Angus heifers with 100% accuracy.

For optimal fetal sexing results, the ultrasound transducer should be manipulated to produce a frontal, cross-sectional, or sagittal image of the ventral body surface of the fetus. In larger-framed cows (ie, Holsteins and continental beef breeds) or older cows, the optimum window for fetal sexing usually is between day 55 and 70 of gestation, whereas for smaller-framed cows (Jerseys and English beef breeds) the ideal window usually is between day 55 and 80 of gestation. There are two limitations that can inhibit the ability of a technician to determine the sex of a fetus: (1) as the fetus increases in size, it becomes more difficult to move the transducer relative to the fetus in order to obtain the desired image; and (2) the gravid horn is more likely to descend ventrally into the abdominal cavity in larger or older cows, making fetal sexing virtually impossible without retracting the gravid horn.

Fetal sexing is an important application in beef production systems (see the beef application section below). In production dairy systems, determination of fetal sex is useful when combined with a management decision or strategy that justifies the expense of fetal sexing [6]. In other words, a dairy producer who pays for information regarding fetal sex must economically justify the usefulness of that information. Fulfilling sales contract obligations regarding the sex of a calf carried by a pregnant cow to be sold is one scenario that may justify this expense. If the sex of a calf is a determining factor for culling decisions regarding a pregnant cow, fetal sexing might also be justified. By contrast, the cost associated with fetal sexing is unwarranted if the information is not used to make a management decision. Because of the economic and management considerations associated with fetal sexing, routine fetal sexing of all pregnant cows in a herd will not likely become a standard reproductive management practice, unless bovine practitioners choose to conduct fetal sexing at little or no additional expense beyond pregnancy diagnosis.

Assessment of embryonic mortality

Before use of ultrasound for pregnancy diagnosis in cattle, practitioners were unable to accurately determine the viability or number of embryos or fetuses. Because the heartbeat of a fetus can be detected at approximately 22 days of age, fetal viability can accurately be assessed. Studies in beef [33,35,36] and dairy [24,37–39] cattle have used ultrasound to assess the incidence of embryonic loss. The number of fetuses can most accurately be assessed at between 49 and 55 days of gestation [20].

Table 2 summarizes the incidence of embryonic loss by study in beef and dairy females. The fertilization rate after artificial insemination in beef cows is 90%, whereas embryonic survival rate is 93% by day 8 and only 56% by day 12 post-AI [35]. The incidence of embryonic loss in beef cattle appears to be significantly less than in dairy cattle. Beal and coauthors [33] report a 6.5% incidence of embryonic loss in beef cows from day 25 of gestation to day 45. Similarly, Lamb and coworkers [36] noted a 4.2% incidence of embryonic loss in beef heifers initially ultrasounded at day 30 of gestation, and subsequently palpated rectally at between day 60 and 90 after insemination. More recent reports [40–42] involving considerably greater numbers of beef cows or heifers indicate that embryonic mortality ranged from 2.7% to 10.8% between 30 and 90 days of gestation.

In lactating dairy cows, pregnancy loss from 28 to 56 days after AI was 13.5%, or 0.5% per day [24]. This rate of pregnancy loss is similar to the 12.4% reported by Smith and Stevenson [37] and the 19.1% reported by

Table 2
Incidence of embryonic/fetal loss in cows after an initial diagnosis of pregnancy by ultrasound, followed by a second diagnosis prior to or at calving

Subjects	Reference	No. pregnant (days of gestation)	No. pregnant (days of gestation)	No. of embryos lost	Embryonic mortality (%)
Beef cattle					
Cows	[33]	138 (25)	129 (45)	9	6.5
		129 (45)	127 (65)	2	1.5
		138 (25)	127 (65)	11	8.0
Cows	[40]	989 (30–35)	955 (80–100)	34	3.4
Heifers	[36]	149 (30)	143 (60)	6	4.0
		271 (35)	260 (75)	11	4.1
		105 (30)	100 (90)	5	4.8
Cows	[41]	701 (30–35)	682 (80–100)	19	2.7
Heifers	[42]	223 (29–33)	199 (54–60)	24	10.8
Dairy cattle					
Cows and heifers	[37]	129 (28–30)	113 (40–54)	16	12.4
Cows	[38]	488 (28)	437 (42)	51	10.5
		437 (42)	409 (56)	28	6.3
		409 (56)	402 (70)	7	1.7
		402 (56)	395 (70)	7	1.7
		488 (28)	395 (98)	93	19.1
Cows	[24]	89 (28)	77 (56)	12	13.5
Cows	[39]	64 (26–58)	52 (Full term)	12	8.6

Vasconcelos and associates [38] during a comparable stage of pregnancy in lactating dairy cows. The greatest occurrences of pregnancy loss were between days 28 and 42 of gestation (10.5%) and between days 42 and 56 of gestation (6.3%). After day 56 of pregnancy, embryonic losses were reduced to 3.4% from 56 to 98 days of pregnancy, and 5.5% from 98 days to calving [38]. Interestingly, the rate of embryonic loss in dairy heifers of 5% to 10% [37,43] is lower than that of lactating cows, and in the range of reported rates for beef cows These studies indicate the usefulness of ultrasonography as a tool to monitor the success of a breeding program by determining pregnancy rates and embryonic survival.

Implementation of ultrasound for reproductive management: dairy cattle

Synergy between new reproductive management technologies holds the key to maximizing reproductive efficiency on dairy farms; however, reproductive management protocols that allow for synchronization of estrus or ovulation and subsequent identification and resynchronization of nonpregnant cows must be practical to implement within the day-to-day operation of a dairy farm, or the protocol will fail because of lack of compliance [44]. This is especially true for larger farms that must schedule and administer AI, hormone injections, and pregnancy tests for a large number of animals on a daily or weekly basis. Identification of nonpregnant cows early post-breeding can only improve reproductive efficiency when coupled with a management strategy to rapidly submit nonpregnant cows for a subsequent AI service. Thus, pregnancy diagnosis using ultrasound must be integrated as a component of the overall reproductive management strategy in place on the farm. The various component technologies of the reproductive management system will in turn determine the timing of the events as they occur on a daily or weekly basis. As stated previously, it has long been accepted that pregnancy status should be determined in dairy cattle as soon as possible after insemination, but without having the diagnosis confounded by subsequent embryonic mortality [45,46]. New research on the practical implementation of early pregnancy diagnosis, using transrectal ultrasonography into a systematic synchronization and resynchronization system, has confirmed this notion, and has illustrated the pitfalls and limitations of early pregnancy diagnosis using transrectal ultrasound [44].

As a pregnancy diagnosis method, transrectal ultrasonography is both accurate and rapid [47], while providing more information at each examination than transrectal palpation; however, because many experienced dairy practitioners can accurately diagnose pregnancy as early as 35 days post-breeding using transrectal palpation, pregnancy examination using transrectal ultrasonography at 26 to 28 days post-breeding only reduces the interval from insemination to pregnancy diagnosis by 7 to 9 days. The rate of embryonic mortality and the efficacy of strategies to rebreed cows at various stages post-breeding also play a role in determining the advantages and disadvantages on the timing of pregnancy diagnosis and resynchronization for dairy systems [44]. Research is needed to clarify these issues and economically assess the decision to displace transrectal palpation with transrectal ultrasonography.

Embryonic mortality diminishes the benefit of early pregnancy diagnosis in two ways. First, because of the high rate of embryonic mortality that occurs around the time during gestation that early diagnosis with ultrasound is performed, the magnitude of pregnancy loss detected is greater the earlier post-breeding that a positive diagnosis is made. Thus, the earlier that pregnancy is diagnosed post-breeding, the fewer nonpregnant cows are identified to which a management strategy can be implemented to rebreed them. Second, and more important, cows diagnosed pregnant earlier post-breeding have a greater risk for embryonic mortality compared with cows diagnosed later post-breeding. If left unidentified, cows diagnosed pregnant early post-breeding and that subsequently loose that pregnancy reduce reproductive efficiency by extending the interval from calving to the conception that results in a full-term pregnancy.

To compensate for embryonic mortality, cows diagnosed pregnant early post-breeding must undergo one or more subsequent pregnancy examinations to identify and rebreed those that experience embryonic mortality. This applies to all methods for early pregnancy diagnosis, including transrectal palpation, conducted before the rate of embryonic mortality decreases at around 70 days in gestation [38]. Thus, implementation of early pregnancy diagnoses must consider the timing and frequency of subsequent pregnancy examinations to maintain the reproductive performance of the herd. Problems caused by embryonic mortality apply to all currently available methods for assessing pregnancy status early post-breeding, and may make pregnancy testing before 30 to 40 days post-breeding an untenable management strategy, unless pregnancy diagnoses can be made continually on a daily basis or at each milking, until the rate of embryonic mortality decreases or until the underlying causes of embryonic mortality are understood and mitigated.

Coupling systematic synchronization with transrectal ultrasonography

Two currently available technologies for reproductive management include hormonal protocols such as Ovsynch [48,49] and Presynch/Ovsynch [50,51] that synchronize ovulation and allow for timed artificial insemination (TAI), and use of transrectal ultrasonography for early identification of nonpregnant cows [6]. A field trial was conducted to compare three intervals from first TAI to resynchronization of ovulation at a dairy incorporating transrectal ultrasonography as a direct method for early pregnancy diagnosis [44]. The objective of this study was to compare fertility to first TAI service with fertility after resynchronization of ovulation using Ovsynch at three intervals after TAI (Resynch protocol), coupled with pregnancy diagnosis using transrectal ultrasonography (Fig. 1). Lactating dairy cows on a commercial dairy farm were enrolled into this study on a weekly basis. All cows received a Presynch/Ovsynch protocol to receive first postpartum TAI as follows: 25 mg $PGF_{2\alpha}$ (day 32 ± 3; day 46 ± 3); 50 μg gonadotropin-releasingt hormone [GnRH] (day 60 ± 3); 25 mg $PGF_{2\alpha}$ (day 67 ± 3); and 50 μg GnRH (day 69 ± 3) postpartum [51]. All cows received TAI immediately after the second GnRH injection of the Presynch protocol (day 0) as per a Cosynch TAI schedule. At first TAI, cows were randomly assigned to one of three treatment groups for resynchronization of ovulation (Resynch) using Ovsynch (50 μg GnRH [day 9]; 25 mg $PGF_{2\alpha}$ [day 2] and 50 μg GnRH + TAI [day 0]) to induce a second TAI for cows failing to conceive to first TAI service. All cows (n = 235) in the first group (day 19) received a GnRH injection on day 19 post-TAI, and continued the Ovsynch protocol if diagnosed nonpregnant using transrectal ultrasound on day 26 post-TAI. Cows (n = 240) in the second group (day 26) and cows (n = 236) in the third (day 33) group initiated the Ovsynch protocol if diagnosed nonpregnant using transrectal ultrasound on day 26 post-TAI or day 33 post-TAI, respectively.

Submission of cows for first postpartum TAI service was scheduled so that the first four injections of the Presynch plus Ovsynch protocol occurred on Tuesdays, followed by the second GnRH injection and TAI occurring on Thursdays (Table 3) (see Fig. 1). Initiation times for Resynch for each of the

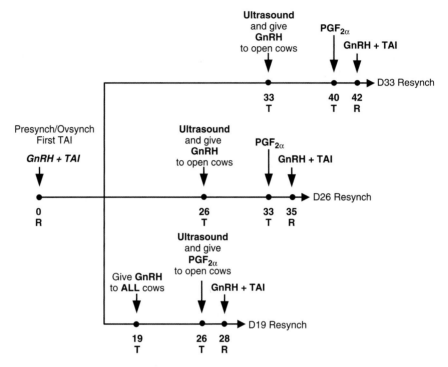

Fig. 1. Diagram of resynchronization treatment groups. Pregnancy rate per artificial insemination (PR/AI) and embryonic mortality from first pregnancy evaluation to a second reconfirmation were evaluated to determine the best method for integration of early pregnancy diagnosis using transrectal ultrasonography. (*Data from* Fricke PM, Caraviello DC, Weigel KA, et al. Fertility of dairy cows after resynchronization of ovulation at three intervals after first timed insemination. J Dairy Sci 2003;86:3941–50.)

three treatment groups in this study were chosen to occur on Tuesdays, so that injection schedules would remain consistent for all cows assigned to weekly breeding groups at any given time. To adhere to the Tuesday/ Thursday schedule, all pregnancy examinations were conducted on Tuesdays. To fit the reproductive management system, the first pregnancy examination using transrectal ultrasound was conducted 26 days after TAI for the day 19 and day 26 cows, and 33 days after TAI for the day 33 cows (see Fig. 1). Thus, the reproductive management systems assessed in this trial allow for administration of all hormone injections, Ovsynch and Resynch TAI services, and for pregnancy examinations to be restricted regularly to either Tuesdays or Thursdays (see Table 3).

Implicit to the experimental design, first assessment of pregnancy status was not conducted at the same interval after the Ovsynch TAI among the three treatment groups (see Fig. 1). Pregnancy status after the Ovsynch TAI was first assessed 26 days after TAI for cows in the day 19 and day 26 groups, whereas pregnancy status was assessed 33 days post-Ovsynch TAI for

Table 3
One possible schedule for administering hormone injections, timed artificial insemination, and pregnancy diagnosis using transrectal ultrasonography for the Presynch/Ovsynch protocol for first timed artificial insemination and Resynchronization for second timed artificial insemination

Sunday	Monday	Tuesday	Wednesday	Thursday	Friday	Saturday
Week 1		PGF				
Week 2						
Week 3		PGF				
Week 4						
Week 5		GnRH				
Week 6		PGF		GnRH + TAI		
Week 7						
Week 8						
Week 9						
Week 10		GnRH				
Week 11		PG + PGF		GnRH + TAI		

All hormone injection, TAI, and pregnancy examinations are restricted to 2 days per week.
Abbreviations: PG, pregnancy diagnosis using transrectal ultrasonography.
Adapted from Fricke PM, Caraviello DC, Weigel KA, et al. Fertility of dairy cows after resynchronization of ovulation at three intervals after first timed insemination. J Dairy Sci 2003;86:3941–50.

cows in the day 33 group. Overall pregnancy rater per artificial insemination (PR/AI) to Ovsynch was 40%, and was greater for day 19 and day 26 cows than for day 33 cows (Table 4). This difference is likely due to a greater period in which embryonic mortality can occur in the day 33 cows, because of the increased interval from TAI to pregnancy diagnosis (26 versus 33 days). When pregnancy status was reassessed for all treatment groups at 68 days after Ovsynch TAI, overall PR/AI to Ovsynch was 31%, and did not differ among treatments (see Table 4). Thus, differences in PR/AI at the first pregnancy examination and pregnancy losses between the first and second pregnancy examinations among treatment groups likely represent an artifact of time of assessment of pregnancy status after TAI inherent to the experimental design, rather than to treatment differences. Overall PR/AI to Resynch was 32%, and was greater for day 26 and day 33 cows than for day 19 cows (Table 5).

Data from Tables 4 and 5 illustrate the limitations of integrating early pregnancy diagnosis into a reproductive management program. First, the system with the most aggressive early nonpregnancy diagnosis and resynchronization schedule (ie, the day 19 treatment) was not a viable management strategy, based on the poor fertility after the Resynch TAI (see Table 5), which was probably due to follicular and luteal dynamics at the stage post-breeding that the synchronization protocol was initiated. Furthermore, these results indicate the counterintuitive notion that delaying pregnancy diagnosis from 26 to 33 days post-TAI may improve reproductive efficiency when using a hormonal protocol for timed AI to program

Table 4
Pregnancy rate per artificial insemination and pregnancy loss after timed artificial insemination to Ovsynch

Item	Treatment group			Overall
	D19	D26	D33	
Interval from Ovsynch TAI to 1st pregnancy exam (d)	26	26	33	—
PR/AI at 1st pregnancy exam, %	46[a]	42[a]	33[b]	40
(n/n)	(108/235)	(101/240)	(77/236)	(286/711)
Interval from Ovsynch TAI to 2nd pregnancy exam (d)	68	68	68	—
PR/AI at 2nd pregnancy exam, %	33	30	29	31
(n/n)	(78/235)	(73/240)	(68/236)	(219/711)
Interval between pregnancy exams (d)	42	42	35	—
Pregnancy loss, %	28[a]	28[a]	12[b]	23
(n/n)	(30/108)	(28/101)	(9/77)	(67/286)

Abbreviations: D, day; PR/AI, pregnancy rate per artificial insemination; TAI, timed artificial insemination.

[a,b] Within a row, percentages with different superscripts differ ($P < 0.01$) among treatment groups.

Adapted from Fricke PM, Caraviello DC, Weigel KA, et al. Fertility of dairy cows after resynchronization of ovulation at three intervals after first timed insemination. J Dairy Sci 2003;86:3945.

nonpregnant cows for rebreeding, due to the high rate of embryonic mortality occurring in cows diagnosed pregnant at 26 versus 33 days post TAI (see Table 4). Further research is needed to develop and optimize strategies for integrating ultrasound into a synchronization and resynchronization system for managing reproduction in lactating dairy cows.

Table 5
Pregnancy rate per artificial insemination after timed artificial insemination to Resynch beginning 19, 26, or 33 days after first timed artificial insemination

Item	Treatment group			Overall
	D19	D26	D33	
Mean ($\pm$ SEM) interval (d) from Resynch TAI to pregnancy exam	27.1 $\pm$ 0.4	26.6 $\pm$ 0.2	33.7 $\pm$ 0.4	—
(range)	(26–54)	(26–40)	(26–75)	
PR/AI, %	23[a]	34[b]	38[b]	32
(n/n)	(28/120)	(41/121)	(54/143)	(123/384)

Abbreviations: D, day; PR/AI, pregnancy rate per artificial insemination; TAI, timed artificial insemination.

[a,b] Within a row, percentages with different superscripts differ ($P < 0.01$) among treatment groups.

Adapted from Fricke PM, Caraviello DC, Weigel KA, et al. Fertility of dairy cows after resynchronization of ovulation at three intervals after first timed insemination. J Dairy Sci 2003;86:3946.

Implementation of ultrasound for reproductive management: beef cattle

Development and rearing of beef cattle involves decisions that impact future production of beef operations. The physiology of reproduction of heifers is critical to the success or failure of the development of genetically superior herd replacements. The majority of factors related to reproductive performance in beef cattle are influenced largely by management, because most components of fertility that influence calving and subsequent reproductive performance are not highly heritable. Use of reproductive technologies such as ultrasonography enables producers to improve breeding performance of heifers during the first breeding season, and during subsequent calving, lactation, and rebreeding. In addition, strategic use of reproductive ultrasound can enhance the overall productivity of the herd. Because of the seasonal nature of the beef industry, the use of ultrasound for reproductive management purposes tends to be concentrated during various stages of the production cycle; however, the extensive nature of the industry also poses cattle-handling issues that tend not to be a factor in dairy operations.

Beef heifers that calve earlier during their first breeding season have greater lifetime calf production than those that calve late [52]. Development of heifers to first calving also affects subsequent breeding and calving performance. Despite these known effects, most beef producers fail to use reproductive management procedures that are known to have significant impact on reproductive performance and overall lifetime productivity. For example, fewer than 30% of beef producers use pregnancy diagnosis, and fewer than 2% of beef producers use some form of reproductive tract scoring. As producers and veterinarians continue to identify and use reproductive ultrasound in beef operations, a few aspects of beef production systems appear to be key areas of emphasis that are improved through the use of ultrasound: (1) reproductive tract scoring (RTS), (2) early pregnancy diagnosis, and (3) fetal sex determination.

RTS is a practical system developed to estimate pubertal status (Table 6) [53]. Scores are subjective estimates of sexual maturity, based on ovarian follicular/corpus luteum development and size of the uterus. An RTS of 1 is assigned to heifers with infantile tracts, as indicated by small, toneless uterine horns and small ovaries without any significant structures. These heifers are likely furthest from puberty. Heifers scored with an RTS of 2 are thought to be closer to puberty than those scoring a 1, due to the larger uterine diameter and larger ovaries. Those heifers with an RTS of 3 are thought to be on the verge of estrous cyclicity, based on uterine tone and palpable follicles. Based on uterine diameter and tone plus the presence of an ovulatory follicle, heifers with an RTS of 4 are considered to be estrous cycling. Heifers with an RTS of 5 are similar to those scoring a 4, except for the presence of a corpus luteum (see Table 6). The use of a 5.0 or 7.5 MHz transrectal transducer is sufficient to locate and identify ovarian structures in the RTS system, plus provide a suitable cross-sectional view of the uterus

Table 6
Reproductive tract scores

RTS	Uterine horns	Ovarian length (mm)	Ovarian height (mm)	Ovarian width (mm)	Ovarian structures
1	Immature, <20 mm diameter, no tone	15	10	8	No follicles >6 mm
2	20–25 mm diameter, no tone	18	12	10	8 mm follicles
3	20–25 mm diameter, slight tone	22	15	10	8–10 mm follicles
4	30 mm diameter, good tone	30	16	12	10 mm follicles, CL possible
5	>30 mm diameter	>32	20	15	CL present

Abbreviations: CL, corpus luteum; RTS, reproductive tract score.
Adapted from Anderson KJ, Lefever DG, Brinks JS, et al. The use of reproductive tract scoring in beef heifers. Agri-Practice 1991;12(4):125.

for measurement. Ultrasound provides a more accurate assessment of ovarian structures and uterine diameter than normal rectal palpation.

A prebreeding examination that includes the RTS, usually performed between 45 and 60 days before the breeding season, furnishes the veterinarian with the opportunity to assess reproductive development of the replacement heifers. With this information, a total herd appraisal of the cycling status and identification of aberrant situations can be done. When performed in a timely fashion, recommendations can be made to ensure that a sufficient number of heifers (greater than 50% receiving an RTS of 4 or 5) are cycling at the initiation of the breeding season.

Early pregnancy diagnosis in beef operations is becoming an increasingly important management practice. Pregnancy diagnosis at 25 to 30 days after insemination provides a tool for many seedstock producers and an increasing proportion of commercial cattlemen to identify AI-impregnated versus cleanup bull-sired calves. Seedstock producers rely on accurate determination of sires and dams of offspring. Therefore, in an AI program or an embryo-transfer program, early pregnancy diagnosis and the ability to age the fetus accurately are excellent tools to enhance reproductive management in beef operations. In addition, the advent of value-based marketing and retained ownership of offspring until after slaughter has increased the focus on genetic merit of beef cattle. Commercial cattlemen now see the value in knowing the genetic base of their cattle, and can identify sires of calves before birth with a high degree of accuracy. As mentioned previously, caution should be noted as to the potential for early embryonic mortality in about 3% to 8% of the pregnancies determined to be viable at about 30 days of pregnancy.

Fetal sexing has tremendous application to the beef industry, and as veterinarians become more comfortable with their ability to make a correct diagnosis, it is becoming more frequently used. The disadvantage of the procedure is the narrow window (day 55 to 85) in which it is feasible to identify the sex of the fetus accurately. In most cases, beef cattle are managed in extensive situations in which handling the cattle an extra time becomes prohibitively costly in time and labor. Nonetheless, seedstock producers use this technology for purchasing females that may be pregnant with either a male or female fetus, and many of the sale catalogs of seedstock producers includes the sex of the fetus. This additional fetal sex information is a selection tool that may add value to both the purchaser and seller. A recent example exists in which fetal sexing has entered the commercial cattle industry. With the drought experienced by the western states during the last 3 to 4 years, many producers had reduced their herd numbers. With the increase in precipitation resulting in more feed, producers in the western states are seeking cows and heifers. The authors recently introduced a Wyoming producer to fetal sexing, and recommend that he pay a premium for heifers that have previously been fetal sexed as carrying female calves. Of the 285 heifers that were pregnancy diagnosed with the sex of the fetus determined, 137 had female pregnancies, whereas 148 had male pregnancies. In this case, the heifers with male pregnancies were sold in an auction at a premium, because all calves were expected to be male. At the same time, the heifers pregnant with female pregnancies were purchased by the Wyoming producer, at a premium!

Scientists have spent some time studying the incidence of twinning in beef operations, and the potential to increase productivity in beef management practices. Cows that produce and raise twins can net a 24% increase in production over input costs, compared with those delivering and raising a single calf [19]. This should merit closer inspection from producers seeking to improve profitability of their cow herd, but has received little attention from the majority of producers. The United States Meat Animal Research Center (MARC), has been selecting for ovulation rate in cattle since 1981, and has attained a twinning rate of greater than 30% [19]. These data confirm that increasing the number of calves born per cow increases total weight weaned per cow, and in spite of the increased costs incurred by raising two calves, results in an additional economic advantage over cows raising a single calf. The MARC has demonstrated the viability of selecting for twins as a possible management practice, although their system required a long-term commitment of greater than 20 years.

The authors have recently reported two additional reliable techniques for inducing twins in beef cattle. The first method is to transfer two demi-embryos to a single recipient [54], and the second method is to transfer a single, whole embryo to recipients 7 days after an AI [55]. From a reproductive ultrasound standpoint, we determined that the most effective time for determining the number of twin fetuses occurs between 45 and 60 days of gestation, with greater than 95% accuracy. For cases in which cows are pregnant with twins, the cows can be managed separately from cows pregnant with single calves, in order to ensure that the nutritional needs are met and that cows receive additional care at calving. With accurate detection of twins using ultrasound during early pregnancy, cows are more likely to raise and support twins at a premium to a producer compared with cows that calve with an unknown status of having either a single calf or twin calves.

Summary

The impact of real-time ultrasound on the study of reproduction has been dramatic, and the further development of portable ultrasound machines has given clinicians an added tool for diagnostic reproductive management. Ultrasound is commonly used to monitor uterine anatomy, involution, and pathology. In addition, it has been used to detect pregnancy, study embryonic mortality, monitor fetal development, and determine fetal sex. Although coupling a nonpregnancy diagnosis with a management decision to quickly reinitiate AI service may improve reproductive efficiency by decreasing the interval between AI services, early embryonic mortality and the effectiveness of hormonal ovulation and estrus control protocols initiated at certain physiologic stages post-breeding may limit the effectiveness of pregnancy examinations conducted before 30 to 33 days post-breeding. The applications of ultrasound used by scientists include the ability to monitor follicular characteristics, ovarian function, and aid in follicular aspirations and oocyte retrieval. As technology improves, technicians will have an opportunity to use the internet or video conferencing for ultrasound image analyses. With every new technological development, scientists, veterinarians, and producers discover new possibilities for the use of reproductive ultrasound to enhance the scientific merit of research or to improve reproductive efficiency in cattle operations.

References

[1] Ginther OJ. Ultrasonic imaging and reproductive event in the mare. Cross Plains (WI): Equiservices, Inc; 1986. p. 1–12.

[2] Pieterse MC, Kappen KA, Kruip TA, et al. Aspiration of bovine oocytes during transvaginal ultrasound scanning of the ovaries. Theriogenology 1988;30:751–62.

[3] Pieterse MC, Vos PLAM, Kruip TA, et al. Transvaginal ultrasound guided follicular aspiration of bovine oocytes. Theriogenology 1991;35:19–24.

[4] Ginther OJ. Ultrasonic imaging and animal reproduction: fundamentals book 1. Cross Plains (WI): Equiservices Publishing; 1995. p. 7–82, 147–55.

[5] Cowie TA. Pregnancy diagnosis tests:a review. Great Britain: Commonwealth Agricultual Bureaux Joint Publication No. 13; 1948. p. 11–17.

[6] Fricke PM. Scanning the future—ultrasonography as a reproductive management tool for dairy cattle. J Dairy Sci 2002;85:1918–26.

[7] Boyd JS, Omran SN, Ayliffe TR. Use of a high frequency transducer with real time B-mode ultrasound scanning to identify early pregnancy in cows. Vet Rec 1988;123:8–11.

[8] Curran S, Pierson RA, Ginther OJ. Ultrasonographic appearance of the bovine conceptus from days 20 through 60. J Am Vet Med Assoc 1986;189:1295–302.

[9] Pierson RA, Ginther OJ. Ultrasonography for detection of pregnancy and study of embryonic development in heifers [abstract]. Theriogenology 1984;22:225.

[10] Kastelic JP, Ginther OJ. Fate of conceptus and corpus luteum after induced embryonic loss in heifers. J Am Vet Med Assoc 1989;194:922–8.

[11] Taverne MAM, Szenci O, Szetag J, et al. Pregnancy diagnosis in cows with linear-array real-time ultrasound scanning: a preliminary note. Vet Q 1985;7:264–70.

[12] Hanzen C, Delsaux B. Use of transrectal B-mode ultrasound imaging in bovine pregnancy diagnosis. Vet Rec 1987;121:200–2.

[13] Pieterse MC, Taverne MA, Kruip TA, et al. Detection of corpora lutea and follicles in cows: a comparison of transvaginal ultrasonography and rectal palpation. Vet Rec 1990;156: 552–4.

[14] Badtram GA, Gaines JD, Thomas CB, et al. Factors influencing the accuracy of early pregnancy detection in cattle by real-time ultrasound scanning of the uterus. Theriogenology 1991;35:1153–67.

[15] Hughes EA, Davies DAR. Practical uses of ultrasound in early pregnancy in cattle. Vet Rec 1989;124:456–8.

[16] Beerepoot GMM, Dykhuizen AA, Mielen M, et al. The economics of naturally occurring twinning in dairy cattle. J Dairy Sci 1992;75:1044–51.

[17] Eddy RG, Davies O, David C. An economic assessment of twin births in British dairy herds. Vet Rec 1991;129:526–9.

[18] Guerra-Martinez P, Dickerson GE, Anderson GB, et al. Embryo-transfer twinning and performance efficiency in beef production. J Anim Sci 1990;68:4039–50.

[19] Echternkamp SE, Gregory KE. Effects of twinning on postpartum reproductive performance in cattle selected for twin births. J Anim Sci 1999;77:48–60.

[20] Davis ME, Haibel GK. Use of real-time ultrasound to identify multiple fetuses in beef cattle. Theriogenology 1993;40:373–82.

[21] Dobson H, Rowan TG, Kippax IS, et al. Assessment of fetal number, and fetal and placental viability throughout pregnancy in cattle. Theriogenology 1993;40:411–25.

[22] Wiltbank MC, Fricke PM, Sangsritavong S, et al. Mechanisms that prevent and produce double ovulation in dairy cattle. J Dairy Sci 2000;83:2998–3007.

[23] Silva Del Rio N, Kirkpatrick BW, Fricke PM. Observed frequency of monozygotic twinning in lactating Holstein cows. J Dairy Sci 2004;87(Suppl 1):65.

[24] Fricke PM, Guenther JN, Wiltbank MC. Efficacy of decreasing the dose of GnRH used in a protocol for synchronization of ovulation and timed AI in lactating dairy cows. Theriogenology 1998;50:1275–84.

[25] Fricke PM, Wiltbank MC. Effect of milk production on the incidence of double ovulation in dairy cows. Theriogenology 1999;52:1133–43.

[26] Fricke PM. Review: twinning in dairy cattle. Professional Animal Scientist 2001;17:61–7.

[27] Nielen M, Schukken YH, Scholl DT, et al. Twinning in dairy cattle: a study of risk factors and effects. Theriogenology 1989;32:845–62.

[28] Day JD, Weaver LD, Franti CE. Twin pregnancy diagnosis in Holstein cows: discriminatory powers and accuracy of diagnosis by transrectal palpation and outcome of twin pregnancies. Can Vet J 1995;36:93–7.

[29] Jost A. Embryonic sexual differentiation. In: Jones HW, Scott WW, editors. Hermaphroditism, genital anomalies and related endocrine disorders. 2nd edition. Baltimore (MD): Williams and Wilkin; 1971. p. 16–67.

[30] Curran S, Kastelic JP, Ginther OJ. Determining sex of the bovine fetus by ultrasonic assessment of the relative location of the genital tubercle. Anim Reprod Sci 1989;19:217–27.

[31] Müller E, Wittkowski G. Visualization of male and female characteristics of bovine fetuses by real-time ultrasonics [abstract]. Theriogenology 1986;25:571.

[32] Wideman D, Dorn CG, Kraemer DC. Sex detection of the bovine fetus using linear array real-time ultrasonography [abstract]. Theriogenology 1989;31:272.

[33] Beal WE, Perry RC, Corah LR. The use of ultrasound in monitoring reproductive physiology of beef cattle. J Anim Sci 1992;70:924–9.

[34] Lamb GC. Reproductive real-time ultrasound technology: an application for improving calf crop in cattle operations. In: Fields MJ, editor. Factors affecting calf crop: biotechnology of reproduction. Boca Raton (FL): CRC Press LLC; 2001. p. 231–53.

[35] Diskin MG, Sreenan JM. Fertilization and embryonic mortality rates in beef heifers after artificial insemination. J Reprod Fertil 1980;59:463–8.

[36] Lamb GC, Miller BL, Traffas V, et al. Estrus detection, first service conception, and embryonic death in beef heifers synchronized with MGA and prostaglandin. Kansas Agricultural Experiment Station Report of Progress 1997;783:97.

[37] Smith MW, Stevenson JS. Fate of the dominant follicle, embryonal survival, and pregnancy rates in dairy cattle treated with prostaglandin F2α and progestins in the absence or presence of a functional corpus luteum. J Anim Sci 1995;73:3743–51.

[38] Vasconcelos JLM, Silcox RW, Lacerda JA, et al. Pregnancy rate, pregnancy loss, and response to heat stress after AI at 2 different times from ovulation in dairy cows [abstract]. Biol Reprod 1997;56(Suppl 1):140.

[39] Szenci O, Beckers JF, Humblot P, et al. Comparison of ultrasonography, bovine pregnancy-specific protein B, and bovine pregnancy-associated glycoprotein 1 tests for pregnancy detection in dairy cows. Theriogenology 1998;50:77–88.

[40] Larson JE, Lamb GC, Geary TW, et al. Synchronization of estrus in replacement beef heifers using GnRH, prostaglandin F$_{2\alpha}$ (PG), and progesterone (CIDR): a multi-location study. J Anim Sci 2004;82(Suppl 1):368.

[41] Larson JE, Lamb GC, Stevenson JS, et al. Synchronization of estrus in suckled beef cows using GnRH, prostaglandin F$_{2\alpha}$ (PG), and progesterone (CIDR): a multi-location study. J Anim Sci 2004;82(Suppl 1):369.

[42] Stevenson JS, Johnson SK, Medina-Britos MA, et al. Resynchronization of estrus in cattle of unknown pregnancy status using estrogen, progesterone, or both. J Anim Sci 2003;81:1681–92.

[43] Rivera H, Lopez H, Fricke PM. Fertility of Holstein dairy heifers after synchronization of ovulation and timed AI or AI after removed tail chalk. J Dairy Sci 2004;87:2051–61.

[44] Fricke PM, Caraviello DC, Weigel KA, et al. Fertility of dairy cows after resynchronization of ovulation at three intervals after first timed insemination. J Dairy Sci 2003;86:3941–50.

[45] Studer E. Early pregnancy diagnosis and fetal death. Vet Med Small Anim Clin 1969;64:613–7.

[46] Melrose DR. The need for, and possible methods of application of, hormone assay techniques for improving reproductive efficiency. Br Vet J 1979;135:453–9.

[47] Galland JC, Offenbach LA, Spire MF. Measuring the time needed to confirm fetal age in beef heifers using ultrasonographic examination. Vet Med (Praha) 1994;89:795–804.

[48] Pursley JR, Mee MO, Wiltbank MC. Synchronization of ovulation in dairy cows using PGF$_{2\alpha}$ and GnRH. Theriogenology 1995;44:915–23.

[49] Pursley JR, Kosorok MR, Wiltbank MC. Reproductive management of lactating dairy cows using synchronization of ovulation. J Dairy Sci 1997;80:301–6.

[50] Moreira F, Orlandi C, Risco CA, et al. Effects of pre-synchronization and bovine somatotropin on pregnancy rates to a timed artificial insemination protocol in lactating dairy cows. J Dairy Sci 2001;84:1646–59.

[51] Navanukraw C, Reynolds LP, Kirsch JD, et al. A modified presynchronization protocol improves fertility to timed artificial insemination in lactating dairy cows. J Dairy Sci 2004;87:1551–7.

[52] Lesmeister JL, Burfening PJ, Blackwell RL. Date of first calving in beef cows and subsequent calf production. J Anim Sci 1973;36:1–6.

[53] Anderson KJ, Lefever DG, Brinks JS, et al. The use of reproductive tract scoring in beef heifers. Agri-Practice 1991;12(4):123–8.

[54] Dahlen CR, Lamb GC, Lindsay B, et al. Pregnancy rates in recipients after receiving either two identical demi-embryos or a single whole embryo. Theriogenology 2002;57:539.

[55] Wasson R, Larson JE, Brown DR, et al. Cow and calf performance in a management system including twinning and early weaning. J Anim Sci 2004;82(Suppl 1):59.

ELSEVIER
SAUNDERS

Vet Clin Food Anim 21 (2005) 437–461

VETERINARY
CLINICS
Food Animal Practice

Embryonic Death in Cattle

E. Keith Inskeep, PhD*, Robert A. Dailey, PhD

Division of Animal and Veterinary Sciences, College of Agriculture, Forestry, and Consumer Sciences, West Virginia University, PO Box 6108, Morgantown WV 26506, USA

Successful calving follows survival of the conceptus through embryonic and fetal development (ovulation rate × fertilization rate × embryonic survival rate × fetal survival rate × perinatal survival rate). To assure that all readers interpret the terms used on the same basis, ovulation rate is herein defined as the proportion of cows ovulating among cows in estrus; fertilization rate is defined as the proportion of recovered oocytes that are fertilized; embryonic survival is based upon the proportion of fertilized oocytes at one stage that remain as viable embryos at a later embryonic stage; and fetal survival is defined as the proportion of fetuses at one stage that are present as viable fetuses at a later stage, which will often be term. Conception rate is defined as the proportion of inseminated cows that are detected pregnant at diagnosis by ultrasound or palpation per rectum, and pregnancy rate is defined as the proportion of cows with successful pregnancies among animals treated or eligible to be bred. Based upon reviews by numerous authors, summarized by Inskeep [1], much of the loss of potential offspring in cattle is concentrated in the embryonic period, the first 42 days after breeding (Fig. 1). This article covers the impact of embryonic mortality on success of pregnancy in cattle, and some of the hormonal factors involved in pregnancy losses during the embryonic period. To establish the relative importance of embryonic death in the final outcome of mating, brief consideration is given to conception rate and fertilization rate.

Conception rate

During the 1950s, records of birth of a live calf to first artificial insemination (AI) in Wisconsin dairy herds [2], showed that bulls in the

---

Work of the authors described in this article was supported by Hatch (WV421) and Hatch Regional Projects (NE-161 and 1007), and USDA grants, including USDA-NRICGP 2002-35203-12230.
* Corresponding author.
E-mail address: einskeep@wvu.edu (E.K. Inskeep).

vetfood.theclinics.com

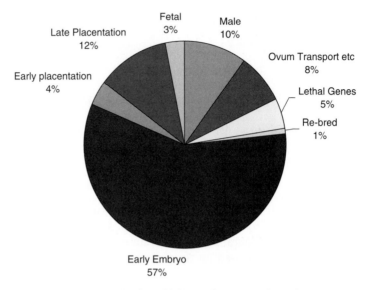

Fig. 1. Distribution of failures of pregnancy in cattle.

service stud had a 65% nonreturn rate, and that 59.5% of the cows delivered live calves. Conception rates in parous dairy cows averaged about 55% in studies by Johnson et al [3] and Mares and coworkers [4]. Conception rates have declined significantly since that time. Nebel [5] found that cows in the 11,667 herds in the Dairy Records Management System North Carolina had average first-service conception rates of 43%, and 39% overall. Others reported conception rates to timed insemination of only 35% or lower [6–8]. From a compilation of the data summarized in reviews by Dailey and associates [9], Santos and colleagues [10] and DeJarnette [11], the decline in fertility over the last 5 decades is depicted in Fig. 2 (see also reviews by Lucy [12] and Washburn and coauthors [13]).

In a recent study in two large herds in California, Chebel et al [14] found that multiparous cows were 13% less likely to conceive than primiparous cows, which might be partially explained by a higher incidence of postparturient diseases, but is consonant with the effects of age of cow on pregnancy losses that are discussed later in this article. In that study, heat stress two cycles before breeding was a major negative factor for conception. In contrast to the negative association of conception rate and milk yield over the years, either no effect of milk production on conception rate [14], or a positive association of conception with milk yield [15] were observed. In the latter study, all cows were on fixed-timed AI protocols. Surprisingly, conception rate was greater with timed AI than with breeding after detected estrus in the study by Chebel and coworkers [14].

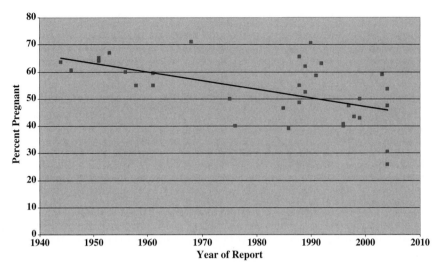

Fig. 2. Compilation of unweighted conception rates for cows artificially inseminated after onset of estrus. Cows were inseminated either in the uterine body or the uterine horn ipsilateral to the ovary with the corpus luteum. (*Data from* Refs. [9–11] for the period 1944–2004).

A major determining factor for conception rate in the cow herd is the postpartum interval at breeding (also referred to as "days in milk" in dairy cows). From a summary of studies in the early literature [1], the pattern of return to fertility showed low conception rates of 33% and 39% in beef and dairy cows, respectively, when cows were inseminated before day 30. Conception rates increased to 58% and 53%, respectively, during days 31 to 60 postpartum, and 69% and 62% during days 61 to 90 postpartum, after which time values reached a plateau. Other factors have been addressed, most recently by Chebel and associates [14] and Starbuck and colleagues [16]. These factors include heat stress, number of the insemination, milk production, incidences of calving difficulty, retained placenta, mastitis, postparturient disease, method of synchronization of estrus, and timing of insemination.

Fertilization rate

Estimates of fertilization rates for both dairy and beef bulls have ranged from 85% to 95% [17–19], and Thatcher and coauthors [20] and Peters [21] generalized that fertilization failure is 10%. When problems associated with ovulation or ovum transport by the uterus (eg, failure to ovulate, empty zonae, adhesions, tubal patency) were accounted for, 75% to 78% of first inseminations resulted in pregnancies [18,22]. On the basis of these data, pregnancy rate to a single breeding should ideally be 75% to 80%. Pregnancy rates should be greater than 93% after two inseminations, and greater than 98% after three $(75\% \times [100\%-75\%] + 75\% = 93.8\%$ pregnant after two inseminations, and by a similar calculation, 98.4% after three inseminations). Cows not pregnant after three inseminations would be classified as repeat breeders or problem breeders [23]. Ideally, only 1% to 2% of the breeding animals should fall into this category.

Fertilization rates may have declined over time in some categories of animals. Santos et al [10] summarized data from several studies performed since 1990, indicating that fertilization rates were 100% in dairy heifers (n = 32), 98% in nonlactating beef cows (n = 73), 88% in beef heifers (n = 125), 76% in lactating dairy cows (n = 165), 78% in nonlactating dairy cows (n = 444), and 75% in early postpartum, lactating beef cows (n = 40). Of the fertilized oocytes, only 88% in beef heifers, 77% and 81% in lactating and nonlactating beef cows, 66% and 74% in lactating and nonlactating dairy cows, and 72% in dairy heifers were considered viable when recovered by flushing the oviduct or uterus or at slaughter. Wiltbank and Parrish [24] showed that conception rates were increased in natural mating by breeding only to bulls with a high proportion of live spermatozoa in semen samples collected for breeding soundness examinations. DeJarnette [11] emphasized the importance of semen quality and handling in obtaining maximum fertilization rates in AI. Based upon their reviews, Dailey and coworkers [9] and Santos and associates [10] used values of 78 and 76%, respectively, to represent fertilization rates (Table 1).

To illustrate the relative importance of fertilization failure and embryonic death, Inskeep [1] cited an example from lactating, early postpartum beef cows studied by Casida and colleagues [25]. Conception rates, calculated from fertilization rates determined on day 3 after insemination and embryos palpated per rectum on days 38 to 44, averaged 15%, 55%, 64%, and 86%, respectively, for cows inseminated at less than 31, 31 to 50, 51 to 90, and greater than 91 days postpartum. The interaction of day postpartum with whether fertility was measured at 3 or 38 to 44 days after insemination had no effect on conception rate. From this observation, Casida and his group concluded that embryonic death was a minimal contributor to early postpartum infertility in beef cows. By combining their data from slaughter

Table 1
Estimates of pregnancy retention (%) in the lactating dairy cow, as compiled and calculated from the literature by contemporary reviewers

Day of gestation	Dailey et al [9]	Santos et al [10]
0–4 (fertilization)	78	76
6		50
20	38	
28–29	36	40
36–42	31	35
90		32
Term	30	28

at 3 days after insemination over all postpartum intervals, however, fertilization rate was 52%, whereas pregnancy rate for cows slaughtered at 15 days or palpated at 38 to 44 days was 35%. Thus, estimated embryonic death would be 17 percentage points, or nearly 33%, of the embryos present at day 3 after insemination. Both fertilization failure (48%) and embryonic death (33% of fertilized oocytes) were significant contributors to low pregnancy rates in the early postpartum cow.

Embryonic loss

Hawk [18] estimated from his review of the literature that embryonic death occurred in 15% of first inseminations. Sreenan and Diskin [26] concluded that much of the pregnancy loss in cattle is due to early embryonic death, after either natural or artificial insemination or embryo transfer. The majority of embryonic mortality occurred within an equivalent of one cycle length [21] after breeding, and, in an early study, with greater frequency in younger animals [27]. In early postpartum beef cows expected to have low pregnancy rates because of short luteal phases, similar proportions of oocytes released at ovulation were fertilized, underwent early embryonic development, and were transported into the uterine horn, as in those cows expected to have normal pregnancy rates because of pretreatment with progestogen [28].

The embryo, which has progressed from a fertilized egg through multiple cellular divisions to reach the morula stage, is transported to the uterus by day 5 [29], and by late day 7, the ball of cells begins to form a cavity within it, termed the blastocoele. Embryos were most susceptible to mortality during development from the morula to blastocyst stage on days 5 through 8 [30]. In multiparous cows, 67% of embryonic loss occurred or was occurring by day 8, whereas 92% of the estimated loss was seen by day 8 in nulliparous females. Similarly, in repeat-breeder cows, the majority of loss occurred 6 to 7 days after breeding [31]. Gustafson and Larsson [32] concluded that slowed embryonic development at day 7 might be a common factor for most repeat breeding heifers. This corroborated a report by Linares [33] of high incidence of embryonic mortality at day 7 for repeat breeder heifers, even when fertilization rate was high (90%).

Tanabe and Almquist [34] demonstrated that even if fertilization rate was compromised, embryonic loss was very high (~35%) in repeat breeder heifers. Tanabe and coauthors [35] concluded that the maternal environment of repeat breeder cows was able to support pregnancy after day 7 by comparing the success rate to day 60 of an embryo implanted into repeat breeder (70%) and normal cows (82%) on day 7. From a meta-analysis of 47 data sets from transfer of one or two embryos into a recipient, McMillan [36] calculated that the embryo and the recipient played approximately equal roles in survival of the embryo.

In their review, Thatcher et al [37] concluded that approximately 30% of repeat breeder cows experienced embryonic loss by day 7 of pregnancy. Additional embryonic losses occurred gradually from days 8 to 17 (approximately 40% of total losses) and between days 17 and 24 (approximately 24% of total losses). In a study in beef heifers in which fertilization rate was 90%, Diskin and Sreenan [19] observed an embryo survival rate of 93% at day 8, but only 56% by day 12. This result shows that factors affecting embryonic survival in that period are independent of fertility of oocytes.

Sreenan and Diskin [26] estimated that 75% to 80% of embryonic loss occurred by day 20. Roche and coworkers [38] surmised that loss of pregnancies occurred gradually between days 8 and 19. Those cows could return to estrus as though they had never conceived. Losses between days 17 and 24 were estimated at 6% to 12% of pregnancies in two studies in which dairy heifers were bred at synchronized estrus after two treatments with prostaglandin (PG) $F_2\alpha$, 11 days apart [39].

Estimates of late embryonic death rate (days 27 to 42) averaged 10% to 12% [1,37,40–42]. Sreenan and Diskin [26] estimated 10% to 15% losses around implantation. An estimated 10% to 12% of pregnancies in dairy cows were lost between days 25 and 60 of pregnancy [39]. Warnick [43] summarized data for loss of pregnancy after first diagnosis of pregnancy by palpation. Loss was 14.8% when diagnosis was made at 30 to 36 days, comparable to values frequently recorded in the summary tabulated for timed-inseminated dairy cows by Inskeep [1]; however, estimated late losses of embryos in timed-insemination programs varied widely, and ranged as high as 45% in lactating cows [1].

Although changes associated with the process begin earlier, attachment of the embryo in the uterus is initiated around day 30 in the cow, with marked development of the placentomes between days 30 and 40 [44,45]. Based upon a review of losses after day 30, Dailey and associates [9] concluded that the processes of attachment and placentation were critical, and that most losses would occur before day 45 (see Table 1), which was indeed the case in the study by Starbuck and colleagues [16].

In contrast to the lactating dairy cow, late embryonic losses in beef cattle and dairy heifers, summarized in detail by Inskeep [42], ranged from 2% to 6%. For example, Dunne and coauthors [46] estimated embryo survival as 68% of ovulations in one sample group of beef heifers at slaughter on day 14, whereas 72% of another sample group calved, and ultrasonography of that sample at day 30 had shown that 76% were pregnant. Thus, they concluded that most losses occurred before day 14, and the estimate of late embryonic and fetal losses together totaled only 4 percentage points, or 5.3%.

Dailey et al [9] summarized data from both beef and dairy cattle indicating that estimated fetal loss after day 40 averaged 3% or less (see Table 1). They concluded that most late embryonic/early fetal losses would have occurred before day 45, and that future research should be concentrated primarily on factors affecting the interval early postinsemination (days 5 through 8), and secondarily on days 30 through 36.

Management variables (poor estrous detection, using semen from low-fertility bulls, inseminating cows not in estrus or cows already pregnant) can be improved upon without research. For example, as many as 7% of pregnant cows show estrus during pregnancy, and insemination of pregnant cows resulted in 17% embryonic loss/abortion [47]. Other factors are either not controllable, or the variety of contributing agents (ie, lethal genes, disease, uncontrollable stressors) is such that improved prediction of successful outcome is unlikely,. Lethal genes have an estimated frequency of 6% in cattle, and losses might occur early or late in embryonic development. In-vitro fertilized oocytes and cultured embryos from cows that genetically were high milk producers yielded lower cleavage rates and fewer blastocysts than those from genetically lower-producing cows [48].

The signal in the cow to maintain the corpus luteum is interferon τ, which is derived from the embryonic trophoblast around day 14 through 17 (eg, Thatcher and coworkers [49]), and is referred to as maternal recognition of pregnancy. A viable embryo during that time is essential for maintenance of the corpus luteum of pregnancy. Luteal tissue might be maintained after embryonic mortality during the maternal recognition process; however, Opsomer and associates [50] reported that in high-producing dairy cows, increased parity, problem calvings, occurrence of puerperal disturbances, health problems during the first month of lactation, and an early resumption of ovarian cycles after calving increased the risk for prolonged luteal cycles before service. Cows could have prolonged luteal phases without clinical signs of causality [51]. Thus in some cases, cows that are inseminated but fail to conceive, and that have prolonged luteal phases, as determined by concentrations of progesterone or ultrasonic evaluation of the ovaries, would be erroneously considered as candidates for early embryonic loss, even though they may not have had a fertile ovulation.

The lactating dairy cow

The lactating dairy cow epitomizes the problems of low conception rate and high rates of embryonic and early fetal death. Authors of recent studies have emphasized the role of low concentrations of progesterone in failures of the reproductive process at several points. First, understanding bases for the occurrence of low progesterone is necessary.

Intuitively, progesterone can be lower because secretion by the corpus luteum is reduced, or because metabolism of progesterone is increased. Feed intake, milk yield, and route of administration of progesterone influenced metabolism and excretion of progesterone in lactating dairy cows in some studies, but neither feed intake nor metabolizable energy had an effect in others [42]. In heifers, greater feed intake increased, decreased, or had no

effect on plasma progesterone. In nonlactating, intact cows or ovariectomized cows injected with progesterone or bearing intravaginal progesterone-
releasing inserts, greater feed intake decreased plasma progesterone. In one
study [52], high-producing cows absorbed more progesterone from an
intravaginal insert, and excreted more progesterone daily in the milk, but
concentrations of progesterone in milk and plasma were not different from
those in low-producing cows. Sartori and colleagues [53] found that
concentrations of progesterone and estradiol-17β in lactating dairy cows
were lower than in heifers in summer, and similar to those in dry cows in
winter, despite the fact that the lactating cows had larger ovulatory follicles
and larger corpora lutea. Several other workers have made similar
observations.

Sangsritavong and coauthors [54] tested the hypothesis that increased
blood flow to the liver, as a result of elevated feed intake, would increase
steroid metabolism. Liver blood flow and metabolic clearance of progesterone reached maximum at 2 hours after feeding in lactating dairy cows,
and persisted longer as cows were given greater amounts of feed. Metabolic
clearance of progesterone was correlated highly with liver blood flow
(r = 0.92). Greater metabolism of progesterone might account for lower
concentrations of progesterone and more frequent ovulation of persistent
follicles in lactating cows than in heifers that received the same intravaginal
inserts containing progesterone [55]. Similarly, this could be responsible, at
least in part, for lower embryo quality in lactating cows than in heifers and
dry cows [56], and for the observation that pregnancy losses between days
30 and 60 were more frequent in lactating cows with lower concentrations of
progesterone at day 30 [16], which is discussed later.

**Embryonic losses before the 16-cell stage in relation to roles of
progesterone, estrogen, follicle stimulating hormone, and luteinizing
hormone in preovulatory follicular development**

The concept that vesicular follicles grow in a wavelike pattern was
proposed originally by Rajakoski [57]. Follicular growth occurs in waves, as
a result of growth of a cohort of follicles, one (or occasionally two) of which
will become the lead follicle, referred to as dominant, while the others
undergo atresia [58]. Two, three, or even four (more frequently in Brahman
cattle) waves may occur during an estrous cycle, but a two-wave pattern has
been predominant in both beef [59] and dairy [60] cattle. Waves emerged on
days 0 (day of ovulation) and 10 of estrous cycles with two waves, and on
days 0, 9, and 16 of cycles with three waves; thus a follicular wave occurred
about every 7 to 10 days.

Frequency of secretion of pulses of gonadotropin releasing hormone
(GnRH) from the hypothalamus and of luteinizing hormone (LH) from
the anterior pituitary are regulated by circulating concentrations of

progesterone (principally) and estrogen [1]. When concentrations of progesterone are low, a high frequency of pulses of LH stimulates continued growth of the lead (dominant) follicle [61], which secretes more estradiol-17β (and all of the follicles in a cohort secrete inhibin). When progesterone is high, a low frequency of pulses of LH fails to support continued follicular growth, and leads to atresia of the largest follicle, with a resultant decrease in secretion of estradiol-17β and inhibin. Thus the lead follicle cannot ovulate during a luteal phase, because the corpus luteum is truly dominant by virtue of secretion of progesterone. When the largest follicle stops growing, an increase in secretion of follicle stimulating hormone (FSH) stimulates development of a new cohort of follicles [62]. The largest follicle present at the onset of luteolysis may ovulate during the ensuing estrus.

Ulberg et al [63] recognized the larger size of follicles in animals completing treatment with low dosages of progesterone. In retrospect, much of the variation in pregnancy rates at synchronized estrus in cattle could be accounted for by whether or not the lead follicle persisted under conditions of low progesterone or progestogen. Concentrations of progesterone during the luteal phase can influence the persistence of a follicle and the number of follicular waves during an estrous cycle; however, concentrations of progesterone and estradiol-17β, in peripheral blood collected every other day from beef animals with two or three follicular waves during normal estrous cycles, differed only in relation to the time that luteal regression occurred, not in mean concentrations [59]. Similar results for progesterone were found in lactating dairy cows [60]. Thus length of the luteal phase appears to determine number of waves, except when very low progesterone leads to persistence of a dominant follicle.

With extensive studies of follicular growth by transrectal ultrasonography, the relationship of lower fertility to persistent follicles began to be recognized [42]. For example, Breuel and coworkers [28] examined fertility of postpartum beef cows with normal luteal phases. Cows with larger dominant follicles 5 days before the surge of LH had greater preovulatory concentrations of estradiol and a lower conception rate (36%) than cows with smaller follicles at that time (91% conception).

Oocytes from persistent follicles were likely to be at a more advanced stage of maturation than those from follicles of normal age and size [42,64]. Although oocytes from persistent follicles had undergone changes characteristic of the early stages of atresia, they were fertilizable, but development of the resultant zygote was retarded, and early embryonic death usually occurred before the 16-cell stage [65,66]. The sequence of relationships of increased pulse frequency of LH, increased preovulatory secretion of estradiol, and aged oocytes provided an explanation for lowered fertility when low dosages of progestogens were used to synchronize estrus. Similarly, fertility was reduced when progesterone was low during the natural estrous cycle before breeding [67,68].

The ovulatory follicle in cows with two waves of follicular development is older and larger than the ovulatory follicle in cows with three waves of follicular development during an estrous cycle. Therefore, greater duration or amount of secretion of estradiol-17β from the ovulatory follicle before breeding could contribute to embryonic losses observed before the 16-cell stage, and could result in lower conception rates in cows with two, rather than three, waves of follicular development. Indeed, conception rate to first service was reduced in lactating dairy cows in which spontaneous ovulation was from the second (63%) compared with the third (81%) wave of follicular development during the estrous cycle before insemination [60], and a similar trend had been seen in spontaneously-cycling beef animals [59]. Ovulatory follicles in the dairy cows were older by 1.5 days and larger by 1.2 mm when originating from the second rather than the third wave. These results were confirmed recently in lactating dairy cows by Bleach and associates [69], who claimed to be the first to show such an effect in spontaneously-cycling animals, and who also showed a linear decline in fertility with increasing intervals from follicular emergence to estrus.

Hormonal mechanisms by which persistent follicles cause low fertility

The sequential relationship of low progesterone, increased frequency of pulses of LH, a persistent largest follicle, increased secretion of estradiol-17β, and decreased fertility has been accepted widely as one of causes and effects. Inskeep [42], however, pointed out that it is not clear whether the reduction in fertility is an effect of estrogen, LH, or both. Patterns of fertility in relation to concentrations of estradiol before breeding have been inconsistent. In cows treated with FSH to produce multiple follicles, which persisted during low progesterone, concentrations of estradiol-17β declined to very low values (<1 pg/mL) during the 7 days immediately before estrus [70]. Even so, follicular oocytes were at a later stage of maturation (meiosis had resumed), just as in animals with high concentrations of estradiol-17β from a single persistent follicle in other experiments.

In most studies, comparisons were made between animals with persistent follicles or control follicles that were younger and smaller. Based upon contemporary comparisons of oocytes collected from follicles on days 8 and 10 of the estrous cycle, in cows with normal or lowered progesterone [42], changes in the oocyte that ultimately led to lowered embryonic survival may have begun very early during exposure to lowered progesterone.

Shaham-Albalancy and colleagues [71] showed that low concentrations of progesterone before estrus (2.1 to 2.3 ng/mL) altered endometrial morphology during the subsequent estrous cycle, and increased subsequent secretion of prostaglandin $F_2\alpha$ ($PGF_2\alpha$) as measured by its major metabolite. These effects might decrease fertility, even though the original oocyte was healthy. Wehrman and coauthors [72], however, showed that development of a persistent follicle before synchronized estrus did not alter rate of survival of control embryos transferred into treated cows on day 7 after estrus.

Follicles can be too small or produce too little estrogen

Several authors have found that premature ovulation of follicles led to reduced ability of fertilized, cleaved oocytes to develop to the blastocyst stage, as well as delayed or inadequate luteal function or premature luteal regression (reviewed by Inskeep [42]). Mermillod et al [73] found a quite variable association of ability of cattle oocytes to develop to the blastocyst stage after in-vitro maturation and fertilization with the endocrine milieu of the follicle. Lower concentrations of progesterone, greater concentrations of estradiol, and more α-subunit of inhibin in follicular fluid sometimes appeared to have predictive value. The study authors concluded that the proportion of developmentally-competent oocytes increased with increasing follicular size, and that an oocyte retained competence to initiate development during early stages of follicular atresia. Lopez and coworkers [74] examined for effects of milk production on diameter of follicle, estrous behavior, and serum concentrations of estradiol in 267 cows that averaged 50 days in milk. Duration of estrus, number of times the cow stood for mounting, and how long she stood were all significantly lower for cows in the upper half of the herd in current milk production. Concentrations of estradiol were lower, but preovulatory follicular diameters were larger, for the high producers.

Smaller follicular diameter has been shown to affect conception rate in several studies. For example, Perry and associates [75,76] monitored preovulatory follicular diameter in beef cows observed for estrus and inseminated 12 hours later, or timed-inseminated after a regimen of GnRH on day 9, $PGF_2\alpha$ on day 2 and GnRH on day 0 (at insemination). Conception rate, measured at days 25 to 39, averaged 72% in control cows compared with 45% in timed-inseminated cows. Much of the difference in fertility was accounted for by the cows with follicles 12 mm in diameter or less in one study, or 11 mm or less in the other study. Concentrations of progesterone rose at a slower rate in cows with smaller follicles at induced ovulation than in cows with larger follicles. Thus, embryos might have been expected to be less advanced [77] and to produce less interferon τ [78,79] in the cows that ovulated small follicles.

Mussard and colleagues [80] arrayed data from studies of effects of follicular diameter, according to the duration of proestrus, in groups of 12 to 54 animals that were induced to ovulate by treatment with GnRH after withdrawal of progesterone. As mean duration of proestrus increased, conception rate increased (for 1.0, 1.0, 2.2, 2.0, 3.3, and 4.7 days, conception rates were 4%, 8%, 57%, 67%, 76% and 100%, respectively). Thus, follicular maturity may be the important variable, and diameter may not reflect maturity as effectively as duration of proestrus. The Mussard group further showed that life span of the corpus luteum was less than 12 days in

74% of 38 animals in which duration of proestrus averaged only 1.3 days before induced ovulation, compared with only 30% of 40 animals in which duration of proestrus averaged 2.3 days. In addition, luteal function was lower on days 8 through 14 in cows with normal luteal life span, when proestrus was shortened by earlier preovulatory treatment with GnRH. Conversely, Baruselli et al [81] observed greater conception rates (52 versus 39%) in primiparous, suckled *Bos indicus* cows treated with 400 international units (IU) of equine chorionic gonadotropin (eCG, which has an FSH-like effect in cows) at withdrawal of controlled internal drug releasing devices, compared with cows that received no eCG, in association with greater concentrations of progesterone on day 12 after ovulation (8.6 versus 6.4 ng/mL).

Follicular maturity relative to fixed-time inseminations might be involved in late embryonic death. In beef cows inseminated at a fixed time after a regimen of progesterone, $PGF_2\alpha$, and estradiol benzoate, Bridges and coworkers [82] found that of 71 cows pregnant at day 39, only one failed to calve. In contrast, the observations by Perry and associates [76] raised the possibility that size of follicle in cows that were timed-inseminated after GnRH might affect late embryonic losses, although numbers were insufficient to be conclusive. Thirteen of 43 timed-inseminated cows with small follicles were pregnant at day 27, but 5 of the 13 (38.5%) lost pregnancy by day 68, leaving a net pregnancy rate of 19%, whereas no late losses occurred in 57 pregnant cows with mature follicles (overall loss 6.7%). In cows inseminated at estrus, 3 of 127 (2.4%) lost pregnancies from first to second diagnosis, but their follicles were 12, 14, and 16 mm or more in diameter. Similarly, Galvão and colleagues [83] observed a trend ($P = 0.08$) for decreased late embryonic loss in lactating dairy cows that were in estrus at timed AI compared with those that were not in estrus. In studies with cultured and cloned embryos, Thompson and Peterson [84] have presented evidence that development of the allantois can lead to failure of late embryonic and early fetal development. Piedrahita and coauthors [85] showed that follicular diameter from which oocytes were obtained affected size of the allantois of cloned embryos at day 27. The involvement of development of the allantois in late embryonic death is worthy of further study.

Overall, one must conclude that fertility can be compromised by either immature or overmature follicles/oocytes. The follicles ovulated at natural estrus in an untreated heifer or beef cow appear to be of more optimum age and size than those ovulated in a high-producing, lactating dairy cow, especially if estrus is synchronized with a less-than-optimum dosage of progestogen or if ovulation is induced prematurely with GnRH.

Early embryonic death associated with short duration of the luteal phase in the postpartum beef cow

The postpartum transition period, during which cyclic occurrence of ovulation is restored, provides an experimental situation in which to determine effects of selected endocrine events. A short luteal phase following first ovulation or first estrus at puberty, after parturition, or after seasonal anestrus is common in ruminants (see reviews by Inskeep [1,42]). Obviously, a corpus luteum that regressed before day 14 in the cow could not support maternal recognition of pregnancy on days 14 to 17. Follicular development and pre-and postovulatory concentrations of gonadotropins and luteal receptors for LH were shown not to affect luteal life span, and it was eventually shown that premature uterine secretion of $PGF_2\alpha$ was responsible for the short luteal phase.

Pretreatment with a progestogen usually led to formation of a corpus luteum with a normal functional life span, in response to weaning or injection of gonadotropins. If the uterus had not been exposed recently to progestogen, secretion of $PGF_2\alpha$ increased prematurely when the first corpus luteum began to secrete progesterone. Progestogen pretreatment prevented the premature increased secretion of $PGF_2\alpha$ on days 4 through 9 postestrus. The effect required both progestogen and the rise in estrogen when it was withdrawn, and was apparently mediated by an increase in numbers of receptors for progesterone in the uterus, which was detected on day 5 after estrus [86,87].

Because there was earlier evidence that ovulation and fertilization occurred at the expected time after estrus preceding a short luteal phase in small numbers of early-weaned cows, researchers at West Virginia University in Morgantown set out to determine the points at which fertility fails in early-weaned postpartum beef cows (reviewed by Inskeep [1,42]). Calves were weaned at about 30 days postpartum, and half of the cows received progestogen pretreatment (6 mg norgestomet implants for 9 days, ending 2 days after early weaning). Control cows that had not formed corpora lutea before calves were weaned were expected to have short luteal phases/estrous cycles in all cases. Cows pretreated with progestogen were expected to have normal luteal phases/estrous cycles in an average of at least 80% of cases. Cows in both groups were at the same stage postpartum when studied.

When oviducts from cows in each group were flushed at day 3 after breeding, fertilization rate (68%), development of fertilized oocytes to the four- to eight-cell stage (100%), and embryo quality did not differ between cows with short or normal luteal phases. When uteri were flushed nonsurgically on day 6, fertilization rate (82%) and development to at least the four-cell stage (90%) again did not differ [28]. Supplemental progestogen therapy did not maintain pregnancy in cows with short luteal phases. In contrast, 41% of all norgestomet-pretreated cows and 50% of those cows that had normal luteal phases maintained pregnancy regardless of whether or not they received supplemental progestogen. Twelve of 13 cows that were deleted from these experiments because of a spontaneous short luteal phase before breeding conceived at the postweaning estrus, at an average of only 33 days postpartum.

Reciprocal embryo transfers between cows expected to have short or normal luteal phases revealed that losses of embryos in cows with short luteal phases involved effects both before and after days 6 and 7 postestrus. Further studies at West Virginia University (Morgantown, West Virginia) and the University of Tennessee (Knoxville, Tennessee), reviewed in detail by Inskeep [1,42], provided strong evidence that the premature uterine secretion of $PGF_2\alpha$ not only regressed the corpus luteum, but also had an embroyotoxic effect, specific to days 4 through 8 postestrus and augmented by additional $PGF_2\alpha$ secreted by the regressing corpus luteum. This scenario fits with the facts that most embryonic mortality in subfertile dairy cows occurred 6 to 7 days after estrus [31], and that 67% of embryonic mortality had occurred or was occurring by day 8 of gestation in beef cows [30].

The preponderance of evidence is that chronic high concentrations of $PGF_2\alpha$ are toxic to the very early embryo in cows and ewes. The effect is direct [88,89] and does not require local transfer from the ovary to the uterus, but a regressing corpus luteum can be a significant source of the $PGF_2\alpha$ involved in the effect.

Oxytocin is released from the corpus luteum by $PGF_2\alpha$ [90], and can increase uterine secretion of $PGF_2\alpha$ [91,92], which in turn can cause luteal regression and early embryonic loss [93]. Thus oxytocin, injected to cause milk letdown, or released by uterine manipulation [94] associated with embryo transfer or by milking, might play a significant role in early embryonic death in cattle, with or without causing complete luteolysis. In fact, Schrick et al [95] and Elli and coworkers [96] found that treatment with agents that inhibit secretion of $PGF_2\alpha$ improved pregnancy rates to nonsurgical embryo transfer. Other factors that increase secretion of $PGF_2\alpha$, such as heat stress [97], uterine infection [98], or mastitis [99–101], might cause very early embryonic death through this mechanism (reviewed by Zavy [102]).

Progesterone secretion during the early luteal phase and treatments designed to prevent early embryonic mortality

Spontaneous luteal regression results in embryonic loss [103], and adequate secretion of progesterone is clearly the major requirement for success of early pregnancy. Indeed, four ovariectomized cows delivered live calves when supplemented only with progestin after embryo transfer [104]. Similarly, Hawk and associates [105] were able to maintain, by exogenous progesterone, pregnancies in 73% of cows ovariectomized between days 5 and 8 (because cows were ovariectomized before determination of pregnancy could be made, nearly all of the predicted pregnancies, based on Hawk [18], were maintained: 73/78 = 93.6%).

Pattern of progesterone secretion early in the estrous cycle has been studied as a possible contributor to early embryonic loss. In subfertile dairy cows, progesterone increased more slowly after estrus than in heifers [106]. Because concentrations of progesterone in peripheral blood were sometimes greater in pregnant dairy cows as early as day 4.5 [107], attempts were made to improve conception rates by increasing progesterone early after breeding. Both GnRH and human chorionic gonadotropin (hCG) have been used extensively as treatments at or near insemination, on the assumption that such treatments might improve luteal function early in the estrous cycle, and thus avoid some of the losses during the first 7 or 8 days, or losses that might be associated with misstiming of embryonic development in relation to maternal recognition of pregnancy. Based upon the data presented and reviewed by Lewis and colleagues [108] and by Chenault [109], one cannot conclude that these treatments are routinely valuable.

In beef cows, Pritchard and coauthors [110] examined conception rates to AI in relation to patterns of peripheral progesterone and estradiol on days 4 through 7 after estrus and found no relationship. Supplementation with progesterone during a similar period appears to be beneficial only if secretion of $PGF_2\alpha$ is not increased and luteal regression is not occurring, based upon the results in postpartum cows with short luteal phases discussed above. Nevertheless, numerous studies of supplemental progesterone have been done over the years. Wiltbank et al [111] used 50 or 200 mg per day from days 3 to 34 after onset of estrus in repeat-breeder cows. Pregnancy rates at day 34 were 42% in treated cows and 30% in controls—a nonsignificant difference. Similarly, Stevenson and Mee [112] used progesterone-releasing intravaginal devices from day 5 to day 13 following estrus in lactating dairy cows that had been inseminated after a single treatment with $PGF_2\alpha$ at 42 to 63 days postpartum. They found no improvement in pregnancy rates to the previous breeding, although pregnancy rate to breeding at the subsequent estrus was improved. Santos and coworkers [10] pointed out in their review that treatment with exogenous progesterone before day 4 would be expected to advance uterine secretion of $PGF_2\alpha$ and cause premature luteolysis.

Role of follicular secretion of estradiol in embryonic mortality during maternal recognition of pregnancy

Patterns of follicular development, and as a result, secretion of estradiol-17β, during days 14 to 17 after breeding may be important in embryonic loss during maternal recognition of pregnancy. This concept, originally presented by Macmillan and associates [113], was supported in studies by Thatcher and colleagues [114] and others, in which ovulation or atresia of the largest follicle during the midluteal phase after breeding sometimes increased pregnancy rate. Numerous studies have been done in which GnRH or hCG has been used to ovulate or luteinize large follicles during this stage after breeding, with considerable variation in response. Based upon the data presented and reviewed by Lewis and coauthors [108], one cannot conclude that routine use of these treatments has value.

Kastelic et al [103] concluded that luteal regression preceded death of the embryo in losses that occurred before day 25 of gestation. Even short periods of deprivation of progesterone can decrease embryo survival during the maternal recognition period. Lulai and coworkers [115] studied the effects of initiation of luteal regression on day 15, either 24 or 36 hours before beginning replacement therapy with norgestomet. Embryo survival was 84% in control heifers and cows, but was reduced to 45% or 13%, respectively, when replacement therapy was delayed for 24 or 36 hours.

Pritchard and associates [110] measured concentrations of progesterone and estradiol in peripheral blood during days 14 to 17 after AI in over 100 lactating beef cows, and obtained evidence for association of embryonic loss with excessive secretion of estrogen during maternal recognition of pregnancy. Cows were divided into three groups according to concentrations of estradiol-17—the lower quartile, middle half and upper quartile—which averaged 1.6, 2.1, and 3.1 pg/mL of estradiol, respectively, during the 4-day sampling period. Conception rate to first service declined as concentration of estradiol increased, averaging 77%, 60%, and 42%, respectively, for the three groups. One might expect that supplemental progesterone would help to decrease estrogen secretion during this period and protect the pregnancy; however, pregnancy rates were not improved by treatment with progesterone-releasing intravaginal devices from days 13 to 21 following estrus, in lactating dairy cows that had been inseminated after a single treatment with $PGF_2\alpha$ at 42 to 63 days postpartum [112].

If secretion of estrogen from a large follicle during days 14 through 17 (or beyond) after breeding can compromise embryo survival, either directly or through interference with mechanisms of maternal recognition of pregnancy and luteal maintenance, then cows with two waves of follicular development during the equivalent of an estrous cycle after breeding would have such a follicle. Ahmad and colleagues [59] found that fewer animals conceived among those that had two (70%) rather than three (96%; $P < 0.05$) waves of follicular development during the equivalent of one estrous cycle after insemination. Surprisingly, however, concentrations of estrogen in peripheral blood on day 14 after estrus and insemination did not differ in animals with two versus three follicular waves.

Although there is a clear association of pregnancy loss during maternal recognition, with higher circulating estrogen in some cases, neither the exact timing of an estrogen effect nor the mechanism by which estrogen may interfere with the developing embryo has been established.

Late embryonic/early fetal mortality: a significant factor in lactating dairy cows during the peri-attachment period

With the recognition that duration of follicular development was a significant factor in determining pregnancy rate at synchronized estrus (reviewed by Inskeep [1]), numerous protocols to regulate follicular development have been devised. In many cases, it has been possible to program the time of AI, without detection of estrus and with greater initial rates of pregnancy than in previous systems [116–120]. Researchers have noted high frequencies of late embryonic and early fetal losses in several studies, both before and after day 25 of gestation [9,10,42]. Cerri and coauthors [121] found no difference in loss rates from 30 to 58 days of gestation between timed-inseminated cows (11%) and those inseminated at detection of estrus (12.4%). Starbuck et al [16] studied lactating Holstein and Ayrshire cows on two farms on which animals were inseminated 12 hours after onset of estrus or bred naturally. Eleven percent of 211 animals that were pregnant at ultrasonography during the fifth week after breeding (days 28 to 36) lost the pregnancy by week 9, and 65% of losses had occurred by week 7. There have been wide variations among individual studies or groups of animals, however [42]. For example, Drost and coworkers [6] estimated late embryonic mortality from the difference in cows pregnant at day 42 and with high progesterone on day 22, which was 65% in cows inseminated artificially and 41% in cows with transferred embryos, when cows were under summer heat stress in Florida.

The observations by Perry and associates [76] raised the possibility that follicle size in cows that were timed-inseminated after GnRH might affect late embryonic losses, but the data were tenuous. Thirteen of 43 timed-inseminated cows with small follicles were pregnant at day 27, but 5 of the 13 (38.5%) lost pregnancy by day 68, leaving a net pregnancy rate of 19%, whereas no late losses occurred in 57 pregnant cows with larger follicles (overall loss 6.7%). In cows inseminated at estrus, 3 of 127 (2.4%) lost pregnancies from first to second diagnosis, but their follicle sizes were 12, 14, and 16 mm or larger. These data illustrate that very large numbers of cows must be sampled to elucidate causes of late embryonic mortality.

In seven of eight heifers in which embryonic death occurred between days 25 and 40 postbreeding, Kastelic and colleagues [103] found that the onset of luteal regression, as detected by ultrasonography, began at least 3 days after embryonic death, as indicated by loss of heartbeat. In another study, in which 7 of 70 pregnancies were lost by day 42, embryonic death preceded luteal regression in each case [122]. Although late embryonic loss preceded luteolysis, the possibility that luteal function was compromised before embryos were lost was not ruled out. Schallenberger and coauthors [90] observed increased secretion of $PGF_2\alpha$ between d 30 and 36 in pregnant heifers, one of which had extremely high values and lost the pregnancy. The placenta may be the source of increased $PGF_2\alpha$, because Eley et al [123] found higher total $PGF_2\alpha$ in allantoic fluid on day 33 than on day 27, 30, 40, 50, 60, or 70.

Lulai and coworkers [124] and Bridges and associates [125] studied the ability of new corpora lutea (CL), induced during the late embryonic and early fetal periods in cows in which the original CL had been removed or induced to regress, to maintain pregnancy. During the period of formation

454 INSKEEP & DAILEY

of the new CL, the animals received exogenous progestogen, which was withdrawn gradually after the presence of new CL was confirmed. When the induced CL was on the ovary contralateral to the pregnant uterine horn, pregnancy usually was lost. If the new CL was induced on the ovary adjacent to the embryo, and was induced later than day 36 after mating, all of 21 pregnancies were maintained; however, when an adjacent new CL was induced on or before day 36 after mating, only 15 of 30 pregnancies were maintained [125].

In one study, Bridges and colleagues [125] removed original CL on day 26 of pregnancy, induced new CL between days 28 and 31, and examined patterns of secretion of $PGF_2\alpha$, progesterone and estradiol-17β during days 31 through 35. Surprisingly, in cows with greater concentrations of $PGF_2\alpha$, induced CL secreted more progesterone and maintenance of pregnancy tended to be higher. The role of prostaglandins in embryonic attachment has not been elucidated in ruminants, but $PGF_2\alpha$ is important in the comparable process of implantation in rodents (reviewed briefly by Inskeep [42]). An additional finding by Bridges and coauthors [125] was a tendency for more pregnancies to continue when concentrations of estradiol were lower.

Because lowered concentrations of progesterone and greater concentrations of estradiol appeared to limit successful maintenance of pregnancy by replacement CL [125], concentrations of these steroids were studied as predictors of pregnancy maintenance in lactating dairy cows followed by routine ultrasonography [16]. In most cases in which cows lost pregnancy, the CL was functional at the last collection of jugular serum before late embryonic or early fetal death was detected, so it was suggested that the embryo died before the CL regressed, in agreement with Kastelic et al [103] and Wolff [122]. Pregnancy loss before day 45 (20%), however, was greater in cows with the lowest 25% of serum concentrations of progesterone at 28 to 37 days of gestation than in cows in the middle 50% (3.8 to 5.9 ng/mL) or upper 25%, each of which had only 8% loss. In contrast to the results of Bridges and coworkers [125], retention of pregnancy to week 7 of gestation increased with increasing classified concentrations of estradiol at week 5 in the study by Starbuck and associates [16], but logistic regression did not reveal an association of retention of pregnancy to week 7 with concentrations of estradiol at either week 5. At this stage of pregnancy supplementation with progesterone may have therapeutic value. Lopez-Gatius and colleagues [126] found that insertion of a progesterone-releasing intravaginal device on days 36 to 42 of gestation for 28 days reduced pregnancy loss through day 90 from 12% in 549 control cows to 5.3% in 549 treated cows.

Embryonic mortality after maternal recognition of pregnancy and during placentation is a major economic problem in the lactating dairy cow. It is associated with lower progesterone during days 28 through 37. Lower progesterone could be due to reduced secretion of progesterone by the CL, or to greater metabolism of progesterone, as pointed out earlier in this article.

Summary

Embryonic mortality is a significant limiting factor to completion of pregnancy in cattle. Some causes and mechanisms involved in loss of embryos have been elucidated, and much of success or failure appears to depend upon circulating concentrations of progesterone at specific time points, and on changes in other hormones as a consequence of patterns of progesterone. Changes in progesterone during the luteal phase immediately before estrus and after insemination can cause losses of embryos during days 4 through 8 after estrus, during maternal recognition of pregnancy on days 14 through 17 after estrus, and during the late embryonic/early fetal period, between days 28 and 42 to 50. Early embryonic, late embryonic, and early fetal losses appear to be greater in lactating dairy cows than in beef cattle and dairy heifers. Management systems designed to limit metabolism of progesterone are needed during the estrous cycle before breeding and during these critical periods after insemination.

Both herd managers and veterinarians servicing herds must be aware that the management required to maximize fertility in the cow is not simple. It can be noted that high fertility was observed in animals in studies that involved frequent ultrasonographic scanning, careful observation of the cows, and breeding in relation to observed estrus. The work of Saacke and coauthors [127] has shown that although insemination later in estrus maximizes fertilization rate, breeding earlier minimizes embryonic death, thus the am:pm rule remains a valid compromise that will maximize ultimate pregnancy rate. Therefore, close observation for estrus in an artificial insemination program, if it is emphasized in educational programs, rather than reliance on timed-insemination protocols, might allow significant improvements in pregnancy rates at term. Treatments for synchronization of estrus must provide relatively high concentrations of progesterone, which will limit LH and estradiol during treatment, leading to development of a highly functional corpus luteum after mating. Early after mating, during maternal recognition of pregnancy, and during the late embryonic period, reduction of luteolytic influences, such as excesses of $PGF_2\alpha$ or estradiol-17β, is important.

References

[1] Inskeep EK. Factors that affect embryonic survival in the cow: application of technology to improve calf crop. In: Fields MJ, Sand RS, Yelich JV, editors. Factors affecting calf crop: biotechnology of reproduction. Boca Raton (FL): CRC Press; 2002. p. 255–79.

[2] Inskeep EK, Tyler WJ, Casida LE. Hereditary variation in conception rate of Holstein-Friesian cattle. J Dairy Sci 1961;44(10):1857–62.

[3] Johnson KR, Ross RH, Fourt DL. Effect of progesterone administration on reproductive efficiency. J Anim Sci 1958;17(2):385–90.

[4] Mares SE, Menge AC, Tyler WJ, et al. Genetic factors affecting conception rate and early pregnancy loss in Holstein cattle. J Dairy Sci 1961;44(1):96–103.

[5] Nebel RL. Optimizing fertility in the dairy herd. Theriogenology 1999;51:443–52.

[6] Drost M, Ambrose JD, Thatcher MJ, et al. Conception rate after artificial insemination or embryo transfer in lactating dairy cows during summer in Florida. Theriogenology 1999;52(7):1161–7.

[7] Cartmill JA, El-Zarkouny SZ, Hensley BA, et al. Stage of cycle, incidence, and timing of ovulation and pregnancy rates in dairy cattle after three timed breeding protocols. J Dairy Sci 2001;84(5):1051–9.

[8] Pancarci SM, Jordan ER, Risco CA, et al. Use of estradiol cypionate in a presynchronized timed artificial insemination program for lactating dairy cattle. J Dairy Sci 2002;85(1):122–31.

[9] Dailey RA, Inskeep EK, Lewis PE. Pregnancy failures in cattle: a perspective on embryo loss. In: Štastný P, editor. Proceedings of the XVIIIth International Conference on Reproduction of Farm Animals. Nitra, Slovak Republic: University of Nitra; 2002. p. 1–8.

[10] Santos JEP, Thatcher WW, Chebel RC, et al. The effect of embryonic death rates in cattle on the efficacy of estrus synchronization programs. Anim Reprod Sci 2004;82–83:513–35.

[11] DeJarnette JM. Sire, semen quality, and technician effects on conception rates of artificially inseminated dairy cattle. In: Proceedings of Taurus 2nd Conference Bovine Reproduction. Buenos Aires: 2004. p. 54–73.

[12] Lucy MC. Reproductive loss in high producing dairy cattle: where will it end? J Dairy Sci 2001;84(6):1277–93.

[13] Washburn SP, Silvia WJ, Brown CH, et al. Trends in reproductive performance in southeastern Holstein and Jersey DHI herds. J Dairy Sci 2002;85(1):244–51.

[14] Chebel RC, Santos JEP, Reynolds JP, et al. Factors affecting conception rate after artificial insemination and pregnancy loss in lactating dairy cows. Anim Reprod Sci 2004;84(3–4):239–55.

[15] Peters MW, Pursley JR. Fertility of lactating dairy cows treated with Ovsynch after presynchronization injections of PGF_2 and GnRH. J Dairy Sci 2002;85(9):2403–6.

[16] Starbuck MJ, Dailey RA, Inskeep EK. Factors affecting retention of early pregnancy in cattle. Anim Reprod Sci 2004;84(1):27–39.

[17] Kidder HE, Black WG, Wiltbank JN, et al. Fertilization rates and embryonic death rates in cows bred to bulls of different levels of fertility. J Dairy Sci 1954;37(6):691–7.

[18] Hawk HW. Infertility in dairy cattle. In: Hawk HW, editor. Animal reproduction (Beltsville symposia in agricultural research 3). Montclair (NJ): Allenheld, Osmun; 1979. p. 19–30.

[19] Diskin MG, Sreenan JM. Fertilization and embryonic mortality rates in beef heifers after artificial insemination. J Reprod Fertil 1980;59(2):463–8.

[20] Thatcher WW, Macmillan KL, Hansen PJ, et al. Embryonic losses: cause and prevention. In: Fields MJ, Sand RS, editors. Factors affecting calf crop. Boca Raton (FL): CRC Press; 1993. p. 135–53.

[21] Peters AR. Embryo mortality in the cow. Animal Breeding Abstracts 1996;64(8):587–98.

[22] Bellows RA, Short RE, Staigmiller RB. Research areas in beef cattle reproduction. In: Hawk HW, editor. Animal reproduction (Beltsville symposia in agricultural research 3). Montclair (NJ): Allenheld, Osmun; 1979. p. 3–18.

[23] Casida LE. Present status of the repeat breeder cow problem. J Dairy Sci 1961;44(12):2323–9.

[24] Wiltbank JN, Parrish NR. Pregnancy rate in cows and heifers bred to bulls selected for semen quality. Theriogenology 1986;25(6):779–83.

[25] Casida LE, Graves WE, Hauser ER, et al. Studies on the postpartum cow. Research bulletin 270. Madison (WI): University of Wisconsin; 1968. p. 23–6; 51.

[26] Sreenan JM, Diskin MG. The extent and timing of embryonic mortality in cattle. In: Sreenan JM, Diskin MG, editors. Embryonic mortality in farm animals. Dordrecht (Netherlands): Martinus Nijhoff; 1986. p. 1–11.

[27] Erb RE, Holtz EW. Factors associated with estimated fertilization and service efficiency of cows. J Dairy Sci 1958;41(10):1541–52.

[28] Breuel KF, Lewis PE, Schrick FN, et al. Factors affecting fertility in the postpartum cow: role of the oocyte and follicle in conception rate. Biol Reprod 1993;48(3):655–61.

[29] McLaren A. The embryo. In: Austin CR, Short RV, editors. Embryonic and fetal development. London: Cambridge University Press; 1972. p. 1–42.

[30] Maurer RR, Chenault JR. Fertilization failure and embryonic mortality in parous and nonparous beef cattle. J Anim Sci 1983;56(5):1186–9.

[31] Ayalon N. A review of embryonic mortality in cattle. J Reprod Fertil 1978;54(2):483–93.

[32] Gustafsson H, Larsson K. Embryonic mortality in heifers after artificial insemination and embryo transfer: differences between virgin and repeat breeder heifers. Res Vet Sci 1985; 39(3):271–4.

[33] Linares T. Embryonic development in repeat breeder and virgin heifers seven days after insemination. Anim Reprod Sci 1982;4(3):189–98.

[34] Tanabe TY, Almquist JO. Some causes of infertility in dairy heifers [abstract]. J Dairy Sci 1953;36:586.

[35] Tanabe TY, Hawk HW, Hasler JF. Comparative fertility of normal and repeat-breeder cows as embryo recipients. Theriogenology 1985;23:687–96.

[36] McMillan WH. Statistical models predicting embryo survival to term in cattle after embryo transfer. Theriogenology 1998;50(7):1053–70.

[37] Thatcher WW, Staples CR, Danet-Desnoyers G, et al. Embryo health and mortality in sheep and cattle. J Anim Sci 1994;72(Suppl 3):16–30.

[38] Roche JF, Boland MP, McGeady TA. Reproductive wastage following artificial insemination of heifers. Vet Rec 1981;109(18):401–4.

[39] Van Cleeff JK, Drost M, Thatcher WW. Effects of postinsemination progesterone supplementation on fertility and subsequent estrous responses of dairy heifers. Theriogenology 1991;36(5):795–807.

[40] Smith MW, Stevenson JS. Fate of the dominant follicle, embryonal survival, and pregnancy rates in dairy cattle treated with prostaglandin $F_2\alpha$ and progestins in the absence or presence of a functional corpus luteum. J Anim Sci 1995;73(12):3743–51.

[41] Vasconcelos JLM, Silcox RL, Lacerda JA, et al. Pregnancy rate, pregnancy loss and response to heat stress after AI at 2 different times from ovulation in dairy cows. Biol Reprod 1997;56(Suppl 1):140.

[42] Inskeep EK. Preovulatory, postovulatory, and post-maternal recognition effects of concentrations of progesterone on embryonic survival in the cow. J Anim Sci 2004; 82(Suppl E):E24–39.

[43] Warnick W. Early embryonic death (EED). Available at: http://www.napoleonvet.com/ dairy.html#Early%20Embryonic%20Death%20(EED). Accessed February 22, 2005.

[44] Melton AA, Berry RO, Butler OD. The interval between the time of ovulation and attachment of the bovine embryo. J Anim Sci 1951;10(4):993–1005.

[45] King GJ, Atkinson BA, Robertson HA. Implantation and early placentation in domestic ungulates. J Reprod Fertil 1982;31(Suppl):17–30.

[46] Dunne LD, Diskin MG, Sreenan JM. Embryo and foetal loss in beef heifers between day 14 of gestation and full term. Anim Reprod Sci 2000;58(1–2):39–44.

[47] Sturman H, Oltenacu EAB, Foote RH. Importance of inseminating only cows in estrus. Theriogenology 2000;53(8):1657–67.

[48] Snijders SEM, Dillon P, Callaghan DO, et al. Effect of genetic merit, milk yield, body condition and lactation number on in vitro oocyte development in dairy cows. Theriogenology 2000;53(4):981–90.

[49] Thatcher WW, Meyer MD, Danet-Desnoyers G. Maternal recognition of pregnancy. J Reprod Fertil 1995;(Suppl 49):15–28.

[50] Opsomer G, Grohn YT, Hertl J, et al. Risk factors for post partum ovarian dysfunction in high producing dairy cows in Belgium: a field study. Theriogenology 2000;53(4):841–57.

[51] Opsomer G, Coryn M, Deluyker H, et al. An analysis of ovarian dysfunction in high yielding dairy cows after calving based on progesterone profiles. Reprod Domest Anim 1998;33:193–204.

[52] Rabiee AR, Macmillan KL, Schwarzenberger F. Excretion rate of progesterone in milk and faeces in lactating dairy cows with two levels of milk yield. Reprod Nutr Dev 2001;41(4): 309–19.

[53] Sartori R, Rosa GJM, Wiltbank MC. Ovarian structures and circulating steroids in heifers and lactating cows in summer and lactating and dry cows in winter. J Dairy Sci 2002a; 85(11):2813–22.

[54] Sangsritavong S, Combs DK, Sartori R, et al. High feed intake increases liver blood flow and metabolism of progesterone and estradiol-17β in dairy cattle. J Dairy Sci 2002;85(11): 2831–42.

[55] Cooperative Regional Research Project. NE-161. Relationship of fertility to patterns of ovarian follicular development and associated hormonal profiles in dairy cows and heifers. J Anim Sci 1996;74(8):1943–52.

[56] Sartori R, Sartor-Bergfelt R, Mertens SA, et al. Fertilization and early embryonic development in heifers and lactating cows in summer and lactating and dry cows in winter. J Dairy Sci 2002b;85(11):2803–12.

[57] Rajakoski E. The ovarian follicular system in sexually mature heifers with special reference to seasonal, cyclical, and left-right variations. Acta Endocrinol (Copenh) 1960;(Suppl 52): 1–68.

[58] Ginther OJ, Wiltbank MC, Fricke PM, et al. Selection of the dominant follicle in cattle. Biol Reprod 1996;55(6):1187–94.

[59] Ahmad N, Townsend EC, Dailey RA, et al. Relationships of hormonal patterns and fertility to occurrence of two or three waves of ovarian follicles, before and after breeding, in beef cows and heifers. Anim Reprod Sci 1997;49(1):13–28.

[60] Townson DH, Tsang PCW, Butler WR, et al. Relationship of fertility to ovarian follicular waves before breeding in dairy cows. J Anim Sci 2002;80(4):1053–8.

[61] Taft R, Ahmad N, Inskeep EK. Exogenous pulses of luteinizing hormone cause persistence of the largest bovine ovarian follicle. J Anim Sci 1996;74(12):2985–91.

[62] Adams GP, Matteri RL, Ginther OJ. Effect of progesterone on ovarian follicles, emergence of follicular waves and circulating follicle-stimulating hormone in heifers. J Reprod Fertil 1992;96(2):627–40.

[63] Ulberg LC, Christian RE, Casida LE. Ovarian response of heifers to progesterone injections. J Anim Sci 1951;10(3):752–9.

[64] Mihm M, Curran N, Hyttel P, et al. Effect of dominant follicle persistence on follicular fluid oestradiol and inhibin and on oocyte maturation in beef heifers. J Reprod Fertil 1999; 116(2):293–304.

[65] Wishart DF. Synchronization of oestrus in heifers using steroid (SC 5914, SC 9880 and SC 21009) treatment for 21 days: the effect of treatment on the ovum collection and fertilization rate and the development of the early embryo. Theriogenology 1977;8(5):249–69.

[66] Ahmad N, Schrick FN, Butcher RL, et al. Effect of persistent follicles on early embryonic losses in beef cows. Biol Reprod 1995;52(5):1129–35.

[67] Folman Y, Rosenberg M, Herz Z, et al. The relationship between plasma progesterone concentrations and conception in postpartum dairy cows maintained on two levels of nutrition. J Reprod Fertil 1973;34(2):267–78.

[68] Meisterling EM, Dailey RA. Use of concentrations of progesterone and estradiol-17β in milk in monitoring postpartum ovarian function in dairy cows. J Dairy Sci 1987;70(10): 2154–61.

[69] Bleach ECL, Glencross RG, Knight PG. Association between ovarian follicle development and pregnancy rates in dairy cows undergoing spontaneous oestrous cycles. Reproduction 2004;127(5):621–9.

[70] Revah I, Butler WR. Prolonged dominance of follicles reduces the viability of bovine oocytes. J Reprod Fertil 1996;106(1):39–47.

[71] Shaham-Albalancy A, Nyska A, Kaim M, et al. Delayed effect of progesterone on endometrial morphology in dairy cows. Anim Reprod Sci 1997;48(2–4):159–74.

[72] Wehrman ME, Fike KE, Melvin EJ, et al. Development of a persistent ovarian follicle during synchronization of estrus does not alter conception rate after embryo transfer in cattle [abstract]. Theriogenology 1996;45(1):291.

[73] Mermillod P, Oussaid B, Cognie Y. Aspects of follicular and oocyte maturation that affect the developmental potential of embryos. J Reprod Fertil 1999;(Suppl 54):449–60.

[74] Lopez H, Satter LD, Wiltbank MC. Relationship between level of milk production and estrous behavior of lactating dairy cows. Anim Reprod Sci 2004;81(3–4):209–23.

[75] Perry GA, Geary TW, Lucy MC, et al. Effect of follicle size at the time of induced ovulation on luteal function and fertility. J Anim Sci 2002;80(Suppl 2):52.

[76] Perry GA, Smith MF, Lucy MC, et al. Effect of ovulatory follicle size at the time of GnRH injection or standing estrus on pregnancy rates and embryonic/fetal mortality in beef cattle [absract]. J Anim Sci 2003;81(Suppl 1):52.

[77] Garrett JE, Geisert RD, Zavy MT, et al. Evidence for maternal regulation of early conceptus growth and development in beef cattle. J Reprod Fertil 1988;84(2):437–46.

[78] Kerbler TL, Buhr MM, Jordan LT, et al. Relationship between maternal plasma progesterone concentration and interferon-tau synthesis by the conceptus in cattle. Theriogenology 1997;47(3):703–14.

[79] Mann GE, Lamming GE, Robinson RS, et al. The regulation of interferon-tau production and uterine hormone receptors during early pregnancy. J Reprod Fertil 1999;(Suppl 54): 317–28.

[80] Day ML. Ovarian follicle maturity at induced ovulation influences fertility in cattle. In: Kastetic J, editor. Proceedings of the Society for Theriogenology. Annual Conference and Symposium. Columbus (OH): Elsevier Science; 2003. p. 179–85.

[81] Baruselli PS, Reis EL, Marques MO, et al. The use of hormonal treatments to improve reproductive performance of anestrous beef cattle in tropical climates. Anim Reprod Sci 2004;82–83:479–86.

[82] Bridges PJ, Lewis PE, Wagner WR, et al. Follicular growth, estrus and pregnancy after fixed-time insemination in beef cows treated with intravaginal progesterone inserts and estradiol benzoate. Theriogenology 1999;52(4):573–83.

[83] Galvão KN, Santos JEP, Juchem SO, et al. Effect of addition of a progesterone intravaginal insert to a timed insemination protocol using estradiol cypionate on ovulation rate, pregnancy rate, and late embryonic loss in lactating dairy cows. J Anim Sci 2004;82(12): 3508–17.

[84] Thompson JG, Peterson AJ. Bovine embryo culture in vitro: new developments and post-transfer consequences. Hum Reprod 2000;15(Suppl 5):59–67.

[85] Piedrahita JA, Wells DN, Miller AL, et al. Effects of follicular size of cytoplast donor on the efficiency of cloning in cattle. Mol Reprod Dev 2002;61(3):317–26.

[86] Zollers WG, Garverick HA, Smith MF, et al. Concentrations of progesterone and oxytocin receptors in endometrium of postpartum cows expected to have a short or normal oestrous cycle. J Reprod Fertil 1993;97(2):329–37.

[87] Kieborz-Loos KR, Garverick HA, Keisler DH, et al. Oxytocin-induced secretion of prostaglandin F$_2$α in postpartum beef cows: Effects of progesterone and estradiol-17β treatment. J Anim Sci 2003;81(7):1830–6.

[88] Scenna FN, Edwards JL, Rohrbach NR, et al. Detrimental effects of prostaglandin $F_2\alpha$ on preimplantation bovine embryos. Prostaglandins Other Lipid Mediat 2004;73(3–4):215–26.

[89] Hockett ME, Rohrbach NR, Schrick FN. Alterations in embryo development in progestogen-supplemented cows administered prostaglandin $F_2\alpha$. Prostaglandins Other Lipid Mediat 2004;73(3–4):227–36.

[90] Schallenberger E, Schams D, Meyer HHD. Sequences of pituitary, ovarian and uterine hormone secretion during the first 5 weeks of pregnancy in dairy cattle. J Reprod Fertil 1989;(Suppl 37):277–86.

[91] Newcomb R, Booth WD, Rowson LEA. The effect of oxytocin treatment on the levels of prostaglandin F in the blood of heifers. J Reprod Fertil 1977;49(1):17–24.

[92] Milvae RA, Hansel W. Concurrent uterine venous and ovarian arterial prostaglandin F concentrations in heifers treated with oxytocin. J Reprod Fertil 1980;60(1):7–15.

[93] Lemaster JW, Seals RC, Hopkins FM, et al. Effects of administration of oxytocin on embryonic survival in progestogen-supplemented cattle. Prostaglandins Other Lipid Mediat 1999;57(4):259–68.

[94] Roberts JS, Barcikowski B, Wilson L Jr, et al. Hormonal and related factors affecting the release of prostaglandin $F_2\alpha$ from the uterus. J Steroid Biochem 1975;6(6):1091–7.

[95] Schrick FN, Hockett ME, Towns TM, et al. Administration of a prostaglandin inhibitor immediately prior to embryo transfer improves pregnancy rates in cattle [abstract]. Theriogenology 2001;55(1):370.

[96] Elli M, Gaffuri B, Frigerio A, et al. Effect of a single dose of ibuprofen lysinate before embryo transfer on pregnancy rates in cows. Reproduction 2001;121(1):151–4.

[97] Malayer JR, Hansen PJ, Gross TS, et al. Regulation of heat shock-induced alterations in the release of prostaglandins by the uterine endometrium of cows. Theriogenology 1990; 34(2):219–30.

[98] Manns JG, Nkuuhe JR, Bristol F. Prostaglandin concentrations in uterine fluid of cows with pyometra. Can J Comp Med 1985;49(2):436–8.

[99] Barker AR, Schrick FN, Lewis MJ, et al. Influence of clinical mastitis during early lactation on reproductive performance of Jersey cows. J Dairy Sci 1998;81(12):1285–90.

[100] Cullor JS. Mastitis and its influence upon reproductive performance in dairy cattle. In: International Symposium on Bovine Mastitis, Indianapolis, Indiana. 1990. p. 176–80.

[101] Stewart AB, Inskeep EK, Townsend EC, et al. Effects of gram-positive bacterial pathogens in ewes: peptidoglycan as a potential mediator of interruption of early pregnancy. Reproduction 2003;125(2):295–9.

[102] Zavy MT. Embryonic mortality in cattle. In: Zavy MT, Geisert RD, editors. Embryonic mortality in domestic species. Boca Raton (FL): CRC Press; 1994. p. 99–140.

[103] Kastelic JP, Northey DL, Ginther OJ. Spontaneous embryonic death on days 20 to 40 in heifers. Theriogenology 1991;35(2):351–63.

[104] Inskeep EK, Baker RD. Successful transfer of bovine embryos into ovariectomized recipients [abstract]. J Anim Sci 1985;61(Suppl 1):409.

[105] Hawk HW, Brinsfield TH, Turner GD, et al. Embryo survival in first service and repeat breeder cattle after ovariectomy and hormone therapy. J Dairy Sci 1963;46(12):1397–401.

[106] Shelton K, Gayerie de Abreu MF, Hunter MG, et al. Luteal inadequacy during the early luteal phase of sub-fertile cows. J Reprod Fertil 1990;90(1):1–10.

[107] Larson SF, Butler WR, Currie WB. Reduced fertility associated with low progesterone postbreeding and increased milk urea nitrogen in lactating cows. J Dairy Sci 1997;80(7): 1288–95.

[108] Lewis GS, Caldwell DW, Rexroad CE Jr, et al. Effects of gonadotropin-releasing hormone and human chorionic gonadotropin on pregnancy rate in dairy cattle. J Dairy Sci 1990; 73(1):66–72.

[109] Chenault JR. Effect of fertirelin acetate or buserelin on conception rate at first or second insemination in lactating dairy cows. J Dairy Sci 1990;73(3):633–8.

[110] Pritchard JY, Schrick FN, Inskeep EK. Relationship of pregnancy rate to peripheral concentrations of progesterone and estradiol in beef cows. Theriogenology 1994;42(2): 247–59.

[111] Wiltbank JN, Hawk HW, Kidder HE, et al. Effect of progesterone therapy on embryo survival in cows of lowered fertility. J Dairy Sci 1956;39(4):456–61.

[112] Stevenson JS, Mee MO. Pregnancy rates of Holstein cows after postinsemination treatment with a progesterone-releasing intravaginal device. J Dairy Sci 1991;74(11):3849–56.

[113] Macmillan KL, Taufa VK, Day AM. Effects of an agonist of gonadotropin releasing hormone (Buserelin) in cattle. III. Pregnancy rates after a post-insemination injection during metoestrus or dioestrus. Anim Reprod Sci 1986;11(1):1–10.

[114] Thatcher WW, Macmillan KL, Hansen PJ, et al. Concepts for regulation of corpus luteum function by the conceptus and ovarian follicles to improve fertility. Theriogenology 1989; 31(1):149–64.

[115] Lulai C, Kastelic JP, Carruthers TD, et al. Role of luteal regression in embryo death in cattle. Theriogenology 1994b;41(5):1081–9.

[116] Burke JM, De La Soto RL, Risco CA, et al. Evaluation of timed insemination using a gonadotropin-releasing hormone agonist in lactating dairy cows. J Dairy Sci 1996;79(8): 1385–93.

[117] Thatcher WW, de La Sota RL, Schmitt EJ-P, et al. Control and management of ovarian follicles in cattle to optimize fertility. Reprod Fertil Dev 1996;8(2):203–17.

[118] Stevenson JS, Kobayashi Y, Shipka MP, et al. Altering conception of dairy cattle by gonadotropin-releasing hormone preceding luteolysis induced by prostaglandin F$_2\alpha$. J Dairy Sci 1996;79(3):402–10.

[119] Pursley JR, Kosorok MR, Wiltbank MC. Reproductive management of lactating dairy cows using synchronization of ovulation. J Dairy Sci 1997;80(2):301–6.

[120] Pursley JR, Wiltbank MC, Stevenson JS, et al. Pregnancy rates per artificial insemination for cows and heifers inseminated at a synchronized ovulation or synchronized estrus. J Dairy Sci 1997;80:295–300.

[121] Cerri RLA, Galvão KN, Juchem SO, et al. Timed AI (TAI) with estradiol cypionate (ECP) or insemination at detected estrus in lactating dairy cows. J Anim Sci 2003;81(Suppl 1):181.

[122] Wolff N. Nachweis embryonaler mortalitat baim rind mit hilfeder sonographie. [Detection of embryonic mortality in cattle using sonography.] Tierarztl Prax 1992;20(4):373–80.

[123] Eley RM, Thatcher WW, Bazer FW. Hormonal and physical changes associated with bovine conceptus development. J Reprod Fertil 1979;55(1):181–90.

[124] Lulai C, Dobrinski I, Kastelic JP, et al. Induction of luteal regression, ovulation and development of new luteal tissue during early pregnancy in heifers. Anim Reprod Sci 1994a; 35(3–4):163–72.

[125] Bridges PJ, Wright DJ, Buford WI, et al. Ability of induced corpora lutea to maintain pregnancy in beef cows. J Anim Sci 2000;78(11):2942–9.

[126] Lopez-Gatius F, Santolaria P, Yaniz JL, et al. Progesterone supplementation during the early fetal period reduces pregnancy loss in high-yielding dairy cattle. Theriogenology 2004; 62(8):1529–35.

[127] Saacke RG, Dalton JC, Nadir S, et al. Relationship of seminal traits and insemination time to fertilization rate and embryo quality. Anim Reprod Sci 2000;60–61:663–77.

VETERINARY
CLINICS
Food Animal Practice

Vet Clin Food Anim 21 (2005) 463–472

Diagnosis of Fetal Loss Caused by Bovine Viral Diarrhea Virus and *Leptospira spp*

Daniel L. Grooms, DVM, PhD[a],*,
Carole A. Bolin, DVM, PhD[b]

[a]*Department of Large Animal Clinical Sciences, College of Veterinary Medicine,
Michigan State University, A100 VTH, East Lansing, MI 48824, USA*
[b]*Department of Veterinary Pathobiology and Diagnostic Investigation,
College of Veterinary Medicine, Michigan State University, 4125 Beumont Road,
East Lansing, MI 48824, USA*

Efficient reproduction is a major contributing factor to the economic viability of the cattle industry [1,2]. Factors that make reproduction less efficient can have a significant economic impact on producers, whose enterprises require that their cattle be able to produce viable and healthy offspring. Causes of reproductive inefficiency are numerous, and range from simple management errors to complicated multifactorial disease complexes.

Infectious diseases can be a significant cause of reproductive inefficiency. Many bacteria, viruses, protozoa, fungi and parasites have been linked to reproductive losses in cattle. Infectious diseases have been associated with infertility, early embryonic deaths, abortions, and congenital defects. Worldwide, bovine viral diarrhea virus (BVDV) and *Leptospira spp* cause two of the most common infectious diseases associated with reproductive losses [3–9] When investigating reproductive inefficiency problems, these two pathogens should be primary considerations and should be ruled out first.

Diagnosis of reproductive loses related to bovine viral diarrhea virus

Epidemiology and reproductive consequences

Reproductive losses form BVDV can present many different clinical pictures, ranging from an insidious reduction in reproductive performance

---

* Corresponding author.
E-mail address: groomsd@cvm.msu.edu (D.L. Grooms).

at the herd level to devastating abortion storms. Because one clinical picture is not pathopneumonic for BVDV, selecting the right diagnostic tests and strategies to rule out BVDV as a cause of reproductive losses is important. To begin, it is important to remember that BVDV has been associated with many different aspects of reproductive inefficiencies, including infertility, early embryonic death, abortion, and congenital defects [9]. Understanding the epidemiology of when various BVDV-related reproductive losses might occur is important to selecting the correct diagnostic tests and strategies (Fig. 1).

Herd screening

If BVDV is suspected of causing reproductive inefficiency, but no diagnostic evidence exists to support the suspicion, an appropriate first step is to determine if it is likely that BVDV is actually circulating on the farm. Several herd-screening tools have been developed as indicators of BVDV presence at the herd level. Bulk tank polymerase-chain-reaction (PCR) assays can be used to rapidly screen the lactating herd for evidence that BVDV is present [10,11]. A positive test is a good indication that BVDV is circulating. A negative test result does not rule out the possibility that BVDV is circulating on the farm, because animals shedding virus may not actually be contributing to the bulk tank on the day of the test; or if they are, the possibility exists that the amount of virus present in milk is below the analytical sensitivity of the PCR assay. PCR should be used on pooled milk samples of no more than 300 cows. Pools of greater than 300 cows reduce the analytical sensitivity significantly. Serial bulk tank screening may be employed to increased diagnostic sensitivity over time.

Serology has historically been used as a diagnostic tool for BVDV. Unfortunately, because of the widespread use of BVDV vaccines in the United States and the relatively common field exposure to the virus, the use of neutralizing BVDV titers can be confusing and difficult to interpret.

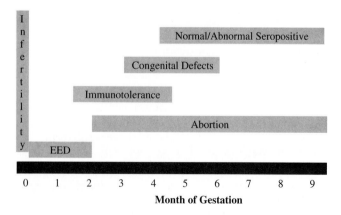

Fig. 1. Potential clinical reproductive outcomes following infection with bovine viral diarrhea virus. EED, early embryonic death.

There are some important things to understand about BVDV neutralizing antibody titers that can make interpretation of single point observations difficult: (1) vaccination titers, especially those induced by modified-live vaccines, can be as high as natural infection titers, thus trying to differentiate between natural exposure and vaccine exposure based on antibody titer can be problematic; (2) antibody titers induced from natural infection and modified-live vaccines can be long-lasting [12], so a high antibody titer today may be indicative of recent or historical virus exposure; (3) neutralizing antibody assay results may vary significantly, depending on the virus exposure and the reference virus used in the assay [13], so when requesting a BVDV virus neutralization assay, it is important to ask for both type 1 and 2 assays to be run.

An application of serology that can indicate if BVDV is circulating on a farm is to use cattle unvaccinated for BVDV as sentinel animals. The strategy involves testing young animals (6–12 months of age) that have not been vaccinated against BVDV. The presence of BVDV-neutralizing antibody titers in these unvaccinated cattle indicates recent virus exposure (presumably natural), and is a strong indicator that BVDV is circulating on the farm [13,14]. It is important to assay for both genotype 1 and 2 neutralizing antibodies when using this approach, because antigenic diversity among isolates of these different genotypes may have limited cross-reactivity [13].

Another use of serology that still has application is looking at acute and convalescent antibody titers in affected individuals or groups of cattle. Looking at BVDV antibody titer levels using a case-control methodology may also be useful.

Diagnosing bovine viral diarrhea virus abortion

Abortions caused by BVDV can occur at any stage of gestation (Fig. 2). Unfortunately, diagnosis of BVDV-related abortion can often be frustrating. A major contributing factor to this frustration is that expulsion of the fetus following BVDV infection is often delayed. Because of this delay, the chance that BVDV is still present in the fetus is significantly reduced. In addition, because of the delayed fetal expulsion, cows have often seroconverted, making acute and convalescent titers of little value. When attempting to identify BVDV in aborted fetuses, it is important to submit fresh tissues for virus isolation or PCR as rapidly as possible. Some laboratories may use immunohistochemistry as the primary means of detecting BVDV in tissues, in which case formalin-fixed tissues should be submitted. Tissues of most value for detecting BVDV include lymphoid tissue such as thymus, spleen, and ileum. Other valuable tissues include lung and liver. A key to diagnosing BVDV-related abortions is timely submission of multiple fetuses. Often, it may take the submission of multiple fetuses before virus is identified.

Months of Gestation	1	2	3	4	5	6	7	8	9	Total
Number of Abortions			1		1	2	4	3	10	21

Fig. 2. Stage of gestation in which BVDV was identified in fetuses in an abortion outbreak on a large dairy farm (D.L. Grooms, DVM, PhD, unpublished data, 1994).

Identifying persistently infected cattle

Once it is established that BVDV is circulating on the farm by the use of herd screening tools or identification of the virus in aborted fetuses, screening the herd for persistently infected (PI) cattle should be considered. This is a significant decision because it may involve a considerable cost to test numerous individual animals. If individual testing is to be undertaken, it should be done as part of a comprehensive BVDV control program that includes the implementation of a biosecurity program to reduce the risk of reintroducing the virus, and a complete immunization program. Several strategies can be employed to screen the herd for PI cattle. The simplest strategy is to screen young stock and use results from those tests as an indicator of the status of that animal's dam. As an example, if a heifer is tested for persistent infection with BVDV and is negative, we can say with near 100% certainty that its dam is not a PI cow. If the calf tests positive, then we must test the dam also to determine if it too is a PI cow. This strategy works well as long as good records are present linking progeny to their dams. Obviously, not all dams are likely to have "sentinel" progeny on the farm at specific times; therefore, to complete the whole-herd screen, individual cattle who have no offspring on the farm need to be tested separately. Tests that can be used to screen cattle for persistent BVDV infection include virus isolation, immunoperoxidase microtiter assay (IPMA), antigen capture ELISA, immunohistochemistry (IHC)/fluorescent (FA) antibody skin test, and PCR. All of these tests have very similar sensitivities and specificities for detecting PI adult cattle. In the face of BVDV colostral antibodies found in neonatal calves, IHC/FA and PCR are the tests of choice. Test selection often comes down to the availability of the test, cost, and ease of sample collection and handling.

Diagnosis of reproductive loses related to leptospirosis

Epidemiology and reproductive consequences

Leptospirosis, caused by infection with any of the more than 200 serovars of *Leptospira*, is recognized as a cause of abortions, stillbirths, and birth of weak calves throughout the world. In addition, infertility and early embryonic death are increasingly being associated with infection with leptospires belonging to serovar Hardjo (either serovar Hardjo type hardjoprajitno or type hardjo-bovis), for whom cattle are the maintenance host. Although the precise prevalence of leptospirosis in cattle in North America is not known, infection with serovar Hardjo has become increasingly recognized, along with a decline in importance of serovar Pomona infections. Recent estimates of the prevalence of leptospiral infection in a sample of US dairies and beef cow-calf operations indicated that the overall herd infection prevalence was approximately 35% to 50%—with most of those infections likely caused by serovar Hardjo (C.A. Bolin, unpublished data, 2004).

Accurate data for the frequency of abortion attributable to infection with serovars Hardjo and Pomona are not readily available in North America. Abortion caused by Pomona has decreased in importance, probably because of vaccination, whereas abortion and stillbirth caused by Hardjo are recognized more commonly. In Northern Ireland, where both types of serovar Hardjo are present, Hardjo was recognized as responsible for nearly half of all bovine abortions in one study [15]. In one large study in Canada, where type hardjo-bovis is prevalent, serovar Hardjo caused about 6% of abortions; Pomona abortions were not recognized [16].

Many leptospiral infections are subclinical, particularly in nonpregnant and nonlactating animals, and are detected only by the presence of antibodies or lesions of interstitial nephritis at slaughter. The subacute to chronic form of disease is most often associated with reproductive sequelae, including fetal infection in pregnant cows presenting as abortion of an autolyzed fetus, stillbirth, or birth of premature and weak, infected calves. Hardjo-infected but apparently healthy calves also may be born [17]. Abortion storms may occur with serovars Pomona or Grippotyphosa infections, but sporadic abortions are more typical of serovar Hardjo infection. Abortions typically occur without premonitory signs and occur 1 or more weeks (Pomona, Grippotyphosa) or months (Hardjo) after infection of the cow.

Infertility and early embryonic death, which has responded to vaccination and treatment, has been described in Hardjo-infected herds [18–21]. The clinical signs include increased services per conception, prolonged calving intervals, delayed returns to heat, and failure to calve. The pathogenesis of these clinical signs is not clear, but is likely related to the persistent localization of leptospires in the uteruses and oviducts of Hardjo-infected cattle.

Diagnosis of leptospiral infections

Diagnosis of leptospirosis is dependent on the clinical and vaccination history and the results of diagnostic testing. Coordination between the diagnostic laboratory and the veterinarian is required to maximize the chances of making an accurate diagnosis. It is advisable to contact the diagnostic laboratory prior to submission of samples, in order to assure that appropriate samples are collected, and that the samples arrive at the diagnostic laboratory in suitable condition. In addition, in problem situations, it may be necessary to consult reference or regional diagnostic laboratories, which have expertise in the diagnosis of this infection.

In general, because *Leptospira* are known to cause reproductive sequelae in cattle, identification of the infection by detection of the organism or significant levels of antibody in the dam or in the herd is considered indicative that leptospirosis may be involved in the reproductive problems seen. Unfortunately, because of the lability of the organism and poor condition of many fetuses presented for examination, identification of the organism in the placenta or fetal tissues is often difficult.

Diagnostic tests for leptospirosis include those designed to detect antibodies against the organism and those designed to detect the organism or its DNA in tissues or body fluids of animals. Each of the diagnostic procedures, for detection of the organism or for antibodies directed against the organisms, has a number of advantages and disadvantages. Some of the assays suffer from a lack of sensitivity, and others are prone to specificity problems. Therefore, no single technique can be recommended for use in each clinical situation. Use of a combination of tests allows maximum sensitivity and specificity in establishing the diagnosis. Serological testing is recommended in each case, combined with one or more techniques to identify the organism in tissue or body fluids.

Serologic assays are the most commonly used technique for diagnosing leptospirosis in animals. Serology is inexpensive, reasonably sensitive, and widely available. The microscopic agglutination test involves mixing appropriate dilutions of serum with live leptospires of relevant serovars [22]. Presence of antibodies is indicated by the agglutination of the leptospires.

Detection of high titers of antibody in animals that have a disease consistent with leptospirosis may be sufficient to establish the diagnosis. This is particularly true in the investigation of abortions caused by serovars Pomona, Grippotyphosa, Canicola, and Icterohaemorrhagiae, in which the dam's agglutinating antibody titer is often ≥1600; however, Hardjo-infected cattle often have a poor agglutinating antibody response to infection. Anti-Hardjo antibody titers may be quite low or negative at the time of abortion. In abortion or stillbirth, it may be useful to do serologic testing on fetal serum, but dilutions should start at 1:10, in contrast to adult studies in which the usual starting dilution is 1:100.

Interpretation of leptospiral serologic results is complicated by a number of factors. These factors include cross-reactivity of antibodies, antibody titers induced by vaccination, and lack of consensus about what antibody titers are indicative of active infection. Antibodies produced in an animal in response to infection with a given serovar of *Leptospira* often cross-react with other serovars of leptospires. Therefore, a cow infected with a single serovar is likely to have antibodies against more than one serovar in an agglutination test. In general, however, the infecting serovar is assumed to be the serovar to which that animal develops the highest titer. Paradoxical reactions may occur with the agglutination test early in the course of an acute infection, with a marked agglutinating antibody response to a serovar other than the infecting serovar.

Widespread vaccination of cattle for leptospirosis also complicates the interpretation of leptospiral serology. In general, cattle develop relatively low agglutinating antibody titers (100–400) in response to vaccination, and these titers persist for 1 to 3 months after vaccination. Some animals, however, develop high titers after vaccination, and although these high vaccination titers decrease with time, they may persist for 6 months or more after vaccination.

The third complication of interpretation of leptospiral serological testing is caused by a lack of consensus as to what titer is significant for the diagnosis of leptospiral infection. An agglutinating antibody titer of >100 is considered significant by many; however, this cutoff level may be exceeded in vaccinated animals, and may not be reached in Hardjo infections. With serovar Hardjo, a significant percentage of cattle that are actively infected and shedding leptospires have anti-Hardjo antibody titers ≤100 [23]. Therefore, a low antibody titer does not necessarily rule out a diagnosis of leptospirosis. Antibody titers are often at a peak at the time of abortion and persist for months following infection, making paired serology around the time of abortion unlikely to demonstrate significant changes in titers.

Leptospires or leptospiral DNA in tissues or body fluids may be detected by immunofluorescence, culture, histopathology with special stains, and PCR assays. Each of these assays is useful in the diagnosis of leptospirosis, and each presents special advantages and disadvantages for routine use.

Immunofluorescence can be used to identify leptospires in tissues (fetal liver, lung, kidney, liver, or placenta) or urine sediment. The test is rapid, has reasonable sensitivity, and can be used on frozen samples. Interpretation of immunofluorescence tests requires a skilled laboratory technician. The fluorescent antibody conjugate currently available for general use is not serovar-specific; serologic examination of the animal is still required to help indicate the infecting serovar. Serovar-specific fluorescent antibody conjugates have been prepared, and are in use in Canada and some research laboratories in the United States.

Bacteriologic culture of urine or tissue specimens is the definitive method for the diagnosis of leptospirosis. Leptospires are usually present in the urine of animals 10 days after the onset of clinical signs. Urine for culture should be collected after injection of furosemide [24]. Furosemide increases the glomerular filtration rate and flushes more leptospires into the urine, producing dilute urine, which enhances survival of the leptospires. Culture of leptospires is difficult, time-consuming, and requires specialized culture medium; however, isolation of the organism from the animal allows definitive identification of the infecting serovar. Diagnostic laboratories rarely culture specimens for the presence of leptospires; however, a few laboratories with a particular interest in leptospirosis can conduct such testing, and can be consulted if leptospiral culture is required.

The use of special stains in histopathology can be effective for identification of leptospires in animal tissues. This common diagnostic technique is the only one that can be used on formalin-fixed tissues. Tissues to be examined include kidney in adults and placenta, lung, liver, and kidney in the case of abortions. Application of silver stains or immunohistochemical stains to tissue sections allows detection of leptospires or leptospiral antigens in the renal tubules and interstitium of the kidney, liver, lung, or placenta. Low sensitivity is a disadvantage of this diagnostic technique. Leptospires are often present in small numbers in affected tissues, particularly in chronic leptospirosis. The infecting serovar cannot be determined by histopathology; serologic studies must also be conducted.

PCR tests are being used for the diagnosis of leptospirosis in cattle [25–27]. A number of PCR procedures are available, and each laboratory running the test may select a slightly different procedure that works well for it. In general, PCR testing of urine is more reliable than testing of tissues. Processing of tissue samples is more difficult, and tissues often contain inhibitors to the amplification reaction, and may therefore cause false-negative results. Most PCR assays are able to detect the presence of leptospires, but are not able to determine the infecting serovar. PCR can be a sensitive and specific technique for the diagnosis of leptospirosis. Unfortunately, the process is complex and exquisitely sensitive to contamination with exogenous leptospiral DNA, and may therefore be prone to false-positive reactions. It is very important that PCR results be interpreted with full knowledge of the quality-control procedures used in the laboratory.

Summary

Determining a cause of reproductive loss in cattle can be difficult. With proper use of diagnostic tools and strategies, the chance of getting a more definitive diagnosis increases significantly. Bovine viral diarrhea virus and *Leptospira* are two common pathogens associated with reproductive losses in cattle. By understanding the disease pathogenesis and the diagnostic tools available, strategies to diagnose and control these important reproductive pathogens are available.

References

[1] Feuz DM, Umberger WJ. Beef cow-calf production. Vet Clin North Am Food Anim Pract 2003;19(2):339–63.
[2] Wolf CA. The economics of dairy production. Vet Clin North Am Food Anim Pract 2003; 19(2):271–93.
[3] Evermann JF, Ridpath JF. Clinical and epidemiologic observations of bovine viral diarrhea virus in the northwestern United States. Vet Microbiol 2002;89(2-3):129–39.

[4] Campero CM, Moore DP, Odeon AC, et al. Aetiology of bovine abortion in Argentina. Vet Res Commun 2003;27(5):359–69.

[5] Murray RD. A field investigation of causes of abortion in dairy cattle. Vet Rec 1990;127(22): 543–7.

[6] Jerrett IV, McOrist S, Waddington J, et al. Diagnostic studies of the fetus, placenta and maternal blood from 265 bovine abortions. Cornell Vet 1984;74(1):8–20.

[7] Agerholm JS, Willadsen CM, Nielsen TK, et al. Diagnostic studies of abortion in Danish dairy herds. Zentralbl Veterinarmed A 1997;44(9-10):551–8.

[8] Kirkbride CA. Viral agents and associated lesions detected in a 10-year study of bovine abortions and stillbirths. J Vet Diagn Invest 1992;4(4):374–9.

[9] Grooms DL. Reproductive consequences of infection with bovine viral diarrhea virus. Vet Clin North Am Food Anim Pract 2004;20(1):5–19.

[10] Renshaw RW, Ray R, Dubovi EJ. Comparison of virus isolation and reverse transcription polymerase chain reaction assay for detection of bovine viral diarrhea virus in bulk milk tank samples. J Vet Diagn Invest 2000;12(2):184–6.

[11] Radwan GS, Brock KV, Hogan JS, et al. Development of a PCR amplification assay as a screening test using bulk milk samples for identifying dairy herds infected with bovine viral diarrhea virus. Vet Microbiol 1995;44(1):77–91.

[12] Cortese VS, Whittaker R, Ellis J, et al. Specificity and duration of neutralizing antibodies induced in healthy cattle after administration of a modified-live virus vaccine against bovine viral diarrhea. Am J Vet Res 1998;59(7):848–50.

[13] Pillars RB, Grooms DL. Serologic evaluation of five unvaccinated heifers to detect herds that have cattle persistently infected with bovine viral diarrhea virus. Am J Vet Res 2002;63(4): 499–505.

[14] Houe H. Serological analysis of a small herd sample to predict presence or absence of animals persistently infected with bovine viral diarrhoea virus (BVDV) in dairy herds. Res Vet Sci 1992;53(3):320–3.

[15] Ellis WA, O'Brien JJ, Bryson DG, et al. Bovine leptospirosis: some clinical features of serovar Hardjo infection. Vet Rec 1985;117(5):101–4.

[16] Prescott JF, Miller RB, Nicholson VM, et al. Seroprevalence and association with abortions of leptospirosis in cattle in Ontario. Can J Vet Res 1989;52(2):210.

[17] Bolin CA, Thiermann AB, Handsaker AL, et al. Effect of vaccination with a pentavalent leptospiral vaccine on Leptospira interrogans serovar Hardjo type Hardjo-bovis infection of pregnant cattle. Am J Vet Res 1989;50(1):161–5.

[18] Dhaliwal GS, Murray RD, Ellis WA. Reproductive performance of dairy herds infected with Leptospira interrogans serovar Hardjo relative to the year of diagnosis. Vet Rec 1996; 138(12):272–6.

[19] Dhaliwal GS, Murray RD, Dobson H, et al. Reduced conception rates in dairy cattle associated with serological evidence of Leptospira interrogans serovar Hardjo infection. Vet Rec 1996;139(5):110–4.

[20] Dhaliwal GA, Murray RD, Dobson H, et al. Effect of vaccination against Leptospira interrogans serovar Hardjo on milk production and fertility in dairy cattle. Vet Rec 1996; 138(14):334–5.

[21] Ellis WA. Effects of leptospirosis on bovine reproduction. In: Morrow DA, editor. Current therapy in theriogenology. 2nd edition. Philadelphia: WB Saunders; 1986. p. 267–71.

[22] Bolin CA. Leptospirosis. In: Manual of diagnostic tests and vaccines for terrestrial animals. Geneva (Switzerland): Office Internationale des Epizooties; 2004. p. 316–27.

[23] Ellis WA. The diagnosis of leptospirosis in farm animals. In: Ellis WA, Little TWA, editors. The present state of leptospirosis diagnosis and control. Dordrecht (Netherlands): Martinus Nijhoff; 1986. p. 13–24.

[24] Nervig RM, Garrett LA. Use of furosemide to obtain urine samples for leptospiral isolation. Am J Vet Res 1979;40(8):1197–200.

[25] Gravekamp C, Van de Kemp H, Franzen M, et al. Detection of seven species of pathogenic leptospires by PCR using two sets of primers. J Gen Microbiol 1993;139(8):1691–700.

[26] Van Eys GJJM, Gravekamp C, Gerritsen MJ, et al. Detection of leptospires in urine by polymerase chain reaction. J Clin Microbiol 1989;27(10):2258–62.

[27] Wagenaar J, Zuerner RL, Alt DP, et al. Comparison of PCR assays with culture, immunofluorescence, and nucleic acid hybridization for detection of *Leptospira borgpetersenii* serovar Hardjo in bovine urine. Am J Vet Res 1998;61(3):316–20.

ELSEVIER
SAUNDERS

VETERINARY
CLINICS
Food Animal Practice

Vet Clin Food Anim 21 (2005) 473–483

Neosporosis in Cattle

J.P. Dubey, MVSc, PhD

Animal Parasitic Diseases Laboratory, Agricultural Research Service,
Animal and Natural Resources Institute, United States Department of Agriculture,
Beltsville Agricultural Research Center, Building 1001, Beltsville, MD, 20705-2350, USA

Neosporosis is caused by the protozoan parasite, *Neospora caninum.* Until 1988, *N caninum* was confused with a closely related parasite, *Toxoplasma gondii* [1,2]. Neosporosis has emerged as a serious disease of cattle and dogs worldwide [3,4]. Additionally, clinical neosporosis has been reported in sheep, goats, deer, a rhinoceros, alpacas, and horses [5]. Until now, viable *N caninum* has been isolated from dogs, cattle, white-tailed deer, water buffaloes and sheep. Antibodies to *N caninum* have been found in the sera of camels, canids, and felids.

N caninum is a coccidian parasite, and its oocysts have been found in feces of dogs and coyotes [6,7]. Thus, dogs are both the intermediate and definitive host for *N caninum* [2,6,8]. The life cycle is typified by three infectious stages: tachyzoites, tissue cysts, and oocysts (Figs. 1,2). Tachyzoites (Fig. 2A, B) and tissue cysts (Fig. 2C) are the stages found in the intermediate hosts, and they occur intracellularly [2]. Tachyzoites are approximately 6 × 2 µm. Tissue cysts are often round or oval in shape, up to 107 µm long, and are found primarily in the central nervous system. The tissue cyst wall is up to 4 µm thick and the enclosed bradyzoites are 7 to 8 × 2 µm. Thin-walled (0.3–1.0 µm) tissue cysts have been reported in muscles of cattle and dogs naturally infected with an *N caninum*-like parasite.

N caninum oocysts are excreted unsporulated in feces and measure approximately 12 µm in diameter; sporulation occurs outside the host (Fig. 2D, E). At the present, little is known regarding the frequency of shedding of oocysts, the survival of the oocysts in the environment, and whether other canids are also definitive hosts for *N caninum* [9]. The parasite can be transmitted transplacentally in several hosts, and vertical route is the major mode of its transmission in cattle [10,11]. There is no cow-to-cow transmission of *N caninum* [11]. Although most *N caninum* infections in cattle are transmitted transplacentally, postnatal rates have been variable,

E-mail address: jdubey@anri.barc.usda.gov

0749-0720/05/$ - see front matter. Published by Elsevier Inc.
doi:10.1016/j.cvfa.2005.03.004

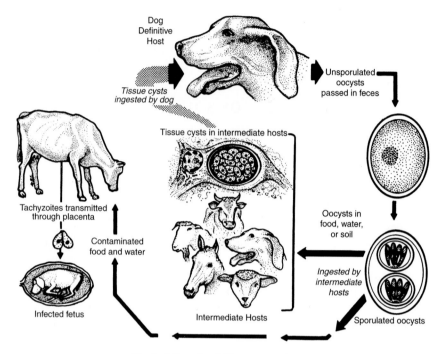

Fig. 1. Life cycle of *Neospora caninum.*

depending on the region of the country, type of test used, and cutoff values used [12]. Although *N caninum* has been found in bovine semen [13], it is unlikely that *N caninum* is transmitted venereally or by embryo transfer from the donor cows. Actually, embryo transfer is even recommended as a method of control to prevent vertical transmission [14,15]; however, it is prudent to test all recipients, and embryos should not be transferred to seropositive cows. Lactogenic transmission of *N caninum* has been demonstrated experimentally in newborn calves fed colostrum spiked with tachyzoites, but there is no evidence that it occurs naturally [12,16–18]. Carnivores can acquire infection by ingestion of infected tissues.

Clinical signs

N caninum causes abortion in both dairy and beef cattle [19–26]. Cows of any age may abort from 3 months of gestation to term. Most neosporosis-induced abortions occur at 5 to 6 months of gestation. Fetuses may die in utero, be resorbed, mummified, autolyzed, stillborn, born alive with clinical signs, or born clinically normal but chronically infected. Neosporosis-induced abortions occur year-round. Cows that have *N caninum* antibodies (seropositive) are more likely to abort than seronegative cows, and this applies to both dairy and beef cattle; however, up to 95% of calves born

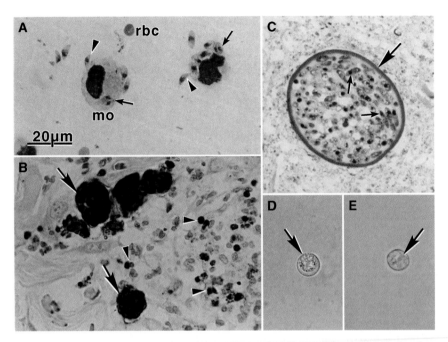

Fig. 2. *Neospora caninum* stages in dogs. Bar = 20 μm and applies to all figures. (*A*) Tachyzoites in an impression smear of lung. Giemsa stain. Note individual organisms (*arrowheads*) and those dividing into two (*arrows*). Compare size with red blood cells (rbc) and a macrophage (mo). (*B*) Tachyzoites in groups (*arrows*) and individuals (*arrowheads*) in sections of skin. Immunohistochemical stain with anti-*N caninum* antibody. (*C*) Tissue cyst in section of brain. Note thick tissue cyst wall (*large arrow*) enclosing bradyzoites (*smaller arrows*). Toluidine blue stain. (*D*) Unsporulated oocyst with an individual sporont (*arrow*). Unstained. (*E*) Sporulated oocyst (*arrow*). Unstained.

congenitally infected from seropositive dams remain clinically normal. The age of dam, lactation number, and history of abortion generally do not affect rate of congenital infection, but there are reports indicating that in persistently infected cattle, vertical transmission is more efficient in younger than older cows [12]. The infected replacement heifers may either abort or transplacentally infect their offspring.

Clinical signs have only been reported in cattle younger than 2 month of age. *N caninum*-infected calves may have neurologic signs, be underweight, unable to rise, or be born without clinical signs of disease [3,27,28]. Hind limbs or forelimbs or both may be flexed or hyperextended. Neurologic examination may reveal ataxia, decreased patellar reflexes, and loss of conscious proprioception. Calves may have exophthalmia or asymmetrical appearance in the eyes. *N caninum* occasionally causes birth defects, including hydrocephalus and narrowing of the spinal cord [29].

Abortions may be epidemic or endemic [23–25]. As many as 33% of dairy cow fetuses have been reported to abort within a few months. Abortions were considered epidemic if more than 10% of cows at risk aborted within 6 to 8 weeks. A small proportion (<5%) of cows have been reported to have repeated abortion due to neosporosis [22]. Cows that have *N caninum* antibodies (seropositive) are more likely to abort than seronegative cows. There is a rise in antibody titers 4 to 5 months before parturition. These observations strongly suggest reactivation of latent infection. Little is known of the mechanism of reactivation. It is likely that there is parasitemia during pregnancy, leading to fetal infection; however, *N caninum* has never been identified in histologic sections of adult cows, and there is a single report of isolation of viable *N caninum* from the brain of an adult cow [30]. Although it is reasonable to speculate that pregnancy-induced immune-suppression or hormonal imbalance may reactivate latent tissue cysts of *N caninum*, such a mechanism has not been demonstrated for neosporosis. *N caninum* DNA has been found in blood of naturally-infected cattle, indicating parasitemia [31].

N caninum is one of the most efficiently transplacentally-transmitted organisms in cattle. In some herds, up to 90% of cattle are infected, and most calves born congenitally infected with *N caninum* remain healthy. Therefore, there is a debate concerning whether *N caninum* causes abortion in cattle or whether it is a bystander [4]. All evidence at the present time indicates that *N caninum* is a primary pathogen.

Prevalence

N caninum infections have been reported from most parts of the world, including Australia, New Zealand, Europe, Korea, Japan, Thailand, and the Americas. Quantitative studies in the United States, New Zealand, the Netherlands, and Germany indicate that 12% to 45% of aborted fetuses from dairy cattle are infected with *N caninum* (Table 1).

Table 1
Diagnosis of *N caninum*-associated abortion in dairy cattle from selected studies

Country	References	No. of fetuses examined	Percent infected
Argentina	[32]	240	12.1
Australia	[33]	729	21.0
Brazil	[34]	46	39.1
Korea	[35]	180	21.2
Germany	[36]	135	12.6
Mexico	[37]	211	77.0
Spain	[38]	80	31.3
Switzerland	[39]	242	21.0
The Netherlands	[40]	2053	17.0
United States	[20]	698	24.4
	[22]	266	45

Serologic prevalence in cattle varies, depending on the country, region, type of serologic test used, and cutoff level used to determine the exposure. In some dairies, up to 87% of cows are seropositive.

In general, less is known of the causes of abortion in beef cattle than in dairy cattle, because of the difficulty of finding small fetuses expelled in the first trimester. Therefore, there are no accurate assessments of *Neospora*-induced losses in beef cattle. Because clinical disease has not been reported in calves older than 2 months of age, there is no direct evidence of *N caninum*-associated morbidity in adult cattle.

Diagnosis

Examination of the serum from an aborting cow is only indicative of exposure to *N caninum*, and histologic examination of the fetus is necessary for a definitive diagnosis of neosporosis. The brain, heart, liver, placenta, and body fluids or blood serum are the best specimens for diagnosis, and diagnostic rates are higher if multiple tissues are examined. Although lesions of neosporosis are found in several organs, fetal brain is the most consistently affected organ [3,21,25]. Because most aborted fetuses are likely to be autolyzed, even semiliquid brain tissue should be fixed in 10% buffered neutral formalin for histologic examination of hematoxylin- and eosin- (H and E) stained sections. Immunohistochemistry is necessary because there are generally only a few *N caninum* present in autolyzed tissues, and these are often not visible in H- and E-stained sections. The most characteristic lesion of neosporosis is focal encephalitis characterized by necrosis and nonsuppurative inflammation [21]. Hepatitis is more common in epizootic than sporadic abortions [40]. Lesions are also present in placenta, but protozoa are difficult to find.

The efficiency of the diagnosis by polymerase chain reaction (PCR) is dependent on the laboratory, stage of the autolysis of the fetus, and sampling procedures [41]. Although immunohistochemical demonstration of *N caninum* in lesions is the best evidence for etiology of abortion at the present time, it is very insensitive. *N caninum* DNA can be detected by PCR in formalin-fixed, paraffin-embedded, aborted bovine brain tissue.

Several serologic tests can be used to detect *N caninum* antibodies, including various enzyme-linked immunosorbent assays (ELISAs), the indirect fluorescent antibody test (IFAT), and the *Neospora* agglutination test (NAT) [42–52]. There are several modifications of the ELISA test used to detect antibodies to *N caninum* in sera or milk, using whole parasite, whole parasite lysate, purified proteins, recombinant proteins, and tachyzoite proteins absorbed on immunostimulating complex (ISCOM) particles, and some of these tests were compared recently in a multicentered study in various laboratories in Europe [53]. Avidity ELISAs designed to distinguish recent and chronic infections in cattle appear promising to distinguish endemic and epidemic abortion. In the avidity ELISAs, sera are treated with urea to release low-avidity (low-affinity) antibodies, and differences in values obtained before and after treatment with urea are used to evaluate recency of infection. In recently acquired infection, avidity values are low [24,48,52]. Another modification of ELISA is antigen-capture (cELISA). This test detects (captures) a 65-kD antigen in sera of infected cattle using a specific monoclonal antibody, and this test is commercially available [54,55]. Immunoblots are useful in detecting *N caninum*-specific antibodies.

Finding *N caninum* antibody in serum from the fetus can establish *N caninum* infection, but a negative result is not informative, because antibody synthesis in the fetus is dependent on the stage of gestation, level of exposure, and the time between infection and abortion. Immunoblotting using *N caninum*-specific antigen improves diagnosis. Although blood serum or any body fluid from the fetus may be used for serologic diagnosis, peritoneal fluid is better than other body fluids. In calves, presuckling serum can be submitted for diagnosis of congenital infection.

The definitive antibody level that should be considered diagnostic for neosporosis has not been established for bovines, because of the uncertainty of serologic diagnosis in chronically infected animals and the availability of sera from noninfected cattle. In serological assays, titer and absorbance values are dependent on antigen composition, secondary antibodies, and other reagents [42,43,47,52]. Further, cutoff levels can be arbitrarily selected to provide sensitivity and specificity requested for a particular application. The age and class of an animal may also affect selection of a cutoff level. Although *N caninum* is closely related to *T gondii*, *Sarcocystis* species, and other apicomplexans, cross-reactivity has not been a major issue. Antibody titers in general are higher in cattle that have aborted due to neosporosis than those who have normal pregnancy; however, titers in individual cows cannot determine etiology of abortions [47].

T gondii and *Sarcocystis cruzi* are two other protozoans that should be considered in the differential diagnosis of protozoal abortion in cattle. Immunohistochemical and detection of parasite DNA by PCR can distinguish them from *N caninum*. *S cruzi* forms schizonts in vascular endothelium and is rarely (<0.1%) found in aborted fetal brains, whereas *N caninum* is usually located in extravascular tissues. Additionally, there are no immature schizonts in *N caninum* infection, in contrast with *S cruzi* infections. Infection by *T gondii* in bovine fetuses is rare [56]. Attempts at isolation of viable *N caninum* by bioassay in mice or cell culture have been largely unsuccessful.

Control

N caninum is efficiently transmitted vertically in cattle, perhaps for several generations. Therefore, culling is one way at present to prevent this transmission from cow to heifer [57,58]; however, culling will not be practical if the prevalence of *N caninum* in a herd is very high. Before making a decision to cull, it is advisable to estimate prevalence of *N caninum* in the herd. Bulk-milk testing can provide the preliminary information about the presence of *N caninum* infection [26,44]. If bulk-milk test is positive, antibody prevalence in dam-heifer samples and cattle of different ages can provide insight to the transmission of *N caninum* in a given herd. In herds that have a high transplacental transmission, prevalence of *N caninum* in cattle of different ages is about the same, and there is high correlation between infection in dams and daughters. To reduce vertical transmission of *N caninum*, culling of seropositive dams or heifer calves from seropositive cows and embryo transfer from seropositive cows to seronegative cows are some of the methods that can be adapted. Drugs that will kill encysted *N caninum* in bovine tissues are unknown.

To prevent horizontal (from outside sources) transmission, it is important to prevent exposure of the cows to feed and water contaminated with oocysts [4,59–61]. Dogs and other canids should not be allowed in cattle barns or pasture, although this is not easy to achieve. How dogs become infected with *N caninum* is not known. Consumption of aborted bovine fetuses does not appear to be an important source of *N caninum* infection in dogs. The consumption of placental membranes may be a source of *N caninum* infection in dogs, because the parasite has been found in naturally-infected placentas, and dogs fed placentas shed *N caninum* oocysts [18]. Little is known at present regarding the frequency of shedding of *N caninum* oocysts by canids in nature, the resistance of the oocysts, and whether dogs shed oocysts more than once. Until more definitive hosts of *N caninum* are found, dogs and coyotes should not be allowed to eat aborted fetuses, fetal membranes, or dead calves. Other factors, such as farm location, can also be risks [61]. Drugs that will prevent transmission of the parasite for the dam to the fetus are unknown, but research is continuing in this area.

There is evidence that cattle can develop protective immunity to subsequent neosporosis abortion [22,24,62,63]. This protective immunity appears to be more effective in cows that are subsequently infected with an exogenous source (oocysts) than in cows in which there is a recrudescence of a persistent infection [64]. Therefore, to elicit protective immunity against abortion in cows that already harbor a latent infection is a problem.

Currently, there is a killed parasite commercial *N caninum* vaccine (Neo Guard, Intervet, Kansas City, Kansas) but there are no convincing data about the efficiency of this vaccine to prevent *N caninum*-associated abortion in cattle [65–67].

Summary

In conclusion, neosporosis is an enigmatic infection of cattle, and inducing immunity to congenital transfer of *N caninum* is a challenge for immunologists, parasitologists, and veterinarians. Further research is needed regarding the pathogenesis of *N caninum* abortion, lifecycle of the parasite in cattle, and sources of infection.

References

[1] Dubey JP, Carpenter JL, Speer CA, et al. Newly recognized fatal protozoan disease of dogs. J Am Vet Med Assoc 1988;192:1269–85.

[2] Dubey JP, Barr BC, Barta JR, et al. Redescription of *Neospora caninum* and its differentiation from related coccidia. Int J Parasitol 2002;32:929–46.

[3] Dubey JP, Lindsay DS. A review of *Neospora caninum* and neosporosis. Vet Parasitol 1996; 67:1–59.

[4] Dubey JP. Neosporosis in cattle. J Parasitol 2003;89(Suppl):S42–56.

[5] Dubey JP. Review of *Neospora caninum* and neosporosis in animals. Korean J Parasitol 2003;41:1–16.

[6] McAllister MM, Dubey JP, Lindsay DS, et al. Dogs are definitive hosts of *Neospora caninum*. Int J Parasitol 1998;28:1473–8.

[7] Gondim LFP, McAllister MM, Pitt WC, et al. Coyotes (*Canis latrans*) are definitive hosts of *Neospora caninum*. Int J Parasitol 2004;34:159–61.

[8] Basso W, Venturini L, Venturini MC, et al. First isolation of *Neospora caninum* from the feces of a naturally infected dog. J Parasitol 2001;87:612–8.

[9] Gondim LFP, Gao L, McAllister MM. Improved production of *Neospora caninum* oocysts, cyclical oral transmission between dogs and cattle, and in vitro isolation from oocysts. J Parasitol 2002;88:1159–63.

[10] Anderson ML, Andrianarivo AG, Conrad PA. Neosporosis in cattle. Anim Reprod Sci 2000;60–61:417–31.

[11] Anderson ML, Reynolds JP, Rowe JD, et al. Evidence of vertical transmission of *Neospora sp* infection in dairy cattle. J Am Vet Med Assoc 1997;210:1169–72.

[12] Dijkstra T. Horizontal and vertical transmission of *Neospora caninum* [PhD thesis]. Utrecht, Netherlands: Universiteit Utrecht; 2002. p. 1–140.

[13] Ortega-Mora LM, Ferre I, del Pozo I, et al. Detection of *Neospora caninum* in semen of bulls. Vet Parasitol 2003;117:301–8.

[14] Baillargeon P, Fecteau G, Paré J, et al. Evaluation of the embryo transfer procedure proposed by the International Embryo Transfer Society as a method of controlling vertical transmission of *Neospora caninum* in cattle. J Am Vet Med Assoc 2001;218: 1803–6.

[15] Landmann JK, Jillella D, O'Donoghue PJ, et al. Confirmation of the prevention of vertical transmission of *Neospora caninum* in cattle by the use of embryo transfer. Aust Vet J 2002;80: 502–3.

[16] Davison HC, Guy CS, McGarry JW, et al. Experimental studies on the transmission of *Neospora caninum* between cattle. Res Vet Sci 2001;70:163–8.

[17] Uggla A, Stenlund S, Holmdahl OJM, et al. Oral *Neospora caninum* inoculation of neonatal calves. Int J Parasitol 1998;28:1467–72.

[18] Dijkstra T, Eysker M, Schares G, et al. Dogs shed *Neospora caninum* oocysts after ingestion of naturally infected bovine placenta but not after ingestion of colostrum spiked with Neospora caninum tachyzoites. Int J Parasitol 2001;31:747–52.

[19] Thilsted JP, Dubey JP. Neosporosis-like abortions in a herd of dairy cattle. J Vet Diagn Invest 1989;1:205–9.

[20] Anderson ML, Blanchard PC, Barr BC, et al. *Neospora*-like protozoan infection as a major cause of abortion in California dairy cattle. J Am Vet Med Assoc 1991;198: 241–4.

[21] Barr BC, Anderson ML, Dubey JP, et al. *Neospora*-like protozoal infections associated with bovine abortions. Vet Pathol 1991;28:110–6.

[22] Anderson ML, Palmer CW, Thurmond MC, et al. Evaluation of abortions in cattle attributable to neosporosis in selected dairy herds in California. J Am Vet Med Assoc 1995; 207:1206–10.

[23] McAllister M, Huffman EM, Hietala SK, et al. Evidence suggesting a point source exposure in an outbreak of bovine abortion due to neosporosis. J Vet Diagn Invest 1996;8: 355–7.

[24] McAllister MM, Björkman C, Anderson-Sprecher R, et al. Evidence of point-source exposure to *Neospora caninum* and protective immunity in a herd of beef cows. J Am Vet Med Assoc 2000;217:881–7.

[25] Wouda W. *Neospora* abortion in cattle, aspects of diagnosis and epidemiology [PhD thesis]. Utrecht, Netherlands: Universiteit of Utrecht; 1998. p. 1–176.

[26] Frössling J. Epidemiology of *Neospora caninum* infection in cattle: evaluation of diagnostic tests and herd studies. Upppsala (Sweden): Swedish University of Agricultural Sciences; 2004.

[27] Barr BC, Conrad PA, Breitmeyer R, et al. Congenital *Neospora* infection in calves born from cows that had previously aborted *Neospora*-infected fetuses: four cases (1990–1992). J Am Vet Med Assoc 1993;202:113–7.

[28] Barr BC, Conrad PA, Dubey JP, et al. *Neospora*-like encephalomyelitis in a calf: pathology, ultrastructure, and immunoreactivity. J Vet Diagn Invest 1991;3:39–46.

[29] Dubey JP, Abbitt B, Topper MJ, et al. Hydrocephalus associated with *Neospora caninum*-infection in an aborted bovine fetus. J Comp Pathol 1998;118:169–73.

[30] Sawada M, Kondo H, Tomioka Y, et al. Isolation of *Neospora caninum* from the brain of a naturally infected adult dairy cow. Vet Parasitol 2000;90:247–52.

[31] Okeoma CM, Williamson NB, Pomroy WE, et al. The use of PCR to detect *Neospora caninum* DNA in the blood of naturally infected cows. Vet Parasitol 2004;122:307–15.

[32] Moore DP, Campero CM, Odeón AC, et al. Seroepidemiology of beef and dairy herds and fetal study of *Neospora caninum* in Argentina. Vet Parasitol 2002;107:303–16.

[33] Boulton JG, Gill PA, Cook RW, et al. Bovine *Neospora* abortion in north-eastern New South Wales. Aust Vet J 1995;72:119–20.

[34] Corbellini LG, Driemeier D, Cruz CFE, et al. Neosporosis as a cause of abortion in dairy cattle in Rio Grande do Sul, southern Brazil. Vet Parasitol 2002;103:195–202.

[35] Kim JH, Lee JK, Lee BC, Park BK, et al. Diagnostic survey of bovine abortion in Korea: with special emphasis on *Neospora caninum*. J Vet Med Sci 2002;64:1123–7.

[36] Söndgen P, Peters M, Bärwald A, et al. Bovine neosporosis: immunoblot improves foetal serology. Vet Parasitol 2001;102:279–90.

[37] Morales E, Trigo FJ, Ibarra F, et al. Neosporosis in Mexican dairy herds: lesions and immunohistochemical detection of *Neospora caninum* in fetuses. J Comp Pathol 2001;125: 58–63.

[38] Pereira-Bueno J, Quintanilla-Gozalo A, Pérez-Pérez V, et al. Evaluation by different diagnostic techniques of bovine abortion associated with *Neospora caninum* in Spain. Vet Parasitol 2003;111:143–52.

[39] Sager H, Fischer I, Furrer K, et al. A Swiss case-control study to assess *Neospora caninum*-associated bovine abortions by PCR, histopathology and serology. Vet Parasitol 2001;102: 1–15.

[40] Wouda W, Moen AR, Visser IJR, et al. Bovine fetal neosporosis: a comparison of epizootic and sporadic abortion cases and different age classes with regard to lesion severity and immunohistochemical identification of organisms in brain, heart, and liver. J Vet Diagn Invest 1997;9:180–5.

[41] Baszler TV, Gay LJC, Long MT, et al. Detection by PCR of *Neospora caninum* in fetal tissues from spontaneous bovine abortions. J Clin Microbiol 1999;37:4059–64.

[42] Álvarez-García G, Collantes-Fernández E, Costas E, et al. Influence of age and purpose for testing on the cut-off selection of serological methods in bovine neosporosis. Vet Res 2003; 34:341–52.

[43] Björkman C, Uggla A. Serological diagnosis of *Neospora caninum* infection. Int J Parasitol 1999;29:1497–507.

[44] Björkman C, Holmdahl OJM, Uggla A. An indirect enzyme-linked immumoassay (ELISA) for demonstration of antibodies to *Neospora caninum* in serum and milk of cattle. Vet Parasitol 1997;68:251–60.

[45] Conrad PA, Sverlow K, Anderson M, et al. Detection of serum antibody responses in cattle with natural or experimental *Neospora* infections. J Vet Diagn Invest 1993;5:572–8.

[46] Dijkstra T, Barkema HW, Eysker M, et al. Evaluation of a single serological screening of dairy herds for *Neospora caninum* antibodies. Vet Parasitol 2003;110:161–9.

[47] Dubey JP, Jenkins MC, Adams DS, et al. Antibody responses of cows during an outbreak of neosporosis evaluated by indirect fluorescent antibody test and different enzyme-linked immunosorbent assays. J Parasitol 1997;83:1063–9.

[48] Jenkins MC, Caver JA, Björkman C, et al. Serological investigation of an outbreak of *Neospora caninum*-associated abortion in a dairy herd in southeastern United States. Vet Parasitol 2000;94:17–26.

[49] Paré J, Hietala SK, Thurmond MC. An enzyme-linked immunosorbent assay (ELISA) for serological diagnosis of *Neospora sp* infection in cattle. J Vet Diagn Invest 1995;7: 352–9.

[50] Schares G, Conraths FJ, Reichel MP. Bovine neosporosis: comparison of serological methods using outbreak sera from a dairy herd in New Zealand. Int J Parasitol 1999;29: 1659–67.

[51] Schares G, Bärwald A, Staubach C, et al. Adaptation of a commercial ELISA for the detection of antibodies against *Neospora caninum* in bovine milk. Vet Parasitol 2004;120: 55–63.

[52] Björkman C, McAllister MM, Frössling J, et al. Application of the *Neospora caninum* IgG avidity ELISA in assessment of chronic reproductive losses after an outbreak of neosporosis in a herd of beef cattle. J Vet Diagn Invest 2003;15:3–7.

[53] von Blumröder D, Schares G, Norton R, et al. Comparison and standardisation of serological methods for the diagnosis of *Neospora caninum* infection in bovines. Vet Parasitol 2004;120:11–22.

[54] Baszler TV, Knowles DP, Dubey JP, et al. Serological diagnosis of bovine neosporosis by *Neospora caninum* monoclonal antibody-based competitive inhibition enzyme-linked immunosorbent assay. J Clin Microbiol 1996;34:1423–8.

[55] Baszler TV, Adams S, Vander-Schalie J, et al. Validation of a commercially available monoclonal antibody-based competitive-inhibition enzyme-linked immunosorbent assay for detection of serum antibodies to *Neospora caninum* in cattle. J Clin Microbiol 2001;39: 3851–7.

[56] Canada N, Meireles CS, Rocha A, et al. Isolation of viable *Toxoplasma gondii* from naturally-infected aborted bovine fetuses. J Parasitol 2002;88:1247–8.

[57] Reichel MP, Ellis JT. Control options for *Neospora caninum* infections in cattle—current state of knowledge. N Z Vet J 2002;50:86–92.

[58] Thurmond M, Hietala S. Strategies to control *Neospora* infection in cattle. The Bovine Practitioner 1995;29:60–3.

[59] Dijkstra T, Barkema HW, Hesselink JW, et al. Point source exposure of cattle to *Neospora caninum* consistent with periods of common housing and feeding and related to the introduction of a dog. Vet Parasitol 2002;105:89–98.

[60] Wouda W, Bartels CJM, Dijkstra T. Epidemiology of bovine neosporosis with emphasis on risk factors. Int J Parasitol 2000;30:884–6.

[61] Schares G, Bärwald A, Staubach C, et al. Potential risk factors for bovine *Neospora caninum* infection in Germany are not under the control of the farmers. Parasitology 2004;129:301–9.

[62] Innes EA, Wright SE, Maley S, et al. Protection against vertical transmission in bovine neosporosis. Int J Parasitol 2001;31:1523–34.

[63] Innes EA, Andrianarivo AG, Björkman C, et al. Immune responses to *Neospora caninum* and prospects for vaccination. Trends Parasitol 2002;18:497–504.

[64] Trees AJ, Williams DJL. Vaccination against bovine neosporosis—the challenge is the challenge. J Parasitol 2003;89:S198–201.

[65] Barling KS, Lunt DK, Graham SL, et al. Evaluation of an inactivated *Neospora caninum* vaccine in beef feedlot steers. J Am Vet Med Assoc 2003;222:624–7.

[66] Choromanski L, Block W. Humoral immune responses and safety of experimental formulations of inactivated *Neospora* vaccines. Parasitol Res 2000;86:851–3.

[67] Romero JJ, Pérez E, Frankena K. Effect of a killed whole *Neospora caninum* tachyzoite vaccine on the crude abortion rate of Costa Rican dairy cows under field conditions. Vet Parasitol 2004;123:149–59.

ELSEVIER
SAUNDERS

Vet Clin Food Anim 21 (2005) 485–501

VETERINARY
CLINICS
Food Animal Practice

Management of Transition Cows to Optimize Reproductive Efficiency in Dairy Herds

Pedro Melendez, DVM, MS, PhD*,
Carlos A. Risco, DVM

Department of Large Animal Clinical Sciences, Section of Food Animal Reproduction and Medicine Service, College of Veterinary Medicine, University of Florida, P.O. Box 100136, Gainesville, FL 32610-0136, USA

The transition period of the dairy cow influences productive and reproductive responses during lactation, and is therefore considered a pivotal time in the production cycle of the cow. During this period, cows are at higher risk of developing diseases related to the metabolic challenges of parturition and the beginning of lactation. At the herd level, the incidence of these diseases can be significantly reduced by appropriate management of the prepartum cow that addresses the metabolic and nutritional needs related to parturition and lactation. This article discusses: (1) the metabolic changes that occur around parturition and their role in disease causation that affect reproduction, and (2) management strategies to prevent calving-related diseases (CRDs).

Definitions

The transition period in dairy cows is defined as the last 3 weeks before and the 3 weeks after parturition [1,2]. This period is characterized by tremendous metabolic and endocrine challenges related to parturition and the onset of lactation [3]. If these challenges are not met by the cow's homeostatic mechanisms, the cow can experience diseases such as, milk fever (MF) or clinical hypocalcemia, ketosis, retained fetal membranes (RFM), metritis, mastitis, and displacement of the abomasum (DA) [1,4]

* Corresponding author.
E-mail address: melendezp@mail.vetmed.ufl.edu (P. Melendez).

0749-0720/05/$ - see front matter © 2005 Elsevier Inc. All rights reserved.
doi:10.1016/j.cvfa.2005.02.008
vetfood.theclinics.com

These diseases primarily affect cows within the first 2 weeks postpartum [4]; however, diseases that become clinically apparent later postpartum, such as laminitis, ovarian cysts, endometritis and anestrus, are related to the early postpartum [1].

Body condition score (BCS) at calving and changes during the postpartum period, milk production, parity, and the incidence of CRD affect the reproductive efficiency of dairy cows during lactation. Collectively, these diseases and conditions suggest that a successful reproductive management of dairy cows must integrate the disciplines of nutrition and herd health programs in order to optimize both milk and reproductive responses.

Physiological changes during the transition period

During late gestation, the dairy cow undergoes a series of complex metabolic and physiological changes as parturition approaches. Mammary gland prepares for lactogenesis, and fetal growth is exponential. Feed intake decreases gradually and parturition is particularly stressful for the cow, with suppression of immune function [1]. CRDs that consequently will affect subsequent fertility of the lactating cow are intimately associated with these changes [1]. Therefore, to properly manage the transition cow, it is important for the clinician to understand how these mechanisms are related to disease causation in order to establish preventive strategies.

Dry matter intake

Dry matter intake (DMI) starts to decrease a few weeks before parturition, with a nadir occurring at calving [5]. Average values for the prepartum transition period have been reported to range between 1.7% and 2.0% of body weight (BW) [6]; however, this is not a constant value, and it can be influenced by the ration that is fed, the stage of the transition period, BCS, and parity [7]. Dry matter intake decreases about 32% during the final 3 weeks of gestation, and 89% of that decline occurs at 5 to 7 days before calving [5,7]. A reduction in DMI and continued fetal growth are mitigating factors for fat mobilization and prepartum ketosis, which can have a deleterious effect on postpartum health.

Glucose and lipid metabolism

Glucose and amino acids are the major fuel supply of the developing fetus in ruminants. Glucose and amino acids are also needed by the mammary gland for lactose and milk protein synthesis, respectively [3,8]. Ruminants are not entirely dependent on dietary glucose; as a result they are in a constant stage of gluconeogenesis [9]. The major gluconeogenic precursor in ruminants is propionic acid produced in the rumen. Its contribution to gluconeogenesis has been estimated to be 32% to 73% [10]. Liver uptake of propionate by portal circulation is almost 100% [9], and its metabolism is modulated during the transition period [11,12]. Amino acids, lactate, and glycerol are secondary substrates for gluconeogenesis in ruminants [9]. The contribution of these secondary precursors is partially dependent upon their supply and metabolic adaptation of transition dairy cows [3].

Non-esterified fatty acids (NEFA) concentrations are maximal at parturition (0.9 to 1.2 mEq/L), with a slow decrease after 3 days postpartum [13]. This finding corroborates the elevated fat mobilization occurring around parturition in dairy cows. Extreme rates of lipid mobilization lead to increased uptake of NEFA by the liver, and increased triglyceride (TG) accumulation [4]. When blood glucose concentrations increase, lipogenesis predominates over lypolysis, NEFA release from adipose tissue is decreased, and ketogenesis is depressed [8]. The effect of glucose on adipose tissue is related to insulin secretion and its role in glycerol synthesis, which is essential for TG assembly [8]. When glucose concentration decreases, NEFA mobilization from adipose tissue is stimulated and ketogenesis is increased [8,14].

Calving-related diseases

The majority of diseases that affect dairy cows during postpartum are consequences of metabolic and immunological events during the peripartal period, and are referred to as CRDs [15]. The most relevant CRDs are MF (clinical hypocalcemia), RFM, metritis, ketosis, DA, mastitis, and lameness [1,15]. In general, these diseases present low heritabilities ($h^2 = 0$–0.05), and management plays a major role in determining their incidence. Some exceptions are lameness ($h^2 = 0.16$) and ketosis ($h^2 = 0.39$), although genetic correlations are low [16].

CRDs result in significant economic losses to dairy producers through reduction in reproductive performance and milk yield during the subsequent lactation, cost of treatments, and increased culling [15].

Several studies that have described the relationship and risk factors among CRDs in dairy cattle are shown in Table 1. Although results in general have been reliable, case or disease definitions have not been consistent. In an effort to homogenize criteria definitions, Kelton et al [17] recommended some guidelines for recording and calculating selected clinical diseases in dairy cattle (Table 2).

Management of the transition period

Management of the transition period must be focused on maintenance of physiological functions during the peripartal period, normocalcemia, adaptation of the rumen to a high-energy diet, and a strong immune

Table 1
Summary of associations and odds ratios among calving-related diseases

Study	Disease	Risk factors	Association
Erb et al [18]	RFM	Milk fever	OR = 2.0
		Parity	Positive
	Milk fever	Parity	Positive
	Metritis	Milk fever	OR = 1.6
		RFM	OR = 5.8
Curtis et al [19]	Milk fever	Parity	Positive
	RFM	Milk fever	OR = 4.0
		Parity	Positive
	Metritis	RFM	OR = 5.7
		LDA	OR = 3.6
	LDA	Ketosis	OR = 11.9
	Ketosis	LDA	OR = 53.5
		RFM	OR = 16.4
		Milk fever	OR = 23.6
Correa et al [20]	RFM	Dystocia	OR = 2.2
		Twinning	OR = 3.4
	Metritis	Dystocia	OR = 2.1
		RFM	OR = 6.0
		Ketosis	OR = 1.7
	Ketosis	Milk fever	OR = 2.4
	LDA	Milk fever	OR = 2.3
		Ketosis	OR = 13.8
		Dystocia	OR = 2.3
Melendez et al [21]	Ovarian cysts	Lameness	Positive
Melendez et al [22]	Ketosis	Displacement of abomasums	Positive
	Displacement of abomasums	Retained fetal membranes	Positive
		Ketosis	Positive
		Parity	Positive
	Metritis	Retained fetal membranes	Positive
		Parity	Negative

Abbreviations: LDA, left displacement of the abomasum; OR, odds ratio.

system. In addition, it is equally important to optimize cow comfort, maintain an appropriate BCS, and provide proper calving assistance. If these conditions are not met, the peripartal cow is at risk of developing metabolic and infectious diseases during the postpartum period [1,15,23,24].

Strategies to prevent milk fever (clinical hypocalcemia)

For many years, the traditional method of preventing MF in dairy cows was the restriction of dietary intake of calcium (Ca) during the prepartum period. Diets with <15–20 g of Ca/d fed during the last 10 days of gestation, followed by a postpartum diet that is high in Ca have been recommended. These diets will greatly reduce the risk of MF [25–28]; however, they are difficult to formulate under present practical conditions.

Table 2
Case definition, incidence and economic losses of calving-related diseases

Disease	Case definition	Incidence	Economic losses
Milk fever	Calcium deficiency causing progressive neuromuscular dysfunction with flaccid paralysis, circulatory collapse, and depression of consciousness	Median 6.5% Range .03%–22.3%	$335 per case
RFM	Fetal membranes visible at the vulva or in vagina or uterus by vaginal examination more than 24 hours after parturition	Median 8.6% Range 1.3%–39.2%	$285 per case
Metritis	Abnormal cervical discharge, vaginal discharge, or both or uterine content. New case if cow did not have a case during the preceding 30 days	Median 10.1% Range 2.2%–37.3%	Treatment, Increased days open and culling
Ketosis	Primary: decreased appetite, elevated milk, urine or breath ketones in the absence of other disease	Median 4.8% Range 1.3%–18.3%	$145 per case
LDA	Decreased appetite accompanied by an audible, high-pitched tympanic resonance (ping) by percussion of the left abdominal wall between the 9th and 12th ribs	Median 1.7% Range 0.3%–6.3%	$340 per case Milk losses 250-2000 kg/lactation
Ovarian cysts	Smooth, rounded structure greater than 25 mm in diameter in one or both ovaries nonpregnant cows	Median 8.0% Range 1.0%–16.0%	$39 per case
Lameness	Episode of abnormal gait attributable to either the foot or leg regardless of etiology or duration	Median 7.0% Range 1.8%–30%	$302 per case
Mastitis	Visually abnormal milk secretion from one or more quarters with or without signs of inflammation of the udder. New case following 8 days of normal milk	Median 14.2% Range 1.7%–54.6%	-

Data from Kelton DF, Lissemore KD, Martin RE. Recommendations for recording and calculating the incidence of selected clinical diseases of dairy cattle. J Dairy Sci 1998;81:2502–09.

Oral and intramuscular doses of vitamin D have also prevented hypocalcemia successfully; however, repeated doses may lead to toxicity [29,30]. Parathyroid hormone (PTH) has been also reported to prevent hypocalcemia in dairy cows [31].

One of the most important determinants of the risk of hypocalcemia is the acid-base status of the animal around parturition. Metabolic alkalosis appears to alter the physiologic activity of PTH so that bone resorption and production of 1, 25(OH)$_2$ D are impaired, reducing the ability of the animal to successfully adjust to increased Ca demands [1,25]. Therefore, diets fed before parturition that induce an acidic response in the animal reduce the risk of MF [27,28]. Dietary cation-anion difference (DCAD) has been defined as the difference in milliequivalents of cations and anions per kilogram of dry matter (DM), and has a direct impact on blood acid base metabolism [32]. Sodium (Na), potassium (K), Ca, magnesium (Mg), chloride (Cl), sulfur (S) and phosphorus (P) are the most important DCAD determinants. The most common equation used to calculate the DCAD has been: DCAD (mEq) = (Na + K) − (Cl + S); however other equations that include Ca, Mg, and P are under study, and theoretically they should be more accurate [28,33,34].

As DCAD decreases, H$^+$ increases, HCO$^-_3$ decreases, and pH decreases. These changes are accompanied by a reduction in urinary HCO$^-_3$ excretion and urinary pH as compensatory mechanisms. Furthermore, low DCAD prepartum increases urinary Ca reabsorption, serum ionized Ca, and responsiveness to Ca homeostatic hormones [27,32]. Unfortunate, typical diets fed to dry cows have a DCAD of about +50 to +250 mEq/kg DM, based on the equation reported above. In common feedstuffs, K is the most variable of the ions, and it is usually the most important determinant of DCAD in nonsupplemented feed [33]. Consequently, K should be reduced at maximum (less than 1.5% DM, if possible). After that, anions can then be added to further reduce DCAD to the desired end point [28]. Commonly used anion sources are CaCl$_2$, NH$_4$Cl, MgSO$_4$, and CaSO$_4$. Anionic salts can be unpalatable and are always accompanied by a cation, which, depending on its rate of absorption, will counteract some of the effects of the anions [33,35]. Other anion sources include mineral acids such as hydrochloric acid mixed into common feed ingredients [28,34,35]. Optimal acidification generally occurs when anions are added to achieve a final DCAD between −50 to −100 mEq/kg DM.

The subclinical expression of hypocalcemia is a common condition that affects about 50% of all adult lactating dairy cows. In this condition, plasma Ca concentration of periparturient cow remains <7.5 mg/dL, but the cow does not present clinical signs such as paresis. Subclinical hypocalcemia has been reported to occur for up to 10 days after calving [23]. This condition may lead to decreased DMI after calving, increased risk of secondary diseases, decreased milk production, and decreased fertility [1]. Subclinical hypocalcemia has been related to uterine prolapse, RFM, uterine atony, and metritis, which can reduce subsequent fertility [1,15,24].

Strategies to prevent retained fetal membranes and metritis

RFMs occur when the detachment of fetal membranes (cotyledons) from the maternal caruncles does not occur within the first 12 to 24 hours after calving [36,37]. Risk factors for RFM are dystocia, parity, abnormal gestation length, season, and sire of the calf [38]. Neutrophils isolated from cows that experienced RFM had significantly lower function than cows without RFM, before calving and during the first 2 weeks postpartum [39]. Considering this, immune system integrity before calving is important to prevent RFM. Immune system activity and RFM occurrence have been related to vitamin E and selenium (Se) prepartum supplementation, BCS dynamic, and energy balance status. Indeed, hyperketonemia has been related to immune system and mammary gland defense mechanisms [40]. Leukocytes from hyperketonemic cows have a lower capacity of phagocytic activity, lower amount of cytokine production, and decreased chemotactic capacity [40]. These mechanisms may also be impaired in the uterus if cows are at higher risk of developing ketosis, increasing the likelihood of uterine infections. A recent study [41] has explored the association of immune response, milk production, and resistance to diseases in dairy cattle. Cows that had a strong response, based on ovalbumin immunization, had a higher milk yield and lower incidence of mastitis. The authors suggest that selection for high immune responses may prove beneficial to herd life by maintaining optimal yield, yet minimizing occurrence of disease. This concept may be applied for future genetic indexes in sire selection.

RFMs are the major factor that predisposes cattle to metritis. Dystocia, improper nutrition, and metabolic disorders also increase the likelihood that a cow develops metritis [22,42,43]. Metritis altered uterine involution, increased calving to first estrus by 6.9 days, calving to first service interval by 7.3 days, first to last service interval by 15.4 days, calving to conception interval by 18 days, and services per conception by 0.20 [44,45].

Prevention of metritis is based on prevention and treatment of RFM (see the article by B. Smith and C. Risco elsewhere in this issue). In addition, metritis may be prevented by proper nutritional management during the dry period, allowing cows to calve in an optimum BCS (3.25 to 3.5), an uncontaminated environment, and employing strict sanitation if assistance is required during parturition [42,43]. Ultimately, the competence of the immune system is important in the prevention of the metritis complex. Uterine trauma, such as dystocia, manual removal of RFM, and intrauterine infusions, reduce the phagocytic activity of uterine and blood neutrophils [46].

Strategies to prevent ketosis and fatty liver

Ketosis may be clinical or subclinical. Subclinical cases are characterized by elevated blood ketone body concentrations without clinical signs [47–49], with more than 90% of the cases occurring during the first 2 months after calving. During this period, approximately 40% of all cows are affected by subclinical ketosis at least once, although the incidence is the highest in the first and second weeks after parturition [48,49]. Cows affected by ketosis were 1.8 and 1.6 times more likely to develop metritis and ovarian cysts, respectively, than normal cows [50]. In addition, ketotic cows had a significantly longer calving-to-conception interval and a higher culling rate than cows that had normal levels of ketones [51].

During early lactation, dairy cows experience a typical negative energy balance characterized by mobilization of NEFA from adipose tissue [1,8,52]. Elevation of plasma NEFA concentrations starts before the DMI depression. Liver TG infiltration does not occur until the concentration of plasma NEFA is maximized on day 1 after calving [53]. Fatty liver can occur very rapidly. Within 48 hours, hepatic TG levels can increase from less than 5% to more than 25% under conditions of extreme adipose mobilization [54]. This condition is typical of cows that have extreme BCS at calving.

To prevent ketosis-fatty liver complex, fat cows at parturition should be avoided. Dry cows should be fed a diet to maintain weight and not to lose weight [54]. Cows overfed during the dry period have higher concentrations of plasma NEFA as a result of greater lipolysis after parturition. Cows experiencing more severe negative energy balance develop a high liver TG concentration [55–57]. Therefore, scoring body condition of cows at dry-off and properly managing the nutrition of transition cows are useful tools to avoid the severe fat mobilization [54]. High BCS at calving negatively affects reproductive responses, milk yield, and health of the cows during lactation [58–62].

Niacin has been suggested as a treatment or preventive for fatty liver in dairy cows during the prepartum period [54]. Propylene glycol is a gluconeogenic compound used to treat and prevent ketosis and fatty liver in postpartum dairy cows, with doses ranging between 250 g and 400 g, given orally twice a day [63–66]. Higher doses may be toxic [67]. Nutritionally, propionate can be supplied orally in the form of sodium or calcium propionate. Calcium propionate is a gluconeogenic precursor as well as a source of calcium, which will be absorbed by the small intestine and may help to prevent clinical and subclinical hypocalcemia [23]; however, transition cows fed anionic salts prepartum, and drenched one dose of calcium propionate (510 g) plus propylene glycol (400 g) neither improve postpartum blood concentrations of Ca, P, Mg, glucose, NEFA, and BHB, nor increase milk yield and reproductive responses [13,22]. The authors suggest that this supplementation might be beneficial for cows that experience complications during delivery.

Ionophores enhance rumen propionate production [68]. Ionophores have been available for use in food animals for over 20 years. Monensin was recently approved for use in lactating dairy cattle in the United States. Monensin has primarily been used as a powder mixed with concentrates. Recently a capsule of slow-release of monensin has been developed successfully in Australia and Canada. Major advantages of monensin have been its antiketogenic effect [69].

Recent evidence suggests that choline or specific fatty acids (linoleic, linolenic) may enhance hepatic export of NEFA and TG in lipoproteins in ruminants and decrease hepatic lipidosis [70].

Strategies to prevent displacement of the abomasum

Left displacement of the abomasum (LDA) is the most regular condition of abomasal disorders, most commonly occurring 2 weeks pre- to 8 weeks postpartum [71]. LDA is a multifactorial disease in which different risk factors have been established. Cows experiencing MF or subclinical hypocalcemia, dystocia, and ketosis are more likely to develop LDA than normal cows [20,72,73]. In one study [74], significant factors associated with an increased risk of LDA included high BCS at calving, winter season, and plasma NEFA concentration >0.3 meq/L between 35 and 3 days prepartum. The risk of LDA decreased as lactation number increased. Other factors associated positively with risk of LDA were predicted transmitted ability for milk production, BCS, winter and summer seasons, and precalving rations containing energy densities >1.65 Mcal of ENl/kg of DM. Feed bunk management considering bunk space, feed availability, and freshness were associated negatively with the risk of LDA.

Nutrition during the transition period has been implicated as one of the most important risk factors in the etiology of LDA [75]. High-concentrate diets, rapid introduction of concentrate in the immediate pre or postpartum period, and rations high in corn silage or low in neutral detergent fiber (NDF) are factors that affect abomasal motility or enhance gas production [71,76,77]. The lack of physical form reduces chewing activity, ruminal fill, motility, and fiber mat formation, and increases ruminal volatile fatty acids (VFA) concentration, all of which may affect the etiology of LDA. Concentrate can be increased at the rate of 0.20 to 0.25 kg/d until peak lactation is reached. Concentrates should be fed three to four times daily. Feeding a total mixed ration (TMR) to control forage-to-concentrate ratio is recommended. A transition-group TMR with a higher effective fiber content for early postpartum cows is also recommended. TMR mixing can alter the physical form of the fiber in the diet. Small particle size reduces chewing activity, ruminal fill, and motility, and increases ruminal VFA concentration, all of which may affect the etiology of LDA. On the other hand, excessively large particle size can allow the cows to sort the TMR in the feed bunk, which can cause the same problem [75,78–84].

Dry cow feeding management and body condition score

BCS is a useful tool for monitoring the nutritional management of dairy cows (energy density and intake). Using a scale of 1 to 5 [85,86], a program can be established. Cows should be dried-off with a BCS 3.0 to 3.25. If BCS is lower, the ration should be adjusted during the last 100 days of lactation and not during the dry period. If many cows are overconditioned, a fat cow group for late lactation should be established and a diet moderate in energy content should be fed [87]. If many cows are underconditioned. a thin cow group should be established and a diet with proper energy content to target the desired weight gain should be fed (one unit BCS $\sim$ 57 kg BW) [87].

Cows should have a dry period length of at least 6 to 8 weeks. A dry period <6 weeks has resulted in lower milk yields in the next lactation [88]; however, more recent evidence has shown that a dry period length of 30 days had no detrimental effects on lactation performance [89]. More information is needed before recommendations are established.

Two groups of dry cows are recommended: the early dry group (8 to 3 weeks before expected calving), and a close-up group (3 weeks to calving). If early dry cows are in proper condition and eating more than predicted to meet their requirements, it may be necessary to lower the energy and nutrient density of the ration by reformulating the diet. Never try to reduce BCS or body weight of dry cows during any stage of the dry period [90]. If BCS is correct at dry-off (3.0–3.25), then cows should gain about 0.3 to 0.45 kg/d to increase BCS by 0.25 to 0.5 units during the period.

Prepartum transition cow feeding management

Critical physiologic events that have to be targeted during the transition period are: adaptation of the rumen to the high energy-density diet that will be fed in early postpartum, maintenance of normal blood calcium concentration, a strong immune system, and maintenance of a slightly positive energy balance up to the time of calving [1,91].

During the transition period, feed intake is decreasing at a time when energy requirements are increasing because of growth of the conceptus. Consequently, to maintain the energy balance, the energy density of the diet should increase [87]. Heifers need higher dietary energy density because of lower feed intakes and growing [87]. A separate close-up group for pregnant heifers might be a beneficial management strategy in farms, if adequate facilities are available [92]. Diet formulation should be based on 10 to 11 kg of DM intake. If cows are overeating, it is not a big problem, because this is a short period of time. Cows should be in a positive energy status and not losing weight. Feed should always be available in the bunk (24 hours a day) in a form of TMR to ensure adequate control of nutrient composition and consumption. Cows should calve having a BCS of 3.5 and heifers should calve having a BCS 3.0 to 3.25 in order to minimize obstetrical problems [90,93].

Grain has to be introduced to the cow's ration for at least 3 weeks before the due date, and for heifers this should be 5 weeks. The energy density should be between 1.56 and 1.62 Mcal/kg of NEl [87]. Crude protein should be between 14% and 15% of the diet [87]. Fiber (NDF content) and particle size should be optimum to stimulate rumination for at least 14 hours a day [79,87].

Minerals and vitamins should be fed to optimize milk production. Most of these nutrient requirements are met through premixes in the TMR or free-choice premixes (Table 3).

Fresh cow feeding management

The primary goal for early fresh cows is to maximize carbohydrate, protein, and nutrient intake, and to provide adequate fiber to meet

Table 3
Nutritional requirements for dry, prepartum and postpartum transition dairy cows

Nutrient	Far-off dry cows[a]	Close-up dry cows[b]	Fresh cows[c]
Dry matter intake (kg/day)	14.4	13.7	15.6
Net energy lactation (Mcal/kg)	0.94	1.54–1.62	1.75
Maximum crude fat (%)	5	6	6
Crude protein (%)	13	14–15	19.0
Undegradable protein (% CP)	25	32	9.0
Acid detergent fiber (%)	21	17–21	17–21
Neutral detergent fiber (%)	33	25–33	25–33
Minimum Forage NDF (%)	30	22	23.7
Maximum NFC (%)	36–43	36–43	36–44
Minimum calcium (%)	0.44	0.45	0.79
Phosphorus (%)	0.22	0.3–0.4	0.42
Ca:P ratio	1.5:1 to 5:1	1.5:1 to 5:1	-
Magnesium (%)	0.20	0.35–0.4	0.29
Potassium (%)	0.55	0.55	1.24
Sulfur (%)	0.11	0.11	0.2
Sodium (%)	0.10	0.10	0.34
Chlorine (%)	0.20	0.20	0.4
DCAD (mEq/kg)	-	< 0	-
Cobalt (ppm)	0.11	0.11	0.11
Copper (ppm)	16	16	16
Iodine (ppm)	0.4	0.4	0.77
Iron (ppm)	26	26	22
Manganese (ppm)	22	22	21
Selenium (ppm)	0.30	0.30	0.3
Zinc (ppm)	30	30	73
Vitamin A (IU/kg)	5500	6500	4795
Vitamin D (IU/kg)	1500	1700	1308
Vitamin E (IU/kg)	80	88	35

Abbreviations: CP, crude protein; NFC, non-fiber carbohydrates.

[a] Far-off dry cow: from 60 to 21 days before expected parturition.

[b] Close-up cow: prepartum transition cow from 21 days before expected parturition to calving.

[c] Fresh cow: postpartum transition cow from calving to 21 days postpartum.

Data from National Research Council. Nutrient requirements of dairy cattle. 7th revised edition. Washington, DC: National Academy Press; 2001.

requirements for increasing milk production [90]. Forage DM intake should be near 2% of the cow's BW. Particle size should be long enough to stimulate 30 minutes of cud-chewing time per kg of DM. Total mixed ration DM content should be between 50% and 65%. Clean water should be provided, expecting cows to drink 2 L for each 0.45 kg of milk. Enough feed bunk space should be also provided [94].

Cows should peak in milk production 8 to 10 weeks after calving. First-calf heifers should peak within 75% the production of older cows. For each extra 1 kg of milk at peak production, the average cow will produce 200 to 220 kg more milk for the entire lactation period. Milk protein-to-fat ratio should be near 0.85 to 0.88 for Holstein cows. Forage intake using good quality roughage should be maximized. Energy density of the top cows should be 1.76 Mcal/kg of ENl. Non-fiber carbohydrates levels should be between 35% and 44%, and starch levels between 25% and 35% of the total ration [87].

Cows should not lose more than 1 BCS during early lactation, otherwise fertility will be highly compromised [59,60]. The last third of lactation should be used to replace lost body condition.

Strategies to monitor transition dairy cow management

Urine pH can be monitored to evaluate effectiveness of anionic salts during the prepartum period, for the prevention of milk fever. A sample of about 10% of precalving cows should be sufficient to determine an accurate and representative urine pH. Urine pH values below 5.5 indicate over-acidification, and DCAD should be increased. The optimal urinary pH is between 6.0 and 6.5 for Holstein cows and between 5.8 and 6.2 for Jersey cows. Over 6.5 is considered inadequate acidification and suggests that a lower DCAD is required [1]. In herds experiencing MF, the urine of close-up dry cows will be very alkaline (pH >8.0). The most accurate results will be obtained by collecting urine samples at a standard time, and not contaminated with manure or vaginal discharges [28,33].

Mammary edema is common in late pregnant heifers. Risk factors for this condition are calving season and gender of the calf. Heifers calving in summer and delivering a female calf were 0.12 and 0.52 times less likely to develop udder edema, respectively, than heifers calving in winter and having a male calf [95]. Monitoring udder edema is important to prevent other conditions. If udder edema is severe, calving induction is recommended.

Calving management is a key point in the prevention of CRD. Proper obstetrical care in parturient cows is critical, requiring proper training and supervision of farm personnel.

A 10- to 14-day postpartum health monitoring program that evaluates body temperature, ketone bodies in urine or milk, metritis, mastitis, and displacement of the abomasums development provides an efficient strategy for early postpartum disease detection and treatment [96].

Summary

Appropriate management of the transition period is of paramount importance to optimize fertility in dairy cattle. Physiological goals are a strong immune system, maintenance of normocalcemia,, positive energy balance, prevention of CRD, and a rumen adapted to a postpartum high energy diet. These goals can be met by feeding an appropriate diet providing cow comfort and proper calving assistance. If these goals are met on a continued basis, they will provide the foundation necessary for a successful reproductive program. Assurance of proper management of transition cows can be achieved by periodic monitoring and evaluation.

References

[1] Goff JP, Horst RL. Physiological changes at parturition and their relationship to metabolic disorders. J Dairy Sci 1997;80:1260–8.
[2] Grummer RR. Impact of changes in organic nutrient metabolism on feeding the transition dairy cows. J Anim Sci 1995;73:2820–33.
[3] Drackley JK, Overton TR, Douglas GN. Adaptations of glucose and long-chain fatty acid metabolism in liver of dairy cows during the periparturient period. J Dairy Sci 2001;84(Suppl E):E100–12.
[4] Drackley JK. Biology of dairy cows during the transition period: the final frontier? J Dairy Sci 1999;82:2259–73.
[5] Ingvartsen KL, Andersen JB. Integration of metabolism and intake regulation: a review focusing on periparturient animals. J Dairy Sci 2000;83:1573–97.
[6] Hayirli A, Grummer RR, Nordheim E, et al. Prediction equations for dry matter intake of transition cows fed diets that vary in nutrient composition. J Dairy Sci 1999;82(Suppl 1):113.
[7] Hayirli A, Grummer RR, Nordheim EV, et al. Animal and dietary factors affecting feed intake during the prefresh transition period in Holsteins. J Dairy Sci 2002;85:3430–43.
[8] Herdt TH. Ruminant adaptation to negative energy balance. Influences on the etiology of ketosis and fatty liver. Vet Clin North Am Food Anim Pract 2000;16:215–30.
[9] Herdt TH. Gastrointestinal physiology and metabolism. Postabsorptive nutrient utilization. In: Cunningham, editor. Textbook of veterinary physiology. 3rd edition. Philadelphia: WB Saunders; 2002. p. 303–22.
[10] Seal CJ, Reynolds CK. Nutritional implications of gastrointestinal and liver metabolism in ruminants. Nutr Res Rev 1993;6:185–208.
[11] Overton TR, Drackley JK, Douglas GN, et al. Hepatic gluconeogenesis and whole-body protein metabolism of periparturient dairy cows as affected by source of energy and intake of the prepartum diet [abstract]. J Dairy Sci 1998;81(Suppl 1):295.
[12] Reynolds CK, Aikman PC, Humphries DJ, et al. Splanchnic metabolism in transition dairy cows [abstract]. J Dairy Sci 2000;83(Suppl 1):257.
[13] Melendez P, Donovan A, Risco CA, et al. Metabolic responses of transition Holstein cows fed anionic salts and supplemented at calving with calcium and energy. J Dairy Sci 2002;85:1085–92.
[14] Nelson DL, Cox MM. Oxidation of fatty acids. In: Lehninger principles of biochemistry. 3rd edition. New York: Worth Publishers; 2000. p. 598–622.
[15] Risco CA, Melendez P. Periparturient disorders. In: Roginski H, Fuquay J, editors. Encyclopedia of dairy science. San Diego: Fox Academic Press; 2002. p. 2309–14.
[16] Van Dorp TE, Dekkers JCM, Martin SW, et al. Genetic parameters of health disorders, and relationships with 305-day milk yield and conformation traits of registered Holstein cows. J Dairy Sci 1998;81:2264–70.

[17] Kelton DF, Lissemore KD, Martin RE. Recommendations for recording and calculating the incidence of selected clinical diseases of dairy cattle. J Dairy Sci 1998;81:2502–9.

[18] Erb HN, Smith RD, Oltenacu PA, et al. Path model of reproductive disorders and performance, milk fever, mastitis, milk yield, and culling in Holstein cows. J Dairy Sci 1985; 68:3337–49.

[19] Curtis CR, Erb HN, Sniffen CJ, et al. Path analysis of dry period nutrition, postpartum metabolic and reproductive disorders, and mastitis in Holstein cows. J Dairy Sci 1985;68: 2347–60.

[20] Correa MT, Erb H, Scarlett J. Path analysis for seven postpartum disorders of Holstein cows. J Dairy Sci 1993;76:1305–12.

[21] Melendez P, Bartolome J, Archbald L, et al. Association between lameness, ovarian cysts and fertility in lactating dairy cows. Theriogenology 2003;59:927–37.

[22] Melendez P, Donovan A, Risco CA, et al. Effect of calcium-energy supplements on calving-related disorders, fertility and milk yield during the transition period in cows fed anionic diets. Theriogenology 2003;60:843–54.

[23] Goff JP, Horst RL, Jardon PW, et al. Field trials of an oral calcium propionate paste as an aid to prevent milk fever in periparturient dairy cows. J Dairy Sci 1996;79:378–83.

[24] Risco CA, Drost M, Thatcher WW, et al. Effects of calving-related disorders on prostaglandin, calcium, ovarian activity and uterine involution in postpartum dairy cows. Theriogenology 1994;42:183–203.

[25] Horst RL, Goff JP, Reinhardt TA. Calcium and vitamin D metabolism in the dairy cow. J Dairy Sci 1994;77:1936–51.

[26] Joyce PW, Sanchez WK, Goff JP. Effect of anionic salts in prepartum diets based on alfalfa. J Dairy Sci 1997;80:2866–75.

[27] Vagnoni DB, Oetzel GR. Effects of dietary cation-anion difference on the acid-base status of dry cows. J Dairy Sci 1998;81:1643–52.

[28] Oetzel GR. Nutritional management of dry dairy cows. Compend Contin Educ Prac Vet 1998;20:391–6.

[29] Jorgensen NA. Combating milk fever. J Dairy Sci 1974;57:933–44.

[30] Markusfeld O. The evaluation of a routine treatment with 1a-hydroxyvitamin D3 for the prevention of bovine parturient paresis. Prev Vet Med 1989;7:1–9.

[31] Goff JP, Kehrli ME, Horst RL. Periparturient hypocalcemia in cows: prevention using intramuscular parathyroid hormone. J Dairy Sci 1989;72:1182–7.

[32] Block E. Manipulation of dietary cation-anion difference on nutritionally related production diseases, productivity, and metabolic responses of dairy cows. J Dairy Sci 1994;77:1437–50.

[33] Goff JP, Horst RL. Factors to concentrate on to prevent periparturient disease in the dairy cow with special emphasis on milk fever. In: Proceedings 31th Conference of American Association of Bovine Practitioners, Spokane, WA, September 24–26, 1998. p. 31:154–63.

[34] Goff JP, Ruiz R, Horst RL. Relative acidifying activity of anionic salts commonly used to prevent milk fever. J Dairy Sci 2004;87:1245–55.

[35] Goff JP, Horst RL. Use of hydrochloric acid as a source of anions for prevention of milk fever. J Dairy Sci 1998;81:2874–80.

[36] Grunert E. Etiology and pathogenesis of retained placenta. In: Morrow DA, editor. Current therapy in theriogenology 2. Philadelphia: WB Saunders; 1986. p. 237.

[37] Eiler H. Retained placenta. In: Youngquist R, editor. Current therapy in large animal theriogenology. Philadelphia: WB Saunders; 1997. p. 340–8.

[38] Joosten I, van Eldik P, van der Mey GJW. Factors affecting retained placenta in cattle. Effect of sire on incidence. Anim Reprod Sci 1991;25:11–22.

[39] Kimura K, Goff JP, Kehrli ME, et al. Decreased neutrophil function as a cause of retained placenta in dairy cattle. J Dairy Sci 2002;85:544–50.

[40] Suriyasathaporn W, Heuer C, Noordhuizen-Stassen EN, et al. Hyperketonemia and the impairment of udder defense: a review. Vet Res 2000;31:397–412.

[41] Wagter LC, Mallard BA, Wilkie BN, et al. The relationship between milk production and antibody response to ovalbumin during the peripartum period. J Dairy Sci 2003;86: 169–73.

[42] Youngquist RS, Shore MD. Postpartum uterine infecctions. In: Youngquist RS, editor. Current therapy in large animal theriogenology. Philadelphia: WB Saunders; 1997. p. 335–40.

[43] Lewis GS. Uterine health and disorders. J Dairy Sci 1997;80:984–94.

[44] Bruun J, Ersbøll AK, Alban L. Risk factors for metritis in Danish dairy cows. Prev Vet Med 2002;54:179–90.

[45] Barlett PC, Kirk JH, Wilke MA, et al. Metritis complex in Michigan Holstein-Friesan cattle: incidence, descriptive epidemiology and estimated economic impact. Prev Vet Med 1986;4: 235–48.

[46] Cai TQ, Weston PG, Lund LA, et al. Association between neutrophil functions and periparturient disorders in cows. Am J Vet Res 1994;55:934–43.

[47] Andersson L, Gustafsson AH, Emanuelson U. Effect of hyperketonaemia and feeding on fertility in dairy cows. Theriogenology 1991;36:521–36.

[48] Duffield T. Subclinical ketosis in lactating dairy cattle. Vet Clin North Am Food Anim Pract 2000;16:231–53.

[49] Geishauser T, Leslie K, Kelton D, et al. Monitoring for subclinical ketosis in dairy herds. Comp Cont Educ Food Anim 2001;23:S65–71.

[50] Gröhn YT, Rajala-Schultz PJ, Allore HG, et al. Optimizing replacement of dairy cows: modeling the effects of diseases. Prev Vet Med 2003;61:27–43.

[51] Cook NB, Ward WR, Dobson H. Concentrations of ketones in milk in early lactation, and reproductive performance of dairy cows. Vet Rec 2001;148:769–72.

[52] Herdt TH, Gerloff BJ. Ketosis. In: Howard J, Smith R, editors. Current veterinary therapy 4. Food animal practice. Philadelphia: WB Saunders; 1999. p. 226–30.

[53] Vazquez-Añon M, Bertics S, Luck M, et al. Peripartum liver triglyceride and plasma metabolites in dairy cows. J Dairy Sci 1994;77:1521–8.

[54] Gerloff BJ, Herdt TH. Fatty liver in dairy cattle. In: Howard J, Smith R, editors. Current veterinary therapy 4. Food animal practice. Philadelphia: WB Saunders; 1999. p. 230–3.

[55] Grummer RR. Etiology of lipid-related metabolic disorders in periparturient dairy cows. J Dairy Sci 1993;76:3882–96.

[56] Rukkwamsuk T, Wensing T, Geelen MJH. Effect of overfeeding during the dry period on regulation of adipose tissue metabolism in dairy cows during the periparturient period. J Dairy Sci 1998;81:2904–11.

[57] Rukkwamsuk T, Wensing T, Geelen MJH. Effect of overfeeding during the dry period on the rate of esterification in adipose tissue of dairy cows during the periparturient period. J Dairy Sci 1999;82:1164–9.

[58] Butler WR, Smith RD. Interrelationship between energy balance and postpartum reproduction function in cattle. J Dairy Sci 1989;72:767–83.

[59] Domecq JJ, Skidmore AL, Lloyd JW, et al. Relationships between body condition scores and milk yield in a large dairy herd of high yielding Holstein cows. J Dairy Sci 1997;80: 101–12.

[60] Domecq JJ, Skidmore AL, Lloyd JW, et al. Relationships between body condition scores and conception at first artificial insemination in a large dairy herd of high yielding Holstein cows. J Dairy Sci 1997;80:113–20.

[61] Markusfeld O, Galon N, Ezra E. Body condition score, health, yield and fertility in dairy cows. Vet Rec 1997;141:67–72.

[62] Heuer C, Schukken YH, Dobbelaar P. Postpartum body condition score and results from the first test day milk as predictors of disease, fertility, yield, and culling in commercial dairy herds. J Dairy Sci 1999;82:295–304.

[63] Studer VA, Grummer RR, Bertics SJ, et al. Effect of prepartum propylene glycol administration on periparturient fatty liver in dairy cows. J Dairy Sci 1993;76:2931–9.

[64] Grummer RR, Winkler JC, Bertics SJ, et al. Effect of propylene glycol dosage during feed restriction on metabolites in blood of prepartum Holstein heifers. J Dairy Sci 1994;77: 3618–23.

[65] Christensen JO, Grummer RR, Rasmussen FE, et al. Effect of method of delivery of propylene glycol on plasma metabolites of feed-restricted cattle. J Dairy Sci 1997;80: 563–8.

[66] Laranja da Fonseca LF, Lucci CS, Rodríguez PHM, et al. Supplementation of propylene glycol to dairy cows in periparturient period: Effects on plasma concentration of BHBA, NEFA, and glucose. J Dairy Sci 1998;81(Suppl 1):320.

[67] Pintchuk PA, Galey FD, George LW. Propylene toxicity in adult dairy cows. J Vet Intern Med 1993;7:150.

[68] Van Maanen RW, Herbein JH, McGilliard AD, et al. Effects of monensin on in vivo rumen propionate production and blood glucose kinetics in cattle. J Nutr 1978;108:1002–7.

[69] Duffield TF, Sandals D, Leslie KE, et al. Efficacy of monensin for the prevention of subclinical ketosis in lactating dairy cows. J Dairy Sci 1998;81:2866–73.

[70] Overton TR, Waldron MR. Nutritional management of transition dairy cows: strategies to optimize metabolic health. J Dairy Sci 2004;87(Suppl E):E105–19.

[71] Trent AM. Surgery of the bovine abomasum. Vet Clin North Am Food Anim Pract 1990;6: 399–448.

[72] Massey CD, Wang C, Donovan GA, et al. Hypocalcemia at parturition as a risk factor for left displacement of the abomasum in dairy cows. J Am Vet Med Assoc 1993;203:852–3.

[73] Fecteau G, Sattler N, Rings DM. Abomasal physiology, and dilatation, displacement, and volvulus. In: Howard J, Smith R, editors. Current veterinary therapy 4. Food animal practice. Philadelphia: WB Saunders; 1999. p. 522–7.

[74] Cameron REB, Dyk RB, Herdt TH, et al. Dry cow diet, management and energy balance as risk factors for displaced abomasum in high producing dairy herds. J Dairy Sci 1998;81: 132–9.

[75] Shaver RD. Nutritional risk factors in the etiology of left displaced abomasum in dairy cows: a review. J Dairy Sci 1997;80:2449–53.

[76] Nocek JE, English JE, Braund DG. Effects of various forages feeding programs during dry period on body condition score and subsequent lactation health, production and reproduction. J Dairy Sci 1983;66:1108–18.

[77] Markusfeld O. The association of displaced abomasum with various periparturient factors in dairy cows. A retrospective study. Prev Vet Med 1986;4:172–83.

[78] Bauchemin KA. Indigestion and mastication of feed by dairy cattle. Vet Clin North Am Food Anim Pract 1991;7:439–64.

[79] Mertens DR. 1992. Nonstructural and structural carbohydrates. In: Van Horn HH, Wilcox CJ, editors. Large dairy herd management. Champaign (IL): American Dairy Science Association; 1992. p. 219–35.

[80] Muller LD. Feeding management strategies. In: Van Horn HH, Wilcox CJ, editors. Large dairy herd management. Champaign (IL): American Dairy Science Association; 1992. p. 326–35.

[81] Varga GA, Dann HM, Ishler VA. The use of fiber concentrations for ration formulation. J Dairy Sci 1998;81:3063–74.

[82] Heinrichs AJ, Buckmaster DR, Lammers BP. Processing, mixing, and particle size reduction of forages for dairy cattle. J Anim Sci 1999;77:180–6.

[83] Melendez P, Rodríguez O, Madrid S, et al. The association between forage particle size at initial feeding and the weigh back and chewing activity in dairy cattle. The Bovine Practitioner 2002;36:66–70.

[84] Melendez P, Back N, Lanhart S, et al. Particle size, feed intake, milk yield and chewing activity in Holstein cows [abstract]. J Dairy Sci 2003;86(Suppl 1):W227.

[85] Edmonson AJ, Lean IJ, Weaver LD, et al. A body condition scoring chart for Holstein dairy cows. J Dairy Sci 1989;72:68–78.

[86] Ferguson JM, Galligan DT, Thomsen N. Principal descriptors of body condition score in Holstein cows. J Dairy Sci 1994;77:2695–703.

[87] National Research Council. Nutrient requirements of dairy cattle. 7th revised edition. Washington (DC): National Academy Press; 2001.

[88] Funk DA, Freeman AE, Berger PJ. Effects of previous days open, previous days dry, and present days open on lactation yield. J Dairy Sci 1987;70:2366–73.

[89] Bachman KC, Schairer ML. Bovine studies on optimal lengths of dry periods. J Dairy Sci 2003;86:3027–37.

[90] Beede DK. Nutritional management of transition and fresh cows for optimal performance. In: Proceedings 34th Annual Florida Dairy Production Conference. University of Florida, Gainesville, FL, April 8–9, 1997. p. 19–25.

[91] Oetzel GR, Goff JP. Milk fever in cows, ewes and doe goats. In: Howard J, Smith R, editors. Current veterinary therapy 4. Food animal practice. Philadelphia: WB Saunders; 1999. p. 215–8.

[92] Grant RJ, Albright JL. Feeding behavior and management factors during the transition period in dairy cattle. J Anim Sci 1995;73:2791–803.

[93] Studer E. A veterinary perspective of on-farm evaluation of nutrition and reproduction. J Dairy Sci 1998;81:872–6.

[94] Mahanna B. Dairy cow nutritional guidelines. In: Howard J, Smith R, editors. Current veterinary therapy 4. Food animal practice. Philadelphia: WB Saunders; 1999. p. 193–8.

[95] Melendez P, Donovan A. Risk factors for udder edema in primiparous Holstein cows. Proc. X International Symposium on Veterinary Epidemiology and Economics. Vina del Mar, Chile, November 17–21, 2003.

[96] Benzaquen M, Risco CA, Archbald LF, et al., Evaluation of rectal temperature and calving related factors on the incidence of metritis in postpartum dairy cows. In: Proceedings of the 37th Annual Conference of the American Association of Bovine Practitioners. Fort Worth, TX, September 23–25, 2004.

ELSEVIER
SAUNDERS

VETERINARY
CLINICS
Food Animal Practice

Vet Clin Food Anim 21 (2005) 503–521

Management of Periparturient Disorders in Dairy Cattle

Billy I. Smith, DVM, MS[a],*, Carlos A. Risco, DVM[b]

[a]Department of Clinical Studies, Section of Field Service,
University of Pennsylvania School of Veterinary Medicine, New Bolton Center,
382 West Street Road, Kennett Square, PA 19348, USA
[b]Department of Large Animal Clinical Sciences,
Section of Food Animal Reproduction and Medicine Service,
College of Veterinary Medicine, University of Florida,
P.O. Box 100136, Gainesville, FL 32610, USA

A major challenge for dairy producers, managers, and veterinarians is to maintain a dairy cow's health during the periparturient period. A basic principle in medicine is that the earlier one can diagnose a sick animal and provide care, the faster that animal will return to a normal state of health. In the past, sick dairy cows were often identified too late, leaving little chance for a successful outcome once care was administered. Many owners, managers, and veterinarians who rely on employees for the identification of sick cows do so without considering proper training, aptitude, or desire of these employees. The reality is that not every employee has the desire or the ability to identify a sick cow in the early stages of a disease process; therefore, the goal of diagnosing and treating sick cows early can be difficult to attain, especially for dairies that become bigger and where a large number of cows require close attention and monitoring.

As dairy herds continue to expand, it becomes clear that a different approach to handling the periparturient dairy cow is needed. Currently, most dairy operations use monitoring programs to aid in the identification of clinically or even subclinically sick animals. These programs are not just for large dairy herds, but are used successfully in even the smallest herds. Their main objective is to use reasonably cost-effective techniques to identify animals in the early stages of disease, thereby allowing routine, reliable treatment methods and the swift return of the animal back to a healthy state.

---

* Corresponding author.
E-mail address: bis@vet.upenn.edu (B.I. Smith).

0749-0720/05/$ - see front matter © 2005 Elsevier Inc. All rights reserved.
doi:10.1016/j.cvfa.2005.02.007   *vetfood.theclinics.com*

This article discusses parameters that can be implemented in a health monitoring program. Particular attention is given to the postpartum period and to identification and management of specific diseases related to bovine theriogenology.

The periparturient period

The periparturient period of dairy cows refers to the time frame near parturition. Although there are many interpretations for this time period, it generally covers the period from approximately 3 weeks before calving to 3 weeks after calving. It is a pivotal time in the production cycle of the cow, in which cattle are at high risk for the occurrence of abnormal events. More specifically, the immediate few weeks following parturition can be particularly problematic, and cattle readily develop diseases related to metabolic disturbances, gastrointestinal upsets, mammary gland infections, and reproductive tract disorders [1,2]. These disorders are costly, with estimated losses ranging from $200 to $400 per case per lactation [3].

Monitoring programs for postpartum dairy cows

History

For years the dairy industry has been experiencing changes related to the size and number of herds. Small dairy herds (<200 cows) are rapidly leaving the industry and are being replaced by larger dairy operations (>500 cows). There are approximately 70,000 dairy herds in the United States, and this number is expected to continue to decline over the next 10 years [4]. Dairy producers are expected to adapt by choosing to expand. As dairy herds become larger, producers and managers are forced to become more involved in managing the daily problems associated with the postpartum period of dairy cows. In the mid 1990s, programs were developed in California that centered on rectal temperatures and attitude of the fresh cow during the first 10 days postpartum [5]. Another program developed around the same time and referred to as "the 100-day contract for dairy cows" was designed to curtail major problems during the periparturient period of dairy cows, thereby allowing dairy producers to be more profitable [6]. Other programs by various companies, dairy producers, and academic institutions have been developed and modified over time. Currently, food animal veterinarians play a significant role in keeping these programs viable. Their primary role as veterinarians is no longer one of solely identifying and treating sick cows, but now also includes developing, instituting, and evaluating monitoring programs.

Goal

The main goal of any monitoring program is to identify any change that occurs from what is considered a normal state. These programs are designed first to prevent disease, and second to allow for early detection and treatment of disease. Monitoring the health status of postpartum dairy cows to minimize costly disorders has become an indispensable action. The ability to continually check and discern change to the normal state of fresh cows has allowed for better management practices to be developed. The early identification of sick cows ensures quick treatment and management intervention. The decisions made based on information gathered from various parameters of monitoring programs ensure the highest level of productivity and profitability by dairy producers.

Parameters

There are various parameters that can be used to monitor the fresh cow's health status. They include milk production, general attitude, blood component analysis, rumenocentesis, urine ketone body levels, and rectal temperature values. The most commonly used parameter by far, however, is evaluation of rectal temperature, and it is therefore the main focus of discussion.

Milk production

Daily production measurements can be obtained by computerized milk machines. Milk production values are closely linked to the normal health of dairy cattle. Therefore, it is safe to assume that any deviation from the normal health status will result in a lower amount of milk produced when comparing day-to-day production values. All dairy cows experiencing a normal postpartum period have a steady progressive day-to-day rise in milk production. Genetic ability greatly influences steepness of the curve for each cow. Many computer data collecting programs used by dairies are capable of monitoring daily milk production values for each cow. Therefore, it becomes easy to identify cows that deviate from their normal daily production or from an accepted average production value. Determining the choice of deviation value to use for identifying these potentially abnormal cattle varies among herds. Many computer programs are programmed to create a list of all cows that deviate from a value equal to or more than a preset value. On most dairies, a 10-pound drop in production is frequently used by dairy managers. Trained employees use this deviation list to individualize these cows and perform a more thorough physical examination. Most farm managers and veterinarians would agree this is a standard monitoring program that has proven to be successful in the early identification and prevention of disease. It is therefore, highly recommended for use as a parameter in monitoring programs.

General attitude

Evaluation of the general attitude of a cow is a strongly subjective measurement. Certain people have a knack for identifying sick cows based solely on their general attitude or appearance. Even the most subtle changes can be identified by such people. Unfortunately, this ability is difficult and usually impossible to teach; some may even say that it is inherent within the individual and cannot be taught. It is, however, usually enhanced by having many years of experience with cows, and by having an acute sense of awareness of the normal dairy cow. With that said, many things about the appearance of the dairy cow can be objectively evaluated. Positioning and appearance of the eyes within the socket to assess level of dehydration or pain are often observed. A scoring system such as 1 (minimal), 2 (mild), 3 (moderate), or 4 (severe) can be used. An animal that has a score of 1 usually will have bright eyes that are positioned normally within the eye socket. An animal that has a score of 2 will have dull eyes that are slightly sunken within the eye socket. An animal that has a score of 3 will have glazed eyes that are moderately sunken, whereas one that has a score of 4 will have dry eyes that are severely sunken within the eye socket. Positioning of the cow's ears is also a good indicator of a cow's attitude. Healthy cattle will have erect ears positioned above a horizontal plane at the level of their attachment to the head. Unhealthy cattle generally have ears that droop down below horizontal, which could be caused by depression, pain, or fever. Basically, happy, bright, and alert cattle have a specific look about them that can be used to separate them from the abnormal animals. Evaluation of attitude is recommended to be used in monitoring programs, especially when the people monitoring cows have the ability to do so.

Blood component analysis (serum haptoglobin and calcium)

Blood component analysis is a measuring tool that is often overlooked. The presence or absence of certain compounds or the significant deviation from a normal value can be valuable. Serum haptoglobin is one blood compound that is either not present or present at a low concentration in normal bovine serum. During inflammation, however, especially from an infectious-related disease process, the presence of this compound in the blood of cattle can be measured. The normal reported value of serum haptoglobin in cattle is less than 10 mg/dl [7]. Smith et al [8] reported the presence of elevated serum haptoglobin in cattle diagnosed with toxic puerperal metritis. The mean concentration value for all cattle included in the study was 19 mg/dl on the first day of diagnosis. The values declined steadily after antimicrobial treatment was initiated, to a mean concentration of 7.5 mg/dl on the final day of treatment [8]. Whether or not serum haptoglobin can stand alone as a monitoring tool to determine severity of disease and therefore influence management options is debatable. Because rectal temperature is considered the gold standard for disease severity, a positive correlation of pyrexia and elevated serum haptoglobin in cattle diagnosed with disease could allow for the use of serum haptoglobin as an indicator of disease severity. Unfortunately, this positive correlation has not been substantiated by research [8,9]. Although identifying cattle that have increased levels of serum haptoglobin concentration can readily be performed, use of the information to determine treatment or management options is limited, and further research is needed to understand how this parameter can be used in monitoring programs.

Periparturient hypocalcemia, or milk fever, is a well-recognized disease of the dairy cow. A single case of milk fever could cost a producer over $300 [10]; however, when combined with the negative effects of subclinical hypocalcemia, such as retained fetal membranes, ketosis, dystocia, uterine prolapse, and displaced abomasums, the cost could be outrageous [1]. Identification of cattle that have subclinical or clinical hypocalcemia by measuring blood calcium values may be helpful. Although measuring blood calcium is not generally needed to correctly diagnose clinical hypocalcemia, it can aid in the identification of cows suffering from subclinical hypocalcemia. There is no specific serum calcium concentration value that is universally accepted to diagnose clinical or subclinical hypocalcemia. The clinical response to varying levels of calcium is different among cows, and is influenced by many factors, including breed, age, health status, and diet [10]. The normal range of calcium for dairy cattle is 8.8 to 10.4 mg/100 mL, and generally a diagnosis of clinical hypocalcemia is made when blood concentration levels are lower than 6 mg/100 mL [11]. A diagnosis of subclinical hypocalcemia using blood concentration levels is more difficult, but measured values in the range of 6.2 to 7.5 mg/100 mL have been suggested [12,13]. Normal smooth-muscle function requires calcium, and cattle that have subclinical hypocalcemia often have clinical signs of disease that are linked to diminished smooth-muscle contractility. Because the postpartum uterus requires normal smooth-muscle contractility to ensure swift involution, abnormalities in this process can lead to uterine prolapse, retained fetal membranes, and uterine infection [1,13]. Because of the negative side effects of hypocalcemia in dairy cattle, monitoring tools to identify these cows should be seriously evaluated. It is no secret that monitoring blood calcium concentration levels in dairy cattle can be difficult. Issues such as handling of samples, time frame in obtaining results, cost of the test, and interpretation of the values have led to skepticism concerning their use as monitoring parameters. Therefore, measuring serum calcium concentrations in postpartum dairy cows is not generally performed.

Rumenocentesis

Subclinical rumen acidosis can be a serious problem in periparturient dairy cow. Cows are subjected to multiple ration changes during transition from being a dry cow to a lactating cow. During this time, cattle generally consume less feed and consume different amounts during each feeding. Also, the diets generally contain high levels of energy to improve milk production. These dietary formulations and consumption changes often result in pH fluctuations in the rumen [14]. Diagnosis of subclinical rumen acidosis can be difficult, and most people rely on secondary clinical signs to make the diagnosis. Rumenocentesis is one diagnostic tool currently used by the industry to determine pH values. The sample should be collected 2 to 8 hours after feeding, depending on what type of feeding system is used (concentrate feeding or total mixed-ration feeding) [15]. A diagnosis of rumen acidosis can be made when 30% of at least 10 cows sampled have results of 5.50 or below [15]. Marginal acidosis should be considered when rumen pH values are 5.6 to 5.8 [16]. It is important to remember that interpretation of a single sample can be problematic, because of the many factors that influence the pH of the rumen at any given time. Use of rumen pH values to assess the rumen health of dairy cows can be valuable; however, because of the invasiveness of obtaining a sample and the multitude of factors influencing the values obtained, including this parameter in a monitoring program needs careful discussion.

Urine or milk ketone body evaluation

Acetonaemia, or ketosis, is a complicated disease of the periparturient dairy cow. Basically, the dairy cow must use body fat as an energy source. This is because her dry matter intake cannot meet the high-energy demands for milk production and maintenance early in lactation. The body has a limit to the amount of body fat that can be converted to an energy source by the liver. Once this limit is reached, certain compounds (acetyl-CoA) are then converted to compounds referred to as ketone bodies. Acetone, acetoacetate, and betahydroxybutyrate are the three major ketone bodies produced during a state of negative energy balance in the cow. These elevated levels of ketone bodies can provide energy to peripheral tissues; however, if these levels rise above a certain baseline, subclinical as well as clinical ketosis may develop. The cost of subclinical ketosis per cow is estimated to be $78 [17]. The estimated cost per case of clinical ketosis to the dairy producer is $145 [18]. Subclinical ketosis has been associated with an increased risk of metritis [19], clinical ketosis [19,20], displaced abomasums [21], and mastitis [22]. The negative side effects of ketosis on the reproductive performance of dairy cattle, including an increase in the interval from calving to first ovulation [23] as well as an increase in calving to first service and cystic ovarian disease [24], have been documented. A negative impact on milk production may also exist, and it has been reported that cattle that produce a positive milk ketone test produce 1.0 to 1.4 kg less milk per day for the lactation [19]. Identification of cattle suffering from subclinical ketosis in the immediate postpartum period could reduce the negative side effects of ketosis.

Identification of postpartum cattle suffering from ketosis is accomplished either by analyzing urine, milk, or plasma ketone body levels.

Urine. Measuring urine ketone body levels is most commonly performed, because the technique to obtain a urine sample is uncomplicated, repeatable, and cost-effective. This test relies on a chemical reaction between acetoacetate and nitroprusside, resulting in a color change which can be measured from negative to severe by use of a color-coded chart. Because this test is highly sensitive (approaching 100%), it is helpful for identifying a cow not suffering from ketoacidosis when a negative result is obtained [25]; however, the urine test will select a higher percentage of positive cows, because of a high probability of false positives [25]. This is a valuable test to use in the screening and identification of animals potentially suffering from ketosis; however, because of the high probability of false positives, one must be cautious in making decisions concerning the treatment and management interventions.

Milk. When monitoring a group of postpartum dairy cows, urine samples may not always be obtained, whereas milk samples are generally always obtainable. This test is similar to the urine test in that it relies on a chemical reaction. The reaction is between not only acetoacetate and nitroprusside, but also acetone and nitroprusside, resulting in a color change that can be measured from negative to severe by use of a color-coded chart. The milk test has a poor sensitivity (<40%) but a high specificity (>90%) [25]. Because of its high specificity, a positive result generally means the animal is positive, whereas a negative result may be a false negative [25]. Again, as with the urine test, one must be cautious in making decisions concerning the results of this test, as well as with the choice of treatment for these animals.

Rectal temperature

Currently, the most commonly used monitoring parameter to identify abnormal periparturient dairy cows is the rectal temperature scores. Numerous disease processes, including infectious ones, complicate the immediate postpartum period in dairy cattle. Metabolic diseases such as periparturient hypocalcemia (milk fever) or acetonaemia (ketosis) are generally identified by classic clinical signs or specific tests. Pyrexia (fever) is a common clinical examination finding in the majority of infectious diseases of the postpartum cow. Quick identification of these animals allows for treatment and management intervention, thereby giving the patient a better chance of improved health and production as well as survival. Because the majority of infectious-related periparturient diseases occur during the first 2 weeks after calving, monitoring rectal temperatures during this time has proven to be a successful tool that aids in the management of disease. Fig. 1 depicts how rectal temperature scores can be used to create an algorithm designed to identify normal and abnormal postpartum dairy cattle. Abnormal cattle identified by rectal temperatures can then be further examined and treated accordingly. Information gained from analyzing dairy farm algorithms may help answer questions concerning how to use a monitoring program based on rectal temperature in dairy cattle.

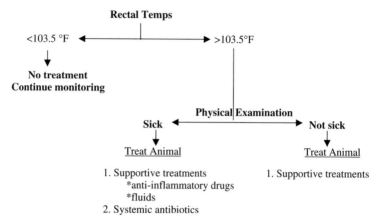

Fig. 1. Example of an algorithm based on rectal temperature scores and designed to identify normal from abnormal cows and provide management guidance.

What is the rectal temperature of dairy cows experiencing a normal periparturient period? There is a wide range of values reported for the normal rectal temperature of the bovine species. A reference range for the normal temperature of cattle can be from 101.5°F to 103°F [26]. Variation in what is considered the normal average bovine temperature is influenced by many factors, including health status, age of animal, production type, season of year, time of day, and many more. Monitoring programs using rectal temperatures will result in a wide range of values from individual cows. Although an individual cow's body temperature will vary, a healthy cow can maintain a narrow range. Kristula and Smith [27] analyzed rectal temperature data taken from 569 normal postpartum dairy cows housed in a free-stall facility in northeast Pennsylvania. Cows in this data set that experienced no clinical problems at the time of calving or for the 10-day monitoring period after calving were defined as "normal," and their average rectal temperature was found to be below 102°F for each day during the first 10 days postpartum [27]. Considering these data, it should be safe to use 102°F or below as the normal rectal temperature in dairy cattle.

What is the rectal temperature of dairy cows experiencing an abnormal periparturient period that may include dystocia, twins, retained fetal membranes, metritis, or mastitis? Normally, one would expect an elevation in rectal temperature scores for cows experiencing an abnormal periparturient period; however, many cows suffering from an acute infectious disease may actually have subnormal temperatures. Therefore, a wide range of temperatures from cows diagnosed with such problems can be expected. Three hundred forty-two rectal temperatures from cows classified as "abnormal" were analyzed [27]. Cows were classified as abnormal if they had a retained placenta, dystocia, metritis, or mastitis evident the first 10 days after calving. These cows tended to have average rectal temperatures above 102°F during days 2 through 8 postpartum. When considering diseases such as metritis, mastitis, dystocia, and retained placenta, there was no difference in daily temperature in animals that had these diseases, except that cows that had metritis had a higher average rectal temperature than cows that had dystocia on day 3, and it was higher than cows that had mastitis on day 4 [27]. Abnormal cows had an average maximum temperature of 103.6°F, and cows diagnosed with mastitis, metritis, retained placenta, or dystocia had an average maximum temperature of 103.9°F, 104.1°F, 103.7°F, and 103.6°F, respectively [27]. Because the average temperature for cows diagnosed with an abnormal periparturient condition exceeded 102°F, it is reasonable to use a rectal temperature score of 103°F or higher to identify cows suffering from an infectious-related disease process in the periparturient period.

At what temperature should one provide treatment intervention? An algorithm using rectal temperature scores was designed by the dairy farm management and veterinarians. It was routinely used to select cattle that had potential systemic involvement that required antibiotic treatment. The data analyzed by Kristula and Smith [27] showed that cows receiving systemic antibiotics had an average temperature of 103.5°F on the first day of treatment intervention; however, it was also noted that 48% of cows classified as normal had at least one temperature greater than 102.5°F, a temperature many would consider abnormal [27]. The algorithm in this study was designed to be more conservative, in that cattle selected for antibiotic treatment required 2 consecutive days of temperatures above the accepted cutoff value of 103.5°F. Because these cows responded with a significant decrease in temperature the day after initiating treatment, cattle that have rectal temperatures above 103.5°F should be considered for treatment.

Does antibiotic treatment intervention work on cows diagnosed with pyrexia? Elevated rectal temperatures indicate an abnormal health status in most animals. More specifically, in postpartum dairy cattle it most likely indicates an infectious disease process for which antibiotic treatment is a logical choice. Several studies have revealed the successful use of antibiotics in cattle that had elevated rectal temperatures [27,28]. Kristula and Smith [27] reported a significant 1.0°F drop in temperature in cattle 24 hours after the initial treatment with antibiotics. Research done by Smith and colleagues [28] also revealed similar findings, in which cattle identified with toxic puerperal metritis and treated with antibiotics responded with a significant decrease in temperature the following day. From these data, it is safe to say that dairy cattle diagnosed with fevers during the postpartum period respond positively by a decrease in temperature 1 day after antimicrobial treatment.

Should all abnormal postpartum cows be treated with antibiotics? If one is to conclude that the majority of cattle suffering from an abnormal event such as metritis, dystocia, retained fetal membranes, or mastitis develop elevated temperatures that respond to antimicrobial treatment, then an argument can be made that all cows categorized as abnormal because they experienced a postpartum disease should be started on antimicrobial treatment. In the data set analyzed by Kristula and Smith [27], 59% of all cows receiving antibiotics because of elevated temperatures that were classified as abnormal (ie, developed metritis, mastitis, retained fetal membranes, or dystocia). Therefore, 41% of cows classified as abnormal never received antibiotics, because their temperatures never registered above the cutoff point. Likewise, 41% of all cows on antimicrobial treatment did not have a postpartum disease [27]. These findings reveal that treating all abnormal cows in the postpartum period would result in overtreating, and that ignoring cows that have a normal parturition could result in missing sick cows that need antimicrobial intervention. Therefore, critically reviewing established monitoring programs for periparturient cows is essential to prevent the unnecessary treatment of these animals.

At what time during the postpartum period are cows most likely to develop a fever and be treated? The use of monitoring programs often involves making tough decisions as to when cows should be treated. Kristula and Smith [27] found that cows classified as abnormal had their highest average temperatures on days 3 through 6, and that 66% of all cows treated were treated between days 2 and 5 postpartum. Kinsel and coworkers [29] reported similar findings when evaluating rectal temperatures for the first 10 days after calving. These findings show that the majority of cows develop pyrexia within 1 week after calving. Therefore, monitoring programs using rectal temperature should be put in place for at least 7 days after calving.

Should primiparous cattle be handled differently from multiparous cattle? It has always been suggested that first-calf heifers are different from mature dairy cows in many aspects. Whether or not they should be treated differently regarding rectal temperature values and treatment interventions is certainly worth discussion. Kristula and Smith [27] found no difference in the average daily rectal temperature scores for the first 10 days of the postpartum period between first calf heifers and mature dairy cows. These data show that it is not necessary to use different algorithms for first-calf heifers and mature lactating dairy cows.

Reproductive disorders of the periparturient dairy cow

Retained fetal membranes

One of the most common and difficult problems seen in the periparturient period of dairy cattle is the retained fetal membrane. It is the major factor predisposing dairy cattle to uterine infection [30–32]. Cattle that have re-tained fetal membranes are six times more likely to develop a uterine infec-tion than cows without retained fetal membranes [31,33]. Specific events, including collagen dissolution within the connective tissue of the placen-tomes, reduction in their blood supply, appearance of polynuclear giant cells, loosening of tissues, and contraction of uterine musculature, must occur in a timely fashion before expulsion of the bovine fetal membranes can occur. A diagnosis of retained fetal membranes is generally made when membranes are retained beyond 24 hours after parturition [34].

The delay in expulsion of fetal membranes has been linked to many factors. Factors reportedly contributing to the development of retained fetal membranes include periparturient hypocalcemia, dystocia, abortion, sex of the calf, twinning, stillbirth, and induction of parturition [31,35]. The overall health status of the cow may also influence the occurrence of retained fetal membranes. It has been reported that impaired neutrophil function before calving and immediately after calving may contribute to retained fetal membranes [36,37].

The overall unsightly appearance of the retained fetal membranes, combined with the negative side effects to the health of the cow, has forced producers and veterinarians to take action. There are several management approaches identified to deal with retained fetal membranes. Many of the approaches are controversial and lack sufficient evidence to support their use. Management options include doing nothing, manual removal of the membranes, hormone therapy, and antimicrobial therapy.

No intervention

The choice to do nothing at the time of diagnosis of retained fetal membranes is common. The membranes at the site of attachment will decay and liquefy until complete separation and expulsion occur within days to weeks after diagnosis. Producers and employees are then expected to monitor these cattle for any systemic changes. If these cattle are going to develop more complicated problems such as septicemia or toxemia, they will likely do so within a few days after diagnosis. Kristula and Smith [27] reported that 72% of all cattle diagnosed with retained fetal membranes were eventually treated with systemic antibiotics, because of the de-velopment of pyrexia of 103.5°F or greater for 2 consecutive days. Because the majority of cattle develop systemic-related signs and more complicated uterine disorders after being initially left untreated, it may not be a wise action to do nothing at the time of diagnosis. Initiating antimicrobial treatment on cows diagnosed with retained fetal membranes, even without other signs of systemic illness, has been advocated by veterinarians in order to prevent uterine infections and related diseases.

Physical removal

The practice of manually removing the placenta within hours after parturition is an old custom performed by many veterinarians, and was often referred to as "cleaning out the cow." Removing the retained fetal membranes, often referred to as "cleanings," is difficult and takes time and patience. Because of the possible trauma to the uterine wall, the high occurrence of leaving membrane tags behind, and the possible iatrogenic contamination of the uterus, it is not a recommended approach to managing retained fetal membranes [38].

Hormone therapy

Several different hormones, including prostaglandin F2α, estrogen, and oxytocin, have been used in an attempt to manage retained fetal membranes in dairy cattle. The physiological limitations of hormonal therapy are addressed in the article by G.S. Frazer elsewhere in this issue. The use of prostaglandin F2α to treat retained fetal membranes is controversial. Postpartum cows have naturally elevated levels of prostaglandin F2α, which decline rapidly during the first 8 days after calving and return to a basal level by 14 days postpartum [39,40]. At present, there is no indication that treatment with prostaglandin F2α aids in the expulsion of retained fetal membranes. Estrogen administration within 24 hours after calving has been suggested as a means to promote the expulsion of fetal membranes [41]; however, this practice is not supported by the physiology of the normal postpartum cow, in which membrane expulsion and uterine involution occur when estrogen levels are basal. The theoretical benefits of using estradiol cypionate for the treatment of retained fetal membranes have not been substantiated by research [32,42]. Although oxytocin has also been used to reduce the incidence of retained fetal membranes, it should be remembered that in most cases the problem is related to disturbances in the loosening mechanism within the placentome [42]. There is no evidence to support the routine use of oxytocin to aid in the expulsion or prevention of retained fetal membranes, but enhancement of uterine motility after assisted vaginal delivery or cesarean section may be valid [32,43].

Intrauterine therapy

Several different intrauterine agents have been used to manage retained fetal membranes. Disinfectants such as iodine or chlorihexidine have been used to aid in the expulsion of retained fetal membranes [44]. These treatments may aid in reducing the incidence of systemic infection caused by retained fetal membranes, but there is no indication that they aid in the expulsion of retained fetal membranes [44]. In fact, there is evidence to show that the use of these compounds can be more detrimental than beneficial to the animal [32,45]. These disinfectant solutions are irritating to the uterine lining and inhibit the cow's own host defense mechanisms [32,45]. Intrauterine antimicrobial agents are also used to manage retained fetal membranes [32]. There is no evidence to show that the use of antimicrobial agents aid in the expulsion of retained fetal membranes [32]. Currently, intrauterine therapy is not recommended for the resolution of retained fetal membranes.

Systemic antimicrobial therapy

Because the majority of cows that have retained fetal membranes develop uterine infections, systemic antimicrobial agents seem warranted. The treatment is not specifically to aid in the expulsion of the membranes, but rather is for the prevention or early treatment of septicemia or toxemia. Current research has shown that the majority of animals that have retained fetal membranes develop fever and are treated with systemic antimicrobial agents [27]. Systemic administration of ceftiofur in dairy cows affected with dystocia, retained fetal membranes, or both has been reported to reduce the incidence of metritis by 70% when compared with cows not treated with antibiotics or those treated with estradiol cypionate [46].

Postpartum uterine infection

The majority of dairy cattle experience bacterial contamination of the uterus at the time of parturition [47,48].When these bacteria are not cleared by the cow's defense mechanisms, a uterine infection ensues. A wide variety of bacteria have been cultured from the dairy cow's postpartum uterus. Many of the bacteria can be considered incidental ones that may or may not be problematic; however, bacteria such as *Arcanobacterium pyogenes, Fusobacterium necrophorum, Clostridium* species, and *Escherichia coli* are considered pathogenic, and produce postpartum uterine infections that can be life-threatening to the animal [49].

Postpartum uterine infections can be categorized according to which layers of the uterus are involved. A classification system using terms such as endometritis, postpuerperal metritis, and toxic puerperal metritis has been described [50].

Toxic puerperal metritis

Inflammation of all the layers of the bovine uterus, with ensuing toxemia or septicemia, is a serious disease condition of the postpartum cow. Clinical signs often include the presence of a large fluid-filled uterus that is located within the abdomen, a copious amount of fetid watery vulvar discharge, and pyrexia. Other clinical signs that may or may not be present include anorexia, dehydration, weakness, and depression. The diagnosis is generally made by performing a thorough physical examination. Management of this disease is critical, because of the life-threatening nature of the infection. Treatment often involves the use of antimicrobial agents and anti-inflammatory agents. Antimicrobial agents can be administered either by intrauterine placement or by systemic injection. Oxytetracycline is the antimicrobial agent most often used for intrauterine treatment [51]. Intrauterine placement of compounds for the treatment of toxic puerperal metritis is controversial and often fails as a treatment [52]. Iatrogenic contamination of the uterus [32,45]; physical trauma to the uterus [32,45]; chemical damage to the uterine lining [32]; negative effects on host defense mechanisms, such as diminished neutrophil function [53,54]; poor absorption of drug by infected uterine tissue [52]; and unknown milk and meat withholding times have made this treatment choice a disputed one [32]. Currently, it is not recommended to use intrauterine placement of various antimicrobial agents for the treatment of toxic puerperal metritis. In contrast, systemic treatment using various antimicrobial agents avoids many of the downfalls of intrauterine treatment. A very important advantage is that it allows for the establishment of milk and meat withholding times [32]. Research has shown that systemic treatment using penicillin or ceftiofur sodium is an effective treatment choice for toxic puerperal metritis [45,52,55,56]. After reviewing the many factors involved in determining treatment success of toxic puerperal metritis, it is the authors' opinion that systemic treatment with penicillin or ceftiofur sodium should be the treatment of choice.

Postpuerperal metritis

Inflammation of multiple tissue layers, including the endometrium and the myometrium that extends beyond the puerperal period, is known as postpuerperal metritis. Clinical signs include enlarged, firm uterine horns, with a significant amount of fetid purulent vulvar discharge that is typically mucoid in consistency [50]. Performing a rectal examination of the uterus allows for the diagnosis of this condition [50]. Other diagnostic procedures that not only help diagnose postpuerperal metritis but also help determine the severity of the inflammation include uterine culture, uterine biopsy, and ultrasonography.

The management approach for endometritis and postpuerperal metritis traditionally has involved hormonal injections, intrauterine antimicrobial therapy, and systemic antimicrobial therapy. Currently, the dairy industry relies heavily on the use of prostaglandins to manage endometritis and postpuerperal metritis. Provided that the cow has ovulated and has a responsive corpus luteum, the induction of estrus takes advantage of natural uterine defense mechanisms [32,45,57]. Luteolysis removes the negative effects of progesterone on these uterine defense mechanisms, and the increasing mucus production and muscle tone of the estrous cow helps to expel the uterine contents [57,58]. There is a lack of objective research to support the theoretical benefits of exogenous estrogen administration in managing postpartum uterine infections [58]. Similarly, research findings regarding the benefits of using prostaglandin F2α in treating postpartum uterine infection are equivocal [59].

Antimicrobial agents have been used to treat cows diagnosed with postpartum uterine infection. Intrauterine placement of nonantibiotic and antibiotic agents has been a long accepted practice; however, the use of nonantibiotic agents such as iodine or chlorhexidine is irritating and potentially damaging to the uterine tissue [57]. Currently, it is not a recommended treatment option. Intuitively, the use of intrauterine antibiotic agents for the

Table 1
Example of parameters that could be included in monitoring programs for periparturient dairy cattle

Parameter	Normal	Abnormal	Intervention
Milk production	Steady rise each day after calving	≥10-pound deviation	Perform physical examination
General attitude	Bright, alert, erect ears	Eyes	Perform physical examination and provide fluid therapy according to percent dehydration
		Score 1 (minimal) = bright eyes positioned normal within eye socket	
		Score 2 (mild) = dull eyes slightly sunken	
		Score 3 (moderate) = glazed eyes moderately sunken	
		Score 4 (severe) = dry eyes severely sunken	
		Ears	
		Ears drooping down below horizontal	
Serum haptoglobin	<10 mg/dl	>10 mg/dl	Perform physical examination
			Provide antibiotics and anti-inflammatory agents
Serum calcium	8.8–10.4 mg/100 ml	Clinical ≤6 mg/100 ml	Provide calcium
		Subclinical = 6.2–7.5 mg/100ml	
Rumenocentesis	pH ≥ 6	Marginal acidosis = pH 5.6 to 5.8	Reevaluate periparturient ration
		Acidosis = pH ≤ 5.50	
Urine or milk ketone levels	Negative	Trace or mild	Provide oral propylene glycol
		Moderate or severe	Provide intravenous dextrose plus oral propylene glycol
Rectal temperature	≤103° F	≥103° F	Provide antibiotic and anti-inflammatory agents

treatment of endometritis or postpuerperal metritis seems to be indicated; however, multiple reasons, such as poor drug absorption locally, potential for drug residue violation, and potential for local tissue irritation, justify not recommending intrauterine antibiotic placement for the treatment of postpuerperal metritis and endometritis [32,52,60,61]. Systemic antibiotic treatment for cows diagnosed with postpuerperal metritis and endometritis could be effective [57]; however, because many of these cattle are showing no clinical signs of systemic involvement, and because there is the potential for the treatment of a large number of animals, it is generally not a recommended method of treatment for endometritis or postpuerperal metritis.

Endometritis

Inflammation of the endometrial lining of the uterus is a common postpartum finding in dairy cattle. No obvious clinical signs are noticed in cows suffering from endometritis. Historically, diagnosis of this condition has been made by rectal palpation or by visual examination (by use of a speculum) of purulent material being discharged from the cervix or located in the cranial vagina [57]. Uterine cultures and biopsies are additional diagnostic methods that can be used [57]; however, because of the high occurrence and mild nature of endometritis, no specific diagnostic measures are generally taken to identify animals that have endometritis.

Summary

Monitoring programs for periparturient dairy cows are essential for the early identification and proper management of abnormal animals. As shown in Table 1, parameters such as milk production, general attitude, serum components, rumenocentesis, ketone levels, and rectal temperature scores can be considered for use in monitoring programs. An appropriately established and critically reviewed monitoring program can be indispensable when managing all disease conditions of the periparturient dairy cow, especially postpartum reproductive disorders.

References

[1] Curtis CR, Erb HN, Sniffen CJ, et al. Association of parturient hypocalcemia with eight periparturient disorders in Holstein cows. J Am Vet Med Assoc 1983;183:559–61.
[2] Curtis CR, Erb HN, Sniffen CF, et al. Path analysis of dry period nutrition, postpartum metabolic and reproductive disorders, and mastitis in Holstein cows. J Dairy Sci 1985;68: 2347–60.
[3] Bartlett PC, Kirk JH, Wilke MA, et al. Metritis complex in Michigan Holstein-Friesian cattle: incidence, descriptive epidemiology and estimated economic impact. Prev Vet Med 1986;4(3):235–48.
[4] Fetrow J, Cady R, Jones G. Dairy production medicine in the United States. Bovine Practitioner 2004;38(2):113–20.

[5] Upham GL. A practitioners approach to management of metritis/endometritis early detection and supportive treatment. In: Proceedings of the 29th Annual Conference of the American Association of Bovine Practitioners. Spokane, WA, September 24–26, 1998. p. 19–21.

[6] Spain JN. The 100-day contract with the dairy cow: 30 days prepartum to 70 days postpartum. Feed Compounder 1999;19:16–9.

[7] Panndorf H, Richter H, Dittrich B. Haptoglobin in domestic mammals 5th communication: plasma-haptoglobin levels in cattle under pathological conditions. Archiv fur Experimentell Veterinarmedizin 1976;30(2):193–202.

[8] Smith BI, Donovan GA, Risco CA, et al. Serum haptoglobin concentrations in Holstein dairy cattle with toxic puerperal metritis. Vet Rec 1998;142:83–5.

[9] Young CR, Wittum TE, Stanker LH, et al. Serum haptoglobin concentrations in a population of feedlot cattle. Am J Vet Res 1996;57:138–41.

[10] Horst RL, Goff JP, Reinhardt TA, et al. Strategies for preventing milk fever in dairy cattle. J Dairy Sci 1997;80:1269–80.

[11] Allen WM, Sansom BF. Parturient paresis (milk fever) and hypocalcemia (cows, ewes, and goats). In: Howard JL, editor. Current veterinary therapy 3 food animal practice. Philadelphia: WB Saunders; 1993. p. 304–9.

[12] Shearer JK, Van Horn HH. Metabolic diseases of dairy cattle. In: Van Horn HH, Wilcox CJ, editors. Large dairy herd management. Champaign (IL): American Dairy Science Association; 1992. p. 358–72.

[13] Risco CA, Reynolds JP, Hird D. Uterine prolapse and hypocalcemia in dairy cows. J Am Vet Med Assoc 1984;185(12):1517–9.

[14] Duffield T, Plaizier JC, Fairfield A, et al. Comparison of techniques for measurement of rumen pH in lactating dairy cows. J Dairy Sci 2004;87:59–66.

[15] Nordlund KV, Garrett EF, Oetzel GR. Herd-based rumenocentesis: a clinical approach to the diagnosis of subacute rumen acidosis in dairy herds. Compendium Contin Educ Pract Vet 1995;17(8):S48–56.

[16] Nordlund KV, Garrett EF. Rumenocentesis: a technique for the diagnosis of subacute rumen acidosis in dairy herds. Bovine Practitioner 1994;28:109–12.

[17] Geishauser T, Leslie K, Kelton D, et al. Monitoring subclinical ketosis in dairy herds. Comp Contin Educ Pract Vet 2001;23(8):S65–71.

[18] Availa 4 from Zinpro. Cost of common diseases in USA. Available at: http://www.availa4.com/technical/tools/commondiseases.html. Accessed September 5, 2004.

[19] Dohoo JR, Martin SW. Subclinical ketosis: prevalence and association with production of disease. Can J Comp Med 1984;48:1–5.

[20] Francos G, Insler G, Dirksen G. Routine testing for milk beta-hydroxybutyrate for the detection of subclinical ketosis in dairy cows. Bovine Practitioner 1997;31(2):61–4.

[21] Geishuaser T, Leslie K, Duffield T, et al. Evaluation of aspartate aminotransferase activity and beta-hydroxybutyrate concentration in blood as tests for left displaced abomasums in dairy cows. Am J Vet Res 1997;58:1216–20.

[22] Syvajarvi J, Saloniemi H, Grohn Y. An epidemiological and genetic study on registered diseases in Finnish Ayrshire cattle. Acta Vet Scand 1986;27:223–34.

[23] Butler WR, Smith RD. Interrelationships between energy balance and postpartum reproductive function in dairy cattle. J Dariy Sci 1989;72:767–83.

[24] Andersson L, Emanuelson U. An epidemiological study of hyperketonaemia in Swedish dairy cows; determinants and the relation to fertility. Prev Vet Med 1985;3:449–62.

[25] Duffield T. Monitoring energy metabolism with NEFAs, beta-hydroxybutyrate, and ketone sticks. In: Proceedings of the Cornell Veterinary Medicine Transition Cows Conference, Canandaigua, NY, 2001. p. 1–11.

[26] Pei Jun Chen. Temperature of a healthy cow. Available at: http://www.hypertextbook.com/facts/1998/PeiJunChen.shtml. Accessed September 11, 2004.

[27] Kristula M, Smith B. The use of daily postpartum rectal temperatures to select dairy cows for treatment with systemic antibiotics. Bovine Practitioner 2001;35(2):117–25.

[28] Smith BI, Donovan GA, Risco CA, et al. Comparison of various antibiotic treatments for cows diagnosed with toxic puerperal metritis. J Dairy Sci 1998;81:1555–62.

[29] Pfizer Animal Health. The 100-day contract fresh dairy wellness plan. Spot problems fast. Available at: http://100daycontract.com/fresh-cow.asp?country = US&Lang = EN&id = temp. Accessed September 4, 2004.

[30] Sandals WCD, Curtiss RA, Cote JF, et al. The effect of retained placenta and metritis complex on reproductive performance in dairy cattle. A case control study. Can Vet J 1979; 20:131–9.

[31] Correa MT, Erb H, Scarlett J. Path analysis for seven postpartum disorders of Holstein cows. J Dairy Sci 1993;76:1305–12.

[32] Paisley LG, Micklesen WD, Anderson PB. Mechanisms and therapy for retained membranes and uterine infections of cows: a review. Theriogenology 1986;25:353–81.

[33] Dohoo IR, Martin SW. Disease, production, and culling in Holstein-Friesian cows. IV. Effects of disease on production. Prev Vet Med 1984;2:755–70.

[34] Heinonen M, Heinonen K. Retained placenta in cattle: the effect of treatment or nontreatment on puerperal diseases and subsequent fertility. Acta Vet Scand 1989;30:425–9.

[35] Stevenson JS, Call EP. Reproductive disorders in the periparturient dairy cow. J Dairy Sci 1988;71:2572–83.

[36] Cai T, Weston PG, Lund LA, et al. Association between neutrophil functions and periparturient disorders in cows. Am J Vet Res 1994;55(7):935–43.

[37] Gunnick JW. Pre-partum leucocytic activity and retained placenta. Vet Q 1984;6:52–4.

[38] Bolinder A, Seguin B, Kindahl H, et al. Retained fetal membranes in cows: manual removal versus nonremoval and its effect on reproductive performance. Theriogenology 1988;30(1): 45–56.

[39] Madej A, Kendahl H, Woyno W. Blood levels of 15-keto-13, 14-dihydro-prostaglandin F2α; during the post partum period in primiparous cows. Theriogenology 1984;21:279–87.

[40] Risco CA, Drost M, Thatcher WW, et al. Effects of calving-related disorders on prostaglandin, calcium, ovarian activity, and uterine involution in postpartum dairy cows. Theriogenology 1994;42(1):183–203.

[41] Bayley AJ. Product monographs. In: Arrioja-Dechert A, editor: Compendium of veterinary products. Port Huron (MI): Adrian Bayley; 2001. p. 1380–1.

[42] Burton MJ, Dzuik HE, Fahning ML, et al. Effects of oestradiol cypionate on spontaneous and oxytocin-stimulated postpartum myometrial activity in the cow. Br Vet J 1990;146(4): 309–15.

[43] Peters AR, Laven RA. Treatment of bovine retained placenta and its effects. Vet Rec 1996; 139(22):535–9.

[44] Arthur GH. Retention of the afterbirth in cattle: a review and commentary. Veterinary Annual 1979;19:26–36.

[45] Smith BI, Risco CA. Therapeutic and management options for postpartum metritis in dairy cattle. Comp Contin Educ Pract Vet 2002;24:S92–100.

[46] Risco CA, Hernandez J. Comparison of ceftiofur hydrochloride and estradiol cypionate for metritis prevention and reproductive performance in dairy cows affected with retained fetal membranes. Theriogenology 2003;60:47–58.

[47] Elliott L, McMahon KJ, Gier HT, et al. Uterus of the cow after parturition: bacterial content. Am J Vet Res 1968;29:77–81.

[48] Griffin JFT, Hartigan PJ, Nunn WR. Non-specific uterine infection and bovine fertility. I. Infection patterns and endometritis during the first seven weeks post-partum. Theriogenology 1974;1:91–106.

[49] Smith BI, Risco CA. Predisposing factors and potential causes of postpartum metritis in diary cattle. Comp Contin Educ Pract Vet 2002;24:S74–80.

[50] Smith BI, Risco CA. Clinical manifestation of postpartum metritis in dairy cattle. Comp Contin Educ Pract Vet 2002;24:S56–63.

[51] Gilbert RO, Schwark WS. Pharmacologic considerations in the management of peripartum conditions in the cow. Vet Clin North Am Food Anim Pract 1992;8:29–56.

[52] Gustafsson BK. Therapeutic strategies involving antimicrobial treatment of the uterus in large animals. J Am Vet Med Assoc 1984;185:1194–8.

[53] Ziv G, Paape MJ, Dulan AM. Influence of antibiotics and intramammary antibiotic products on phagocytosis of Staphylococcus aureus by bovine leukocytes. Am J Vet Res 1983;41:385–8.

[54] Jayappa H, Loken KI. Effect of antimicrobial agents and corticosteroids on bovine polymorphonuclear leukocyte chemotaxis. Am J Vet Res 1983;44:2155–9.

[55] Drillich M, Beetz O, Pfutzner A, et al. Evaluation of a systemic antibiotic treatment of toxic puerperal metritis in dairy cows. J Dairy Sci 2001;84:2010–7.

[56] Masera J. Gustafsson BK, Afiefy MM. Blood plasma and uterine tissue concentrations of sodium penicillin G in cows at intramuscular vs intrauterine administration. In: Proceedings from the 9th International Congress of Animal Reproduction and Artificial Insemination, Madrid, Spain, June 16–20, 1980. p. 687–90.

[57] Bretzlaff K. Rationale for treatment of endometritis in the dairy cow. Vet Clin North Am 1987;3(3):593–607.

[58] Carson RL, Wolfe DF, Klesius PH, et al. The effects of ovarian hormones and ACTH on uterine defense to Corynebacterium pyogenes in cows. Theriogenology 1988;1:91–8.

[59] Olson JD. Metritis/endometritits: medically sound treatments. In: Proceedings of the 29th Annual Convention of American Association of Bovine Practitioners, San Diego, CA, September 12–14, 1996. p. 8–14.

[60] Masera J, Gustafsson BK, Afiefy MM, et al. Disposition of oxytetracycline in the bovine genital tract: systemic vs intrauterine administration. J Am Vet Med Assoc 1980;176:1099–102.

[61] Bretzlaff KN, Ott Rs, Koritz GD, et al. Distribution of oxytetracycline in genital tract tissues of postpartum cows given the drug by intravenous and intrauterine routes. Am J Vet Res 1983;44:764–9.

VETERINARY
CLINICS
Food Animal Practice

Vet Clin Food Anim 21 (2005) 523–568

A Rational Basis for Therapy in the Sick Postpartum Cow

Grant S. Frazer, BVSc, MS, MBA

College of Veterinary Medicine, The Ohio State University,
A100 Sisson Hall, 1920 Coffey Road, Columbus, OH 43210, USA

The periparturient period is perhaps the most critical few weeks in the whole reproductive process. Infectious disease and nutritional errors in late gestation can result in complications such as dystocia, stillbirth, uterine prolapse, fetal membrane retention, or metritis. The veterinarian's role is to not only attend to the cow's immediate health, but also to ensure the future production and fertility of the affected animal and the entire herd. Veterinary advice should focus on prevention through appropriate breeding practices (calving-ease sires), vaccination and biosecurity protocols, optimal nutrition and transition management programs, and an emphasis on calving hygiene. Several articles in this issue address appropriate management strategies.

Prompt uterine involution and elimination of the inevitable calving-related bacterial contamination is the key to optimal first-service conception rates and reduction of days open. Pharmaceutical agents can only be used effectively when the natural process is fully understood. The intimate cellular and molecular events that regulate myometrial functions during gestation, parturition, and uterine involution are extremely complex [1]. Despite extensive research efforts spanning several decades, our level of understanding of these intricate processes is rudimentary at best. Unfortunately, our knowledge about the pathophysiology of the diseased postpartum uterus is even more deficient. The purpose of this article is to present a review of peripartum physiology, and to use this scientific

---

This material was to have been presented at the combined annual meetings of the American Association of Bovine Practitioners and the Society for Theriogenology, in Vancouver, Canada, September 2001. The terrorist attacks of 9/11 severely disrupted the planned Bovine Reproduction Symposium. The content of the paper has since been extensively revised, and the reference list updated.

E-mail address: frazer.6@osu.edu

information to justify appropriate therapy for fetal membrane retention and postpartum metritis. The author has endeavored to point out that caution should be exercised when extrapolating in-vitro effects on myometrial cells or muscle strips to the in-vivo environment. Likewise, suggestions that a certain therapeutic agent has a desired effect in vivo may only hold true if the time frame, frequency, and route of administration (intravenous [IV] versus intramuscular [IM]) is replicated. The scientific evidence suggests that this is especially true of hormones. Cellular receptor dynamics, the method of metabolism, and the biological half-life are all important variables. Although intrauterine medication has been a mainstay of veterinary practice for decades, there is an increasing body of evidence that suggests that such intervention does not enhance fertility, and that it is generally contra-indicated. Likewise, several hormonal therapies have questionable scientific validity in the immediate postpartum period.

Normal physiology

The parturient cascade is initiated by activation of the fetal hypotha-lamic-pituitary-adrenal axis through the release of adrenocorticotrophic hormone (ACTH) [2,3]. It is thought that when the combined fetal mass and volume of fetal fluids approach the inherent capacity of the uterus, a stress response by the mature fetus initiates its delivery [4]. In the fetal lamb, it is now known that fetal cortisol acts on glucocorticoid receptors in the placental trophoblast cells. This results in upregulation of prostaglandin synthase, and subsequent production of prostaglandin E_2 (PGE_2). The PGE_2 acts by an autocrine/paracrine route to cause upregulation of the microsomal cytochrome P_{450} enzyme system (hydroxylase, lyase, and aromatase) in the placenta [5–8]. The activated P_{450} enzyme systems within the cotyledons increase the capacity of the bovine placenta to convert C-21 steroids (progesterone, pregnenolone) into C-19 estrogen precursors (androstenedione, dihydro-epandrostenedione) and estrogen as the partu-rient cascade progresses [4,9–11]. The enzymatic changes result in a dramatic prepartum elevation of plasma estrogen, estrone sulfate, and estrogen precursors. The decline in progesterone and increasing estrogen levels are known to stimulate endometrial prostaglandin synthase expression [12–14]. The caruncular tissue is a very active site of prostaglandin $F_{2\alpha}$ ($PGF_{2\alpha}$) synthesis [15]. $PGF_{2\alpha}$ metabolite (PGFM; 15-keto-prostaglandin $F_{2\alpha}$) con-centrations gradually increase in maternal plasma approximately 1 week before parturition (Fig. 1).

Despite decades of research, our understanding of the intimate cellular and molecular events that regulate myometrial function is very limited [1]. Whether exogenous prostaglandins have a direct effect on periparturient uterine activity in cattle has been a contentious issue amongst researchers [15–31]. Prostanoids (prostaglandins and thromboxanes) are metabolites of

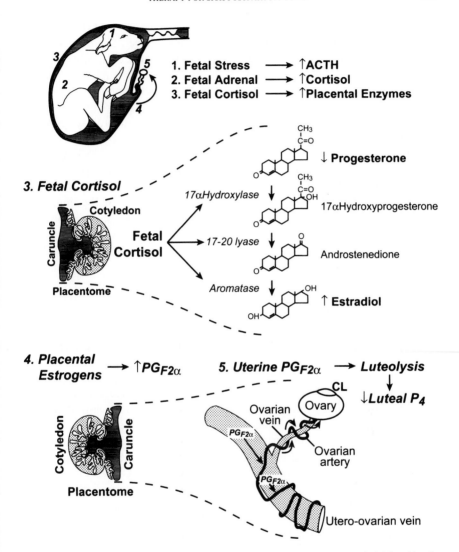

Fig. 1. Birth of a calf is the culmination of an intricate hormonal cascade that is initiated by the mature fetus. The placentome (cotyledon and caruncle) plays a vital role in this process. Ration imbalances during the dry period can affect placental separation (Stage III of labor). Retention of the fetal membranes predisposes the cow to uterine infection and the development of toxic metritis.

the cyclo-oxygenase (COX) pathway of arachidonic acid metabolism, and $PGF_{2\alpha}$ itself is very rapidly metabolized [32–35]. The myometrial response to prostaglandins ($PGF_{2\alpha}$; PGE_2) depends on the presence of different receptors in different uterine regions, and their activation may promote relaxation or contraction [36]. In the rat model, PGE_2 receptors are located in the cervical region, and are responsible for myometrial relaxation and cervical dilation [37]. Myometrial contraction occurs when $PGF_{2\alpha}$ binds to its receptor and the phosphatidylinositol pathway is activated. This results in calcium mobilization from intracellular stores and extracellular fluids [36,38]. Obviously, the stimulatory effect on the myometrium may be quite different depending on the route of delivery. Exogenous prostaglandins have to pass through the lungs (site of metabolism) during delivery via the systemic circulation, whereas endogenous production in apposing tissues (endometrium, allantochorion) permits a direct, paracrine route to the myometrium. Enhanced production within the myometrium itself may play an important role [39]. The total concentration of PGF receptors on rat myometrial cell membranes (circular and longitudinal smooth muscle) is high in late gestation, but the numbers fall significantly in the immediate postpartum period [40,41]. Immunostaining patterns suggest an association with myofibrils (the contractile cell mechanism), thus reinforcing the role of $PGF_{2\alpha}$ in uterine contractility at term [40]. It has been proposed that the term myometrium may have an enhanced sensitivity to prostaglandins, and that this leads to contractions and labor [42].

In an in-vitro study [18], prostaglandin-desensitized uteri responded significantly to oxytocin challenge, and vice versa, suggesting that there are separate uterine receptors for oxytocin and prostaglandin. This is, in fact, the case. $PGF_{2\alpha}$ is integrally involved in a feedback loop with oxytocin, even though the molecules have different receptors on the myometrium, and different second messengers within the cells [18,43–45]. Oxytocin appears to stimulate myometrial contraction by two parallel mechanisms—direct activation of receptors on myometrial cells, and indirect stimulation of contraction through the release of stimulatory prostaglandins from the endometrium [46,47]. In periparturient ruminants, circulating oxytocin binds to myometrial receptors, leading to rapid uterine contraction and a rise in $PGF_{2\alpha}$ levels [45,47–50]. Recent data reveal that bovine parturition is associated with a marked induction of COX-2 in the uterus [34]. Research in ewes and rats has indicated that $PGF_{2\alpha}$ stimulates the release of more oxytocin (ovary, pituitary?) and also enhances the sensitivity of the myometrium to oxytocin [51–54]. This complex interaction is demonstrated by the fact that whereas a prostaglandin synthase inhibitor (meclofenamic acid) can block corticosteroid induced parturition in sheep, uterine motility can be reactivated by administration of oxytocin. It appears that by inhibiting $PGF_{2\alpha}$ production the meclofanamic acid indirectly blocks uterine activity. The low $PGF_{2\alpha}$ levels do not promote further release of oxytocin, and thus there is an indirect inhibitory effect on the myometrium [42,55,56]; however, in the presence of prostaglandin synthase inhibitors, the myometrium will still respond if exogenous oxytocin is administered [18,51].

Recent studies in sheep have revised our understanding of the parturient process, and it seems likely that a similar process holds true in cattle [5,6]. Challis [57] has proposed that the fetal genome impacts on delivery by two separate but interdependent pathways. The developing pregnancy causes progressive uterine stretch, but the presence of progesterone maintains uterine quiescence. The structure of smooth muscle permits the uterus to assume the shape and size necessary to accommodate the fetus [33]. As the PGFM level peaks, there is an abrupt decline in progesterone levels associated with regression of the corpus luteum [11,58–60]. This eliminates the "progesterone block" on myometrial activity, and as estrogen becomes the dominant steroid hormone, parturition ensues [39,61,62]. In the absence of progesterone, the uterine stretch effect causes activation of myometrial function by upregulating a cassette of genes that are referred to as "contraction-associated proteins." One is the major gap-junction protein (connexin-43), and others include the receptors for oxytocin and prostaglandin $F_{2\alpha}$ [33,63–69]. Gap junctions are intercellular connections with low electrical impedance [70]. They serve to synchronize myometrial function via conduction of electrophysiological stimuli during labor [33]. Enhanced movement of electrolytes and small molecules between adjacent myoepithelial cells leads to increased contractility [2,66,71–74]. As parturition approaches, a rapid membrane depolarization results in the onset of strong, coordinated uterine contractions that characterize the first stage of labor. Oxytocin activates phospholipase C to produce inositol 1,4,5-triphosphate, which releases calcium ions from intracellular stores [75]. When oxytocin binds to receptors on myometrial cells, there is a change in intracellular calcium concentrations, and increased myometrial contractility results [76].

It appears that fetal movement results in localized myometrial contractions (contractures), possibly associated with positioning of the fetus in preparation for delivery [16,24,77]. There is minimal uterine activity during the final week of gestation [16,24,39,78–81]. The concentration of relaxin-like factor—a proteohormone produced by the corpus luteum—may have a significant impact in the preparturient cow [82]. In nonruminant species, relaxin has a mostly suppressive impact on uterine motility, possibly by increasing the efflux of calcium ions out of the myometrial cells [82,83]. The high relaxin levels may serve to increase collagenase activity in the uterus and other tissues (cervix, pelvic symphysis, and ligaments) [82,84]. Connective tissue remodeling within the placentome may be an essential feature of the placental maturation process, facilitating rapid detachment of the fetal membranes following fetal expulsion [85–88]. Macrophages in the placentomes of cows that have fetal membrane retention have decreased lysosomal enzyme (acid phosphatase) activity [89].

In the last 18 to 20 hours before fetal expulsion, there are tubocervical waves of increasing frequency [24]. The amount of uterine work (force and frequency of contractions) increases markedly during the 12 hours before delivery of the calf [16,24,78,79,90,91]. As parturition approaches, the falling levels of progesterone and high levels of estrogen result in regular, strong waves of uterine contraction, each lasting 5 to 15 minutes [11,16]. After the onset of regular uterine contractions, the cervix starts to dilate in response to the repeated increases in intrauterine pressure [92]. In the final

6 hours of Stage I, uterine activity is present about 70% of the time [16]. Oxytocin, which is mainly secreted into the blood stream in the expulsion phase, increases the contractile activity of the myometrium [68]. This occurs subsequent to an increased influx of calcium ions into the smooth muscle cells, and also increased calcium availability within the cells [76,93–97]. Maternal straining (contraction of the abdominal muscles) is almost always associated with large sustained uterine contractions that are most commonly associated with the uterine body. Rupture of the amnion, and loss of the remaining fetal fluids, leads to a transient reduction in uterine activity until the calf itself enters the cervico-vaginal canal. The frequency and amplitude of the contraction waves then increase markedly. The speed of wave propagation (propagation time) down the horn is about twice as rapid as that before the onset of the second stage of labor, and is probably the result of oxytocin binding following its reflex release. Although propagated contractions always start at the tip of the uterine horn, the rate of propagation is so rapid that all parts of the uterus tend to contract simultaneously, approaching one contraction every 2 minutes [16,24].

The postpartum period is a unique combination of both physiological and pathological processes (bacterial infections and inflammation) [23]. It involves contraction of the uterine musculature, sloughing of excess caruncular tissue, and regeneration of the endometrial epithelium—uterine involution [39]. This process occurs during three distinct phases with respect to the hormonal milieu. The puerperal period has traditionally been defined as that period extending from calving until the pituitary gland becomes responsive to GnRH [98]. It may be more meaningful to designate it as being the first 8 to 10 days postpartum. It is the period when fetal membrane retention may occur, when most of the uterine fluid (lochia) should be expelled, and when uterine infections can become a problem; thus the term "puerperal metritis." The second phase of uterine involution—the intermediate period—persists up until the first postpartum ovulation has occurred. In most studies, the number of bacteria that can be isolated from uterine fluid begins to decrease after the second week [23,99–101]. Phagocytosis in the uterine lumen is mainly accomplished by polymorphonuclear leukocytes (PMN) [102,103]. Although endometritis with fetid, sanguine-purulent lochia persists longer than milder cases that have mucopurulent to purulent lochia, the profiles of blood and uterine leukocytes may not be significantly different. In susceptible cows, there may be a deficiency in the ability of the PMN to "kill" engulfed bacteria [102,104]. Spontaneous recovery from endometritis may not be completed until 20 to 25 days postpartum [105]. Uterine infections (endometritis) carried over from the intermediate period tend to result in chronic infertility problems. The time to first ovulation varies tremendously, depending on many factors, including nutrition and energy balance [106–113]. Activity of the reproductive axis appears to be controlled by the negative energy state through various metabolic signals, most likely insulin-like growth factor 1

(IGF-1) and leptin [107,112,114–117]. In one study of well-managed cows (N = 90) [113], the negative energy balance nadir was reached at 7.2 days, but the first ovulation was not detected until 23.9 days. In an evaluation of over 1800 postpartum cows [118], only 42% had a palpable corpus luteum by 33 days-in-milk. The postovulatory period is self-explanatory, and extends until about 45 days postpartum, when uterine involution is complete. It is only in this latter period, when luteal tissue is present on the ovary, that it is widely accepted that exogenous administration of prostaglandin appears to have a beneficial effect in the postpartum cow. Removal of the immunosuppressive effects of luteal progesterone may aid in the resolution of chronic postpartum endometritis [118–121].

In a healthy postpartum cow the PGFM levels peak by day 3, then gradually decline to baseline by the end of the second week (Fig. 2) [15,26,60,105,122–124]. The physiologic role of this elevated postpartum prostaglandin level is unclear, and the levels are even higher in cows that have infected uteri [124–130]. Cows that had fetid sanguine-purulent lochia at up to day 15 postpartum had significantly higher concentrations of plasma PGFM than cows that had mucopurulent to purulent lochia; however, the uterine fluid PGFM concentrations in these same animals was not different between the two endometritis groups [105]. This suggests that the intensity of inflammation in the uterine tissues may impact on the plasma levels of PGFM—be it from a myometrial contribution, or merely

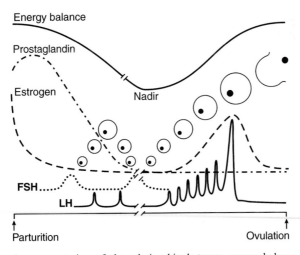

Fig. 2. Schematic representation of the relationship between energy balance and the first postpartum ovulation. The time line of the X axis varies tremendously, depending on when the negative energy balance nadir is reached. Increasing luteinizing hormone (LH) pulses can then drive a dominant follicle to maturation. Rising estrogen levels promote an LH surge that brings about ovulation, the formation of a corpus luteum, and a return to progesterone dominance. If chronic endometritis is present, exogenous prostaglandin may then be administered to cause luteolysis and promote resolution of the infection. FSH, follicle-stimulating hormone.

due to increased uterine blood flow to an inflamed endometrium. Either way, elevated plasma levels may be a useful indicator of the severity of uterine infection [105,121,125,128,130]. It should be noted that, although high plasma levels of the PGFM are negatively correlated with uterine involution time in cows that have a normal puerperium (high levels mean a shorter involution time), this does not hold true for cows that have experienced obstetrical complications or retention of the fetal membranes. In animals that have puerperal uterine infections, the duration of endometrial $PGF_{2\alpha}$ release is positively correlated with the time for completion of uterine involution—high levels mean a high number of days to complete uterine involution [105,124,125,128]. If a hysterectomy is performed within 8 hours of parturition, the PGFM levels fall dramatically and become undetectable within 5 hours. This conclusively demonstrates that the uterus is the source of the postpartum prostaglandin production [15]. In postpartum cows that have been treated with a COX inhibitor (flunixin meglumine) the response to a low dose of oxytocin (5 international units [IU] IV) is attenuated, but the rate of uterine involution is not affected [31]. This study suggests that although the action of oxytocin is closely associated with prostaglandin levels, high levels of $PGF_{2\alpha}$ are not a prerequisite for uterine involution. Flunixin meglumine does not appear to affect the metabolism of $PGF_{2\alpha}$ into PGFM, but does inhibit the COX enzymes that form $PGF_{2\alpha}$ itself from arachidonic acid [14,23,131]. Endometrial $PGF_{2\alpha}$ causes luteolysis through an endocrine signaling mechanism. Attention to both dosage and frequency of administration of flunixin meglumine is required to suppress $PGF_{2\alpha}$ release sufficiently to prevent its luteolytic effect [23,132]. Even when large doses are administered, $PGF_{2\alpha}$ production is not totally abolished [23]. This could have significant relevance in the postpartum uterus, where $PGF_{2\alpha}$ likely works through a paracrine signaling mechanism from the endometrium to the myometrium.

The systemic estrogen levels fall precipitously at parturition, and are at baseline levels (< 5 pg/ml) within 2 to 3 days (see Fig. 2) [59,60,122]. Follicle-stimulating hormone (FSH) secretion resumes within the first week, and cohorts of follicles begin to emerge. The first dominant follicle may be selected as soon as 10 to 12 days postpartum [107,108,115,133,134]. This dominant follicle acquires luteinizing hormone (LH) receptors on its granulosa cell layer, and thereby attains enhanced steroidogenic capacity compared with the other members of the cohort; however, continued growth and increased estradiol production from the dominant follicle depends on LH pulse frequency, otherwise it will become atretic. There is a clear relationship between the timing of the negative energy balance nadir and the LH pulse frequency [107,108,111–113,115,133–135]. Fresh cows experience a period of negative energy balance because the increase in dry matter intake lags behind the increased nutrient requirements for high milk production. Once the negative energy nadir is passed and energy levels rise, there is an increasing LH pulse frequency that is able to support dominant follicle growth and steroidogenesis. Thus, if a dominant follicle is selected during the recovery period from negative energy balance, the frequency and magnitude of LH pulses can drive the follicle to maturity. Finally, the increasing estradiol synthesis may be sufficient to induce a gonadotrophin surge, and from 40% to 75% of the time ovulation will result (see Fig. 2) [106,108,134–139]. The first ovulation postpartum may occur 7 to 14 days after the energy balance nadir. Thus if the lowest point of the negative energy balance occurs between the first and second weeks postpartum, then well-fed cows may ovulate by 21 to 30 days [109,113,140]. Often this is not the case, and the severity and duration of negative energy balance can delay the return of normal estrous cycles by several weeks, or even months [115,141–144].

The postpartum uterus

One has to be cautious when extrapolating uterine activity data obtained from nonpregnant, cycling cows [145]. Likewise, although laboratory studies using myometrial strips may provide useful new knowledge, these in-vitro experiments cannot be assumed to mimic the response of the postpartum uterus in vivo [29]. For example, it has been known since the 1930s that strong uterine contractions are present during estrus, and that these become very weak during the progesterone-dominated diestrous period [146]; however, the postpartum uterus is a vastly different organ in both size and activity, and data from periparturient studies have been quite variable. There are three reasons for this: differences in the recording equipment employed, variability in the duration of recording sessions, and the limitations inherent when small numbers of animals are studied [16,20,24,25,31,77–79,90,91,147–150]. One often-cited study [27] monitored involution in three cows, and the conclusions were based on palpation per rectum. Any attempt to critically evaluate uterine tone has been hampered by the lack of any reliable, noninvasive methodology to quantitate the texture of the uterine wall [20]. Assessment by palpation per rectum is very subjective, and open to investigator bias. Multiple intraluminal balloons (pressure data), as well as strain gauges or electrodes (electromyographic data) can capture the frequency and direction of contraction waves [16,20,24,25,77–79,90,91,146–153]. More recent studies have incorporated ultrasonography [20,154,155]. Some of these methods for documenting uterine activity are prone to artifacts attributable to respiration, rumination, or postural or excretory activity, as well as local myometrial irritation around the surgical site of tissue implants. One major disadvantage that most of these experiments have in common is that the animals being studied were healthy postpartum cows. It is impossible to say what, if any, of the conclusions actually apply to the atonic uterus that characterizes the toxic metritis cow. Unfortunately, very little is known about the pathophysiology of the diseased postpartum uterus. A prerequisite for scientifically based therapeutic intervention is a thorough understanding of the pathologically disrupted mechanisms.

Immediately after delivery of the calf, there is a significant change in the activity of the uterus. Almost all tubocervical waves end with a contraction of the uterine body [16,78,79,90]. The frequency of contractions becomes extremely regular, slowing to approximately 1 every 2.5 minutes [16,24,90]. The contraction size increases quadratically as parturition progresses, and continues to increase after the calf is expelled. The frequency of contractions declines steadily as their size increases. Frequency, amplitude, and duration of contractions are highest at 1 hour postpartum and decrease progressively thereafter [149]. The strong propagated postpartum contractions serve to rapidly involute the uterus and promote placental expulsion [16,24,77,90]. Early in Stage III, these organized postpartum contractions are still prop-agated mainly (70% to 90%) in a tubocervical direction [16,24,77,79,90,147]. The greater frequency of contractions at the tip of the uterine horn, compared with the uterine body, may serve to invert the apices of the fetal membranes, and lead to a gradual peeling of the cotyledonary villi from the caruncular crypts in a progressive tubocervical direction, such that the membranes are expelled "inside-out" [16,77]. Passage of the fetal membranes by 3 to 8 hours causes a rapid decrease in uterine activity [20,24]. Although discrete myometrial contractions can be detected up until at least 7 days postpartum, the frequency of contractions and the rate of contrac-tion propagation (propagation index) decreases with time [16,20,24,77–79, 90,91,147,149].

Clinicians should appreciate that, despite what is promulgated by some pharmaceutical companies (ie, the need for uterine contractors), the retention of fetal membranes itself actually doubles the rate and increases the frequency of uterine contractions. This results in a higher relative percentage of uterine activity and a larger amount of uterine work [16,149]. By 24 hours postpartum, the amount of uterine work normally decreases by over 50%, but if the membranes are retained, then uterine work remains at approximately 80% of the activity at 6 hours postpartum [16]. On day 1 postpartum, a third of the uterine body contractions form at the end of a tubocervical wave, whereas two thirds occur in cows that have retained membranes. By day 3, the cows that have retained membranes still have a third of the uterine body contractions forming at the end of a tubocervical wave, whereas only about 6% occur in normal cows. On days 2 to 5 postpartum, the amount of relative uterine work is twice as great, and the frequency of contractions at the body of the uterus is 3.5 times as great in cows that have fetal membrane retention. On day 5, this tubocervical wave propagation has ceased in normal cows, but 13% of the waves in cows that have retained fetal membranes still propagate through to the uterine body [16].

Although dry cow ration imbalances and dystocia will predispose a cow to postpartum uterine problems, overcrowded and unhygienic calving facilities can exacerbate the level of infection, especially when the fetal membranes are retained [141,156–163]. The lochia of cows that have fetal membrane retention have a rapidly multiplying population of coliform bacteria, and the endotoxin levels are related proportionately to the numbers of pathogenic bacteria [164,165]. Some animals that have no fetid or purulent lochial discharge may still have a heavy pathogenic bacterial population (*Escheria coli, Arcanobacterium pyogenes, Fusobacterium necrophorum, Bacteroides melaninogencus*) in the postpartum uterine fluid [102]. The systemic response is quite variable, possibly related to the amount of birth trauma (endometrial integrity) and the cow's metabolic (transition ration) status at the time [166]. The clearance time for coliform-derived endotoxin (after experimental IV administration) was only 30 minutes in healthy cows; however, cows that had hepatic lipidosis were not able to clear the endotoxin [167]. The efficiency of both hepatic and blood detoxification mechanisms is obviously important in determining the clinical outcome following an endotoxin insult. The normal physiologic blood profile of the periparturient cow is characterized by a prepartum leukocytosis (cortisol peak), followed by a variable postpartum decrease as leukocytes migrate toward the uterine lumen and mammary gland [102,168].

Endotoxins are potent inducers of prostaglandin release, and they play an important role in the development of postparturient disease [164,166,169]. Even when cows that exhibited systemic signs of metritis were eliminated from a study, the remaining animals that had severe endometritis (fetid, sanguine-purulent lochia) had a significantly higher concentration of endotoxin in the uterine fluid than those that had a more mucopurulent discharge. The presence of endotoxin in plasma was detected in one of six mild cases of endometritis, but in all eight cows that had a fetid, sanguine-purulent lochial discharge. The peak plasma endotoxin concentrations (in the cows that did not develop systemic signs) occurred between days 1 and 12 postpartum [105]. Further research is needed to better understand what facilitates extension of the inflammatory process beyond the endometrial barrier, and what makes an individual animal susceptible to endotoxemia and bacteremia. Endotoxins are reported to activate the COX-2 pathway and induce the specific production of PGE_2 [105,170]. It is interesting that cows that have retained fetal membranes have higher PGE_2 synthesis in placental tissue than $PGF_{2\alpha}$ synthesis [126,171]. Uterine fluid PGE_2 concentrations are significantly higher in cows that have fetid, sanguine-purulent lochia than in cows that have mucopurulent to purulent lochia [105]. Intrauterine PGE_2 reduced intrauterine immunoglobulin concentrations, slowed the rate of uterine involution, and increased the incidence and severity of uterine infections in cows. It is a potent vasodilator, with myorelaxant action and immunosuppressive effects [105,172]. In cases of chronic endometritis that have extended into the postovulatory period, the immunosuppressive effects may be compounded by progesterone. Pyometra may be the end result [105,121,173,174]. There is little doubt that the significance of PGE_2 in the pathophysiology of postpartum metritis warrants further investigation.

Under normal circumstances, the outer longitudinal muscle layer serves to shorten the uterine horns and the inner circular muscle layer decreases the luminal size [175]. Metritis, by definition, means that all layers of the uterine wall are inflamed, not just the endometrium (endometritis) [160,173, 176–178]. Unresolved uterine infection and inflammation tend to be associated with the presence of a flaccid, atonic uterus (delayed involution) [100,173,179]. Toxic puerperal metritis is usually diagnosed within the first week postpartum, and is characterized by fever, depression, fetid watery uterine discharge, and ultimately dehydration. The flaccid, fluid-filled uterus cannot be retracted. Toxemia or bacteraemia cause the affected cow to become inappetant, and milk production declines [173,178–182]. Decreased rumen fill in the postpartum period predisposes the cow to abomasal displacement. Although most animals recover, cows that have severe toxic metritis may become recumbent, and susceptible to all of the negative features that are associated with the "downer cow" syndrome [183].

Clinical management of a toxic metritis case poses quite a dilemma for veterinarians, because there are numerous anecdotal reports, testimonial type papers, and book chapters that espouse the benefits of a particular drug or protocol. Unfortunately, the lack of controls makes it impossible to verify their efficacy [184–187]. Even the scientific literature contains peer-reviewed papers that report conflicting results and diametrically opposed conclusions. Major problems are the variable time frame (days postpartum), and the variability in what evidence of infection (type of vaginal discharge, fever, uterine size and tone) is used to classify a case as being either "metritis" or "endometritis" [102,105,128,160,179,188]. This makes interpretation and comparison of data extremely difficult. The end point, uterine involution, is typically determined by palpation per rectum, and that is subjective by its very nature [27].

Does hormonal therapy have a place?

Cows that have experienced an assisted delivery, a twin birth, or have retention of the fetal membranes are most at risk for development of "toxic metritis" [127,164,189]. Strong myometrial contractions promote the mechanical separation of the cotyledonary villi from the caruncle, by intermittently spreading the maternal tissue so that the crypts are distended. Connective tissue remodeling within the placentome is of paramount importance, however, and incomplete maturation of the placentomes plays an important role in fetal membrane retention [190–194]. One study [195] suggested that an abnormal hormonal milieu in the preparturient cow may be involved. Despite pharmaceutical company "fresh-cow management literature" that recommends injection with a uterine contractor to aid in expulsion of retained placenta, suboptimal uterine contraction in the nontoxic cow is seldom the underlying problem (unless there is concurrent hypocalcaemia) [127,156,157,196–199]. In fact, several research groups have demonstrated that the frequency of uterine contractions and their rate of propagation along the length of the uterus are significantly greater in cows that have retained fetal membranes. Because it is known that fetal membrane retention causes an overall increase in myometrial contractile effort, it seems illogical to advocate hormone use in affected cows on the pretext that this therapy will enhance uterine activity. Uterine effort is already greater than normal in these animals! Manual removal of fetal membranes is an historic treatment that can damage the endometrium and suppress natural uterine immunological processes [28,200,201]. If the procedure is performed, the perineal region should be thoroughly cleansed before any vaginal intervention. The attached membranes should be left intact if gentle twisting and traction do not result in their immediate release. Aggressive intrauterine manipulations probably increase the amount of endotoxin that is subsequently absorbed into the systemic circulation, and an elevated body temperature can be expected to follow such intervention. Fetal membrane retention facilitates secondary bacterial uterine infections, and thus a high prevalence of this condition can have a significant negative impact on the economic well-being of a dairy farm [159,164,165,202–204]. Addressing imbalances in the dry cow ration is very important when managing a herd problem [156–158,162,163,199,205].

A conservative approach to treatment requires close supervision of postpartum cows (temperature, demeanor, and appetite). Although pyrexia is an indicator of postpartum inflammation, additional clinical signs are necessary to identify those animals that have a significant uterine bacterial infection (metritis) [206]. Despite the tendency of some pharmaceutical companies to promote "recipe book" therapy directly to farmers, antibiotics should not be administered simply because a cow's rectal temperature exceeds some threshold "fever" level. Apart from other considerations, such blanket recommendations have the potential to create resistance problems with pathogens such as *Salmonella*. It should be remembered that rectal temperatures of healthy cows may be elevated on hot days, and recent research has confirmed that reliance on body temperature alone can result in overmedication of lactating animals [206]. It is important that the animals are watched closely during the first 7 to 10 days postpartum, because the objective is to detect and treat cows before the effects of toxic metritis take hold. Healthy cows should be bright and alert, whereas a sick animal will have dropped ears, dry caked nostrils, and dull eyes that sink as dehydration develops. Mastitis and respiratory infections are not uncommon during this period, and thus should always be considered as a possible differential diagnosis for metritis. If the characteristic muscular tone and longitudinal folds (linear rugae) of a normally involuting uterus are not palpable, then metritis should be suspected. When early signs of systemic illness become apparent, prompt intervention with supportive measures (anti-inflammatory medication, systemic antibiotics, and fluid therapy) is appropriate [101, 120,164,178,188,207–213]. Although nonsteroidal anti-inflammatory drugs (NSAIDs) are widely used, routine use in all cows that have fetal membrane retention does not appear to be beneficial [188,207]; however, administration to cows that look sick, and that have a fever, does tend to improve their demeanor. It may help to maintain the cow's appetite and rumen motility, and thus may prevent the additional complication of abomasal displacement [214]. Although widely practiced, the efficacy of intrauterine treatments is poorly documented. Claims are usually based on personal experience, or on incorrectly designed studies (lack of controls; insufficient numbers). Known negative effects of uterine infusions include tissue irritation and suppression of the local immune response. Milk residues from extra-label use of antibiotics are always a cause for concern [28,119,178,184,210,215–217]. Unfortunately, very little is known about the pathophysiology of the inflamed bovine myometrium (metritis). The purpose of the following discussion is to summarize the known scientific facts about the efficacy, or lack thereof, of postpartum hormonal therapy.

Oxytocin

Oxytocin is the strongest uterotonic agent known [46]. Oxytocin formulations typically contain 20 United States Pharmacopeia (USP) units/ml, and package inserts recommend dosages of up to 100 USP units (5 mL) [218]. That amount is excessive considering that treatment with as little as 1.0 IU oxytocin will achieve blood concentrations that are comparable with those that occur physiologically during milking. Although a suckling calf will stimulate more oxytocin release than with mechanical milking, the resulting blood levels are still less than those that result from treatment with 10 to 20 USP units oxytocin [219–224]. In other words, an oxytocin dosage of 10 IU is still supra-physiologic. When 50 IU oxytocin was administered IM, the blood levels were increased within 1 minute, and were still above baseline 2 hours later. It appears that absorption of oxytocin from muscle is a slow and continuous process [224]. When oxytocin was given IV at a rate of 0.5 IU/min and at 1.0 IU/min for a period of 60 minutes, there was an initial rapid ($T_{1/2}$ 3.5–4.0 min) then slower ($T_{1/2}$ 26 min) elimination phase [225].

As little as 2.5 IU of oxytocin IV will cause the proximal ends of the uterine horns to respond within 30 to 50 seconds when progesterone levels are low (2 days before to 2 days after estrus). The increased frequency of myometrial activity persists for up to 80 minutes. If the same dose is administered during estrus itself, the latency period is reduced to 10 seconds, and the frequency of the prolonged rhythmic activity is doubled for about 2 hours [146]. Studies such as this in cycling cows have supported the belief that the myometrium is only responsive to oxytocin when estrogen is dominant. Whether this hormone is effective in cows that have already developed toxic metritis remains to be determined [226,227].

The pain (endorphins) and fear (adrenaline) associated with dystocia manipulations are known to impede uterine motility via an oxytocin block [39,228,229]. In fact, a slow IV infusion of epinephrine (10 mL of 1:1,000) can be used to facilitate manual prolapsing of the postpartum uterus. Relaxation of the uterus is detectable within 1 to 2 minutes of initiating the infusion [15]. The same inhibitory effect on myometrial activity has been demonstrated when adrenaline is administered IV to a cow in estrus [146]. Adrenaline exerts a beta-mimetic effect on the estrogen primed uterus (beta2-receptors), thereby suppressing motility [77,230,231]. The pain- and fear-induced uterine atony that is associated with dystocia manipulations can be reversed by the administration of 20 IU oxytocin. Post-cesarean section fetal membrane retention was reduced from 35% (controls) to 7% (treatment group) when cows received 20 IU oxytocin IM immediately following surgery, and again in 2 to 4 hours [228].

Although some authors suggest that an injection of oxytocin immediately after a routine calvings (not dystocias) may reduce the incidence if fetal membrane retention, there are limited data to support this approach, and the reports are contradictory [192,193,232–237]; however, one report on 175 multiparous cows [238] did indicate that there was a significant reduction in placental retention at 24 hours when cows were treated with 30 IU immediately after calving, and again in 2 to 4 hours. Studies have shown that the mere presence of retained fetal membranes doubles the rate and increases the frequency of uterine contractions [16]. As little as 5 IU of oxytocin IV will initiate a more intense rhythm of contraction in these cows [25]. In two fetal membrane retention studies that reported no beneficial effect of postpartum oxytocin therapy [16,233–235], the authors used what has been demonstrated to be a "spasm-inducing" dose of 60 to 100 IU. Few studies have attempted to determine what is the most physiologic uterotonic dose of oxytocin [16,19,25].

During the first 6 days postpartum, IV doses of oxytocin ranging from 2 USP units up to 40 USP units will increase the frequency of myometrial contractions, with the onset of response occurring approximately 30 seconds after injection. The magnitude of this increase is dependent on both dose and day of treatment [16,25]. Each successively larger dose produces a significantly greater increase in contraction frequency, ranging from 1 every 6.5 minutes (2 USP units) up to 1 every 3 minutes (40 USP units). The last detectable responses to doses of 2, 5, 10, 20, and 40 USP units of oxytocin were observed on postpartum days 6, 7, 8, 9, and 10, respectively. The percentage of uterine body contractions that formed at the end of a propagated tubocervical wave (propagation index) was also increased by all doses of oxytocin. An IV injection of 25 USP units oxytocin at 12 hours postpartum increases the propagation index to 80%—up from the baseline 50% of contractions reaching the uterine body. The same dose of oxytocin (25 USP units) consistently caused an increased contraction frequency ($P < 0.01$) and higher tubocervical wave propagation ($P < 0.01$) on treatment days 1 to 5. The initial response to oxytocin (during the first hour after injection) was similar on days 1 to 5 [16].

On postpartum days 1 to 6, the mean overall duration of response following injection of 20 or 40 USP units of oxytocin (approximately 2 hours and 25 minutes) was significantly greater than that following the lower doses (approximately 1.5 hours). When 25 USP units oxytocin was injected IV, the uterine response lasted at least 2.0 hours on days 1 to 4, but had decreased to 1.5 hours on day 5. Although the overall duration of response was similar following injection of either 20 or 40 USP units, the higher dose caused an initial tetaniclike spasm that lasted 6 to 10 minutes. This tetanic effect was only observed at the 40 USP units dose, and was most marked on the first 3 days postpartum. Three independent studies [16,20,25] have reported that oxytocin's effect is to not only increase the frequency of uterine contractions, but also the percentage of these contractions that travel completely down the horn to the uterine body. It has been shown that an IV dose of only 5 IU oxytocin resulted in a rapid and strong increase in contractility during the first 2 to 3 days postpartum, but that by days 4 and 5, the amplitude and duration of the response began to decrease [25]. Because the 40 USP units dose causes an initial tetanic spasm, it would appear that most cows are currently being overdosed. The overall duration of response at 2 days postpartum is approximately 3 hours, decreasing and plateauing to 1.5 hours by days 5 to 6 [16]. Thus, the most efficacious oxytocin therapy may need to be adjusted with days postpartum. It has been suggested that a suitable day 2 to 3 protocol may be repeated 20 USP units (1.0 mL) oxytocin injections, administered at least 3 hours apart, or three doses evenly spaced between milkings [187]. By day 4, the dose could be increased to 30 USP units and the frequency increased to every 2 hours. Although this frequent low-dose therapy may be impractical, it certainly would be more physiologic than the widely used, infrequent, tetany-inducing doses [239]. Further studies are required to determine if the long-acting oxytocin formulations could have therapeutic benefit. These products are not currently available in the United States. Because flunixin meglumine attenuates the uterine response to an IV injection of 5 IU oxytocin, doses lower than 20 IU are probably not appropriate when sick cows are being concurrently treated with anti-inflammatory medication [31]. It must be emphasized, however, that in cows that have been treated with flunixin meglumine, uterine involution progresses normally [31].

Prostaglandins

A study in the 1980s [240] reported that routine administration of prostaglandin $F_{2\alpha}$ immediately after dexamethasone-induced calving could be used to reduce the incidence of retained fetal membranes; however, numerous subsequent studies have failed to confirm these results, and many actually suggest that exogenous prostaglandin has no effect. Although several authors do report that prostaglandin therapy may enhance uterine involution and promote the passage of fetal membranes, the results are far from conclusive [17,19,22,23,27,28,128,184,241–252]. In many instances, the reports must be considered anecdotal because of the small number of animals used, lack of controls, and the concurrent use of other medications. Controlled field studies are difficult to perform, because it is usually not acceptable to the owner that a group of cows receive no treatment at all. Concurrent use of intrauterine medication, or traction on the membranes, is a common study flaw. A study that alluded to a beneficial effect of $PGF_{2\alpha}$ administration after cesarean section [241] was clouded by the concurrent use of a smooth muscle relaxant (isoxsuprine) during surgery.

There is no relationship between PGFM profiles and uterine involution in cows that have an abnormal puerperium [128]. This author believes that it is unlikely that an IM prostaglandin injection before the formation of a functional corpus luteum will have any beneficial effect in the postpartum cow [16,25,120,243,249,252]; however, one often-cited study (N = 3 healthy cows) [27] claimed that high doses, administered twice daily for 10 days, could hasten uterine involution, as determined by palpation per rectum. Another study [128] reported that 1 mg fenprostalene subcutaneous (SQ) at 7 to 10 days postpartum in cows that had dystocia or retained placenta hastened uterine involution by 5 days. A more recent investigation [179] specifically selected cows for treatment if they had retained fetal membranes for at least 24 hours. These animals were treated with ceftiofur hydrochloride (2.2 mg/kg) for 5 days, starting from 3 to 7 days postpartum, if there was a foul-smelling uterine discharge and an enlarged, flaccid uterus. Interestingly, severe cases of toxic puerperal metritis—characterized by fever ($>39.5\,°C$), dehydration, and depression—were eliminated from the study. The experiment itself started on day 8 postpartum, when these "ceftiofur-primed" cows (N = 100) received two doses (25 mg) of $PGF_{2\alpha}$, 8 hours apart. On day 12, the dimensions of the previously gravid uterine horn were measured by ultrasound in a random subsample of treated cows. Although there was a 7 mm difference in uterine horn diameter between the treatment (n = 20) and control (n = 22) primiparous cows, there was no treatment effect in the multiparous animals. There was also no significant treatment effect when the day 8 and day 12 haptoglobulin concentrations were compared [179]. Haptoglobulin is a major acute-phase protein that has been associated with the inflammatory process in bovine metritis [253–256].

Certainly a single IM injection of 25 mg prostaglandin $F_{2\alpha}$ (dinoprost) has no effect on uterine motility [16,25]. Even when the prostaglandin dose was doubled (50 mg $PGF_{2\alpha}$), there was still no uterotonic effect detected [16]. This is not really surprising when one considers that there is already a high endogenous level of prostaglandins in the postpartum cow [58,123,128]. The concentration of PGFM drops slowly after the first 2 days postpartum, reaching baseline levels by day 11 [23,31,128]; however, luteolytic doses of $PGF_{2\alpha}$ (25 mg dinoprost) administered by rapid IV (bolus) injection are uterotonic in postpartum cows, increasing both the frequency of contractions and the amount of tubocervical wave propagation [16,20]. When 15 mg of dinoprost was injected IV, it resulted in a strong, but delayed (10–20 minutes), stimulation. If repeated on day 4 postpartum, the stimulatory effect was markedly diminished [25,31]. IV prostaglandin therapy would be impractical in a toxic cow, because there are dramatic side effects (uneasiness, dyspnea, frequent urination, milk ejection, and salivation) [25]. Dogs tend to experience similar side effects at a much higher subcutaneous dose rate of $PGF_{2\alpha}$ (0.1–0.25 mg/kg) when being medicated to expel pyometra contents [257,258].

In contrast to the natural prostaglandin (dinoprost), an IV injection of the synthetic $PGF_{2\alpha}$ derivative (cloprostenol 0.25 mg) resulted in a minimal increase in uterine activity on day 1 [25]. The minimal uterotonic effect from cloprostenol has been confirmed by other investigators [19]. Fenprostalene, a synthetic analog of $PGF_{2\alpha}$ with a prolonged plasma half-life, has also been recommended as a treatment for fetal membrane retention [246]. Peak plasma levels of fenprostalene concentrations are reached approximately 10 hours after injection, and the elimination half-life is reported to be 18 to 23 hours [16,243,259]. Interestingly, SQ injections of this long-acting synthetic prostaglandin have not been shown to produce any significant changes in the percentage of recording time that is occupied by uterine activity (activity index), the percentage of contractions of the uterine body that form at the end of a tubocervical contraction wave (propagation index), or the amount of time taken for propagated tubocervical contraction waves to pass along the length of the uterus (propagation time) [16]. Repeated SQ injections of fenprostalene (1 mg) at 12, 36, 60, and 84 hours postpartum did not produce any cumulative uterotonic effects, and did not promote passage of the fetal membranes [16]. Even when the fenprostalene dose was doubled (2 mg) there was still no uterotonic effect detected [16]. It was not uterotonic after IV injection either [18]. When fenprostalene (1 mg SQ) was administered at 7 to 10 days postpartum, the endogenous release of $PGF_{2\alpha}$ was not affected in cows that had dystocias or retained placenta [128].

The metabolism of $PGF_{2\alpha}$ is very rapid, and thus its half-life is short—reportedly less than 1 minute [32,33,260]. IM injections of $PGF_{2\alpha}$ may not be uterotonic because the $PGF_{2\alpha}$ is metabolized almost entirely into PGFM upon a single passage through the lungs [261]. Thus, gradual absorption of $PGF_{2\alpha}$ from an injection site, followed by immediate metabolism by the lungs, may mean that levels equivalent to the bolus IV effect are never achieved. The half-life of PGFM itself is approximately 18 minutes [15]. The myometrial response to IV prostaglandin $F_{2\alpha}$ may explain why in-vitro studies have demonstrated a uterotonic effect of $PGF_{2\alpha}$ [29,30,36,262]. These studies may mimic the in-situ environment, where the local release of $PGF_{2\alpha}$ from the endometrium is able to impact directly upon the overlying myometrium through a paracrine signaling mechanism. Readers should be aware that there are two optically active isomers of cloprostenol. Both DL- and D-cloprostenol are synthetic analogs of $PGF_{2\alpha}$ [36]. Certainly the scientific evidence suggests that neither IM or SQ injections of either natural or synthetic prostaglandin appear to have any significant uterotonic effect in the postpartum cow [16,18,19,24,25,31]; however, what is especially intriguing is that prostaglandin does appear to have a uterotonic effect in the nonpregnant cow if estrogen is dominant (follicular phase; estrogenized ovariectomized cows) [16–19,263,264]. A more recent intrauterine pressure study using cows in the diestrus phase [265,266] did report an effect following IM injections.

Another factor that speaks against a direct uterotonic effect for exogenous $PGF_{2\alpha}$ in the postpartum cow is that although the administration of the COX inhibitor, flunixin meglumine (days 1–10 postpartum) will significantly decrease the levels of PGFM, the rate of uterine involution is not affected [21,31,267]. Even if large doses of flunixin meglumine are administered, prostaglandin production is not totally abolished [23]. In one study [31], the overall reduction in prostaglandin production exceeded 80%. These studies indicate that partial suppression of prostaglandin synthesis early in the postpartum period does not affect the rate of decrease in the cervical and uterine horn diameter, nor the location of the uterus within the pelvic canal [21,31]. It appears that high levels of $PGF_{2\alpha}$ are not an essential factor for normal uterine involution. The physiologic processes involved in uterine involution (vasoconstriction, myometrial contractions, collagen tissue reorganization) seem to progress normally even if anti-inflammatory medication has lowered the normal endogenous prostaglandin level. This is despite the fact that spontaneous uterine motility and the response of the myometrium to oxytocin and IV $PGF_{2\alpha}$ are attenuated [31]. When eight cows were treated twice daily with flunixin meglumine for 10 days, uterine involution was actually completed in significantly less time than the control animals [31]. A study suggesting that a large dose of flunixin meglumine (1.5 g) after cesarean sections increases the incidence of fetal membrane retention [251] may have been compromised by the fact that a smooth muscle relaxant (isoxsuprine) was administered before surgery.

Phagocytosis by neutrophils and subsequent killing of ingested bacteria are important in the elimination of infection [102,104]. Advocates may argue that exogenous prostaglandins could have beneficial effects on the postpartum uterus that do not relate to the uterine motility controversy [28]. Eicosanoids ($PGF_{2\alpha}$, leukotrienes, and other arachidonic acid metabolites) do influence immune functions [121]. Leukotrienes are formed from arachidonic acid by lipoxygenase. In-vitro studies with mouse peritoneal macrophages have investigated a possible effect of prostaglandins on phagocytic ability [268]. Similar experiments with neutrophils from ovariectomized cows indicate that $PGF_{2\alpha}$ is a chemo-attractant, and that it increases the ability of cells to engulf bacteria [269]. Whether these in-vitro experiments have any relevance to exogenous prostaglandin therapy in the immediate postpartum period remains to be proven.

Estrogens

The administration of exogenous estrogens as a treatment for metritis has been in vogue off and on for many years. Advocates claim that estrogen therapy will improve uterine tone [226,227,232,270,271]; however, because estrogen levels fall dramatically once the calf is expelled, it appears that uterine involution can actually progress without estrogenic influence in the normal cow. A 1987 field study that involved 374 postpartum cows was not able to demonstrate a beneficial effect of 6 mg estradiol cypionate (ECP), prostaglandin and ECP, or oxytocin and ECP. Despite this earlier work, broadly disseminated claims of efficacy in the mid-1990s led to widespread adoption of estrogen therapy for delayed uterine involution and metritis [272–275]. Unfortunately, solid scientific evidence was lacking to support the use of this estrogen product, even at the lower 4 mg dose that was being advocated by the pharmaceutical company [274–276]. Four studies [211,277–279] have since demonstrated that administration of 4 mg ECP does not have beneficial effects on metritis prevention or reproductive performance, and that it may have a detrimental effect on subsequent fertility. In another study [280], intrauterine administration of 10 mg estradiol benzoate did not enhance postpartum involution.

The rationale for ECP therapy is based on an unsubstantiated belief that estrogens will enhance the response of the postpartum bovine uterus to uterotonic agents such as oxytocin. Because serum estrogen levels decline rapidly in the postpartum period, however, it appears that the dogma about estrogen-primed receptors warrants serious questioning [122]. Perhaps the estrogen-induced oxytocin receptors persist on the postpartum uterus for several days, because there is no inhibition from rising progesterone levels that would characterize the early luteal phase [65,281–285]. There is no scientific evidence that estrogen therapy stimulates the type of rhythmic tubocervical contractions required to empty the postpartum uterus. The claims of a beneficial effect of estrogen on myometrial activity in the postpartum cow are subjective, based on clinical impression [16,90,272]. This author believes that the expectation of a beneficial postpartum effect results from an over-extrapolation of the data from nonpregnant, cycling cows [284,286]. Estradiol has a positive effect on the ability of the endometrium to secrete $PGF_{2\alpha}$ in response to oxytocin, but the nonpregnant uterus must have been exposed to progesterone first (luteal phase) [46,282,287–290]. The role of estradiol in the regulation of oxytocin receptor synthesis remains controversial, and the exact mechanism of oxytocin receptor upregulation in the endometrium remains unknown [282]. In the late gestation ewe (130 days) the number of myometrial oxytocin receptors begins to increase, possibly due to the effect of mechanical stretch. It is the rate of stretch, rather than the degree of stretch, that might be the important factor [69]. The concentration of myometrial oxytocin receptors was five times higher in pregnant compared with nonpregnant myometrial samples

[76]. Although the oxytocin responsiveness of cultured human myometrial cells was upregulated in the presence of estradiol, the estrogenic effect on the oxytocin pathway was thought to be at a postreceptor level [75]. Although estradiol will induce an increase in oxytocin receptors, uterine oxytocin receptor concentrations have been shown to be high in ovariectomized ewes [69,291]. Concentrations decline soon after progesterone replacement therapy is initiated. This work supports the notion that removal of the "progesterone block" may be more important than stimulation by estrogen [285,292]. Studies on the cyclic bovine endometrium have demonstrated that estradiol speeds up the spontaneous upregulation of oxytocin receptor expression via the estradiol receptor, but it is not essential for this process. Although endometrial oxytocin receptors were elevated in ovariectomized cows, oxytocin-induced release of PGFM is reduced [284,289]. Local factors from the endometrium may be necessary to regulate oxytocin receptor expression via interaction with the estradiol receptor [293]. Myometrial estradiol receptors may well be downregulated in the postpartum cow [294,295]. Certainly spontaneous upregulation of endometrial oxytocin receptors occurs in the absence of estradiol. In fact, some now believe that estradiol may not the primary regulator of oxytocin-receptor gene expression [69,292,293].

Observations on the uterine motility of sheep and rabbits have confirmed some interesting features about the nongravid, estrogen-dominated uterus. In estrous rabbits, the majority of uterine contractions move from the cervix toward the oviducts [296]. This cervicotubal contraction pattern has also been reported in estrous ewes [297–299]. In early estrus, at least two thirds of the contractions originate in the uterine body and progress anteriorly, but by late estrous, only a third of the contractions originate in the uterine body. In contrast, 2 days after estrus, some three quarters of the contractions originate at the tip of the horns and move in a tubocervical direction [300,301]. These tubocervical contractions are possibly an extension of the oviduct contractions that carry the embryo down into the uterus [146,302]. Administration of estradiol-17β during late estrous prevents the change in direction of the contractions. Ovariectomies performed during the luteal phase of the cycle, in conjunction with estradiol injections, will initiate the onset of typical cervicotubal estrus contractions within 48 hours [300].

Hormonal control of the direction of uterine contractions has been confirmed in the cycling cow as well [303,304]. Open-tipped catheters have been employed to demonstrate a relationship between the motility pattern of the uterine horn and the phases of the estrous cycle. It was shown that maximal rhythmic activity occurs during estrus, with contractions running from the cervix toward the oviduct (cervicotubal). The direction was reversed at the end of estrus [305]. Another study showed that in the 48 hours before the onset of estrus, there is a gradual transition from local, nonpropagating electrical activity to propagating electrical activity with an increase in the duration of contractions, and then of their amplitude [146].

This transition coincides with a rapid decrease in progesterone level, from 5 to 10 ng/ml to less than 0.1 to 0.4 ng/ml. Bursts of activity (5 minutes) start near the cervix, then progress toward the oviduct. The prevailing direction of uterine contractions through until late estrus is cervicotubal [306].

The catecholamine (dopamine, noradrenaline, adrenaline) content in the bovine oviduct varies by region (infundibulum, ampulla, isthmus), and with phase of the estrous cycle [307,308]. The bovine oviduct is an important target tissue for the sex steroids, and the fine-tuned differences in the expression of steroid receptors in the muscular layer suggest an interaction with oviduct motility [302]. There appear to be selective time- and region-specific effects during the estrous cycle [302]. These findings are not unexpected, because cervicotubal contractions during estrus will assist with sperm transport. In fact, vaginal stimulation during estrus leads to a myometrial response that spreads over the whole of the uterus and into the lower part of the oviduct. These contractions last from 5 to 30 minutes beyond the time of stimulation [146]. Oxytocin activates contractions in both the ampulla and isthmus during the follicular phase [146,307]. Estrogen-induced reverse peristalsis is probably the reason for the high incidence of salpingitis reported when the 10 mg labeled dose of ECP was widely used to treat metritis (C. Callahan, personal communication, 1998) [239,276]. In metestrus, the majority of contractions appear to originate in the oviduct near the uterotubal junction, and to propagate toward the cervix. Perhaps this facilitates expulsion of extraneous foreign protein (sperm) before the arrival of the embryo. The strength, but not the frequency, of activity diminishes progressively for 2 to 3 days after estrus, and then relative inactivity ensues [146]. It is interesting to speculate that the characteristic tone of the estrus uterus is rapidly lost not so much because of a fall in postovulatory estrogen concentrations, but rather because of the inhibitory effect of a rising progesterone level.

Research to date does not support the theory that ECP enhances the myometrial response to oxytocin or prostaglandin. The myometrial effects of an IM injection of 5 mg ECP at 18 hours postpartum have been compared with baseline motility, and with oxytocin responses before, and on the first day after injection of ECP [16,90]. The estrogen treatment had a statistically significant and negative impact on uterine motility. Contraction frequency was reduced from 9.6/hour to 2.9/hour ($P < 0.01$), and duration of each contraction was increased from 2.35 minutes to over 7 minutes ($P < 0.05$). The ECP treatment changed the normal motility pattern from predominantly single-peak contractions into a sustained contraction pattern with multiple superimposed small peaks. The uterus could be best described as in spasm, because all parts of the uterus tended to contract simultaneously. Despite this, the contractile force was probably reduced, because the mean amplitude of contraction curves was lowered significantly ($P < 0.05$). These uterine effects of ECP became apparent by approximately 4 hours after treatment, and they persisted until day 5. Only then did some discrete, single-peak contractions return [16,90]. The 5-day time frame fits with this author's unpublished observations (2004) of the artificially elevated estradiol-17β levels following ECP administration. When 4 mg ECP was administered to ovariectomized beef heifers, the estradiol-17β levels did not fall to near maximal estrus levels until day 5 (Fig. 3).

When 25 USP units oxytocin was administered (IV) on day 2 postpartum (6 hours after the ECP treatment), the myometrial activity returned to the normal, single-peak, propagated contraction waves. The effect of 25 USP units oxytocin on the contraction frequency (17.5/hour) in this ECP-primed uterus was not different to the 6-day mean (17.3/hour) for 20 USP units oxytocin on the normal uterus [16,90]. This tends to dispel the notation that ECP enhances the myometrial effect of oxytocin. Estrogen priming actually caused a slight suppression in the post-oxytocin mean contraction duration (119 seconds) and propagation index (72%). The mean duration of myometrial response to oxytocin in the ECP-primed uterus was not significantly different from that of the normal postpartum uterus. Burton [90] concluded that there were no detectable differences between myometrial response to oxytocin administered before and 6 hours after the ECP (5 mg) injection. Oxytocin was then administered daily following the ECP (5 mg) priming to determine whether there was any delayed positive effect on postpartum myometrial activity. No changes were detected. Thus, these studies [90] clearly demonstrate that there can be no valid argument with respect to the oxytocin receptors that would support the use of exogenous long-acting estrogen formulations in the postpartum dairy cow [16,20,24,25].

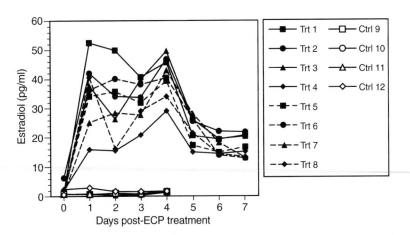

Fig. 3. Unpublished data from the author's laboratory. Eight ovariectomized beef heifers received 4 mg ECP intramuscularly. Four ovariectomized control animals received a saline injection. Note the tremendous variability (concentration and day) between animals in the plasma levels achieved. A biphasic clearance pattern appears to be characteristic for this long-acting estrogen. Ctrl, control animal; Trt, treated animal.

Furthermore, pretreatment with ECP (5 mg) did not result in either $PGF_{2\alpha}$ (25 mg IM) or fenprostalene (1 mg SQ) becoming uterotonic. There were no significant changes in postpartum myometrial activity. The prostaglandin injections were repeated daily for 5 days to determine if there was an effect of the ECP treatment, but no effect was detected [16].

Another proposed benefit of estrogen therapy is stimulation of natural uterine defense mechanisms [104,232,309–313]. Advocates hypothesize that exogenous estrogens may improve uterine blood flow and thus bring more neutrophils to the site of infection; however, one recent experiment [314] found that although endogenous estradiol-17β levels had no significant influence on a diapedesis model, the addition of exogenous estradiol-17β did have an adverse effect. Another study [315] demonstrated that administration of estradiol-17β may actually reduce PMN chemotaxis. This in vitro study investigated the ability of PMNs to migrate from the endothelial wall of a blood vessel into the lumen, following a chemoattractant gradient to the site of infection [316]. It has also been suggested that exogenous estrogens will improve the phagocytic capacity of these neutrophils. Yet again, the evidence is inconclusive, and the variability in the methods used to assess neutrophil function makes it difficult to reach a definitive answer. The antibacterial action of neutrophils recovered from the uterine lumen has been measured by their chemotactic activity, phagocytic capacity, and bacterial killing ability [315,317,318]. A recent study [315] reported that there was no consistent influence of the reproductive state on the resistance of the uterus to infection, as measured by differences in either peripheral or intrauterine neutrophil function. Comparisons were made between responses obtained at estrus and diestrus, and following the administration of exogenous estradiol and progesterone to ovariectomized cows. Leukotriene B4 (LTB4) may play an important role in both placental separation and uterine involution in cattle [319]. It is a metabolite of the 5-lipoxygenase pathway of arachidonic acid metabolism, and is a potent chemoattractant of PMNs. This association with prostaglandin metabolism may explain why oxytocin has been shown to stimulate LTB4 synthesis during the early postpartum period in cattle [320]. Perhaps that is why repeated small doses of oxytocin may have some therapeutic merit. Caruncular tissue taken from the previously gravid horn produces less LTB4 if it is treated with progesterone, but estrogen treatment has no effect, neither increasing or decreasing LTB4 synthesis [319]. Once again, it may be the absence of progesterone's inhibitory action rather than the presence of estrogen that enhances the uterine defense mechanisms when a cow is in estrus [321,322]. The inhibitory effect of progesterone may also explain the increased incidence of clinical endometritis in cows if the first ovulation occurs early in the postpartum period [174,313,318,323,324]. Luteolytic doses of prostaglandin in the postovulatory period are beneficial to return the cow to estrus. In this instance, the estral uterine tone and characteristic mucus flow appear to be therapeutic [325].

Veterinarians should consider the tissue half-life of long-acting estrogens when using these products. Because estradiol-17β has a very short half-life (<5 minutes), it is marketed in commercial preparations (cottonseed or sesame oil) in one of several esterified forms (E2-17B benzoate, E2-17B valerate, and E2-17B cypionate) [326,327]. Although ECP is an old drug (from the 1950s), there is limited information available on its pharmacokinetics for any of the veterinary species [218]. Esterified estrogens such as ECP have delayed absorption after IM administration. Estrogens are distributed throughout the body and accumulate in adipose tissue [218]. ECP is highly fat-soluble [276]. Only after slow hydrolysis in the liver is the active estradiol-17β released [327]. The eventual elimination of the steroidal estrogens occurs principally by hepatic metabolism. Thus this author believes that there is cause for concern if a treated animal has compromised liver function, a not-uncommon problem in sick cows during the early postpartum period. Estrogens and their metabolites are primarily excreted in the urine, but are also excreted into the bile, where most is then re-absorbed from the gastrointestinal (GI) tract [218]. In short, the various esterified forms are long-acting formulations of estrogen.

When the progestogen ear implant (Syncro-Mate B, Merial Limited, Iselin, NJ) was available for commercial use in the United States, it was only approved for synchronization of breeding in cycling beef cattle and in nonlactating dairy heifers. The package insert specifically warned that the product was not to be used in cows producing milk for human consumption [328]. The protocol included an IM injection that is administered at the time of insertion of the 6 mg norgestomet ear implant. The 2 ml injection contained 5 mg estradiol valerate and 3 mg norgestomet. In a study that investigated the impact of progestins on luteinizing hormone release [329], it was determined that the estradiol valerate resulted in elevated estradiol-17β levels that persisted for several days. Levels peaked at over 80 pg/ml estradiol-17β on day 2 and then slowly declined to what are maximal follicular estrogen derived levels by day 5 [329]. There is one report that specifically looked at the plasma estradiol-17β concentrations in the cow during induced estrus and after injection of estradiol-17β benzoate and ECP [327]. The objective of that study was to use plasma estradiol-17β levels attained during the normal estrous cycle as a baseline in making withholding recommendations for esterified estrogens. The maximal estradiol levels in some cycling cows have been reported to be in the range of 25 to 28 pg/ml, but with population mean values of approximately 16 pg/ml [327,330–332]. In fact, a recent study [137] reported that lactating Holsteins had a maximal mean serum estradiol concentration preceding ovulation of only 7.3 to 7.8 pg/ml, even with multiple ovulations included. An IM injection of 10 mg ECP (5 ml) resulted in maximal estradiol-17β levels of 56 to 128 pg/ml over a range from 13 hours and 5 days. The concentrations then decreased steadily to estrual levels by 5.6 to 9.6 days (135 to 231 hours). In some cows, there were two peaks in the E2-17B plasma concentration following an ECP injection. This biphasic curve warrants further investigation because it may be a reflection of an initial redistribution of the mobilized ester, followed by an elimination phase [327]. Estradiol benzoate (10 mg) caused a higher initial E2-17B peak level (82 to 320 pg/ml) but also a more rapid decline, with a return to estral levels within 3.6 to 6.0 days (87 to 143 hours) [327]. The marked variability in the peak levels and in the return to estrus levels warrant further investigation. Only five cows were evaluated in this study [327]. It may be that there is substantial biological variation in how cows metabolize these estrogen esters, possibly related to the level of body fat and liver function [218]. The work needs to be repeated in postpartum dairy cows, especially because the long-acting steroids may well be concentrated in the butterfat component of the milk [333–339]. A recommendation for a 10-day withdrawal period was proposed for the 10 mg (5 ml) ECP injection, based on adding twice the standard error of the mean to the average time taken for concentrations of E2-17B to return estral levels [327].

It has been reported that estradiol-17β and estrone are located predominantly in the lipid fraction of milk [337–340]. Although this suggests that milk fat content is an important factor when determining estradiol-17β concentrations, another laboratory did not find a difference between whole and defatted milk. The issue is further confounded by the fact that there appears to be a high degree of cow-to-cow variability in the association between plasma and milk estradiol-17β concentrations [341]. Milk estradiol-17β concentrations have been reported to be lower than, equivalent to, or higher than plasma values, but some studies specifically reported on defatted milk [333,336–338,340–354]. Obviously there is considerable variation in sensitivity and specificity among estrogen assays (eg, radioimmunoassay [RIA], enzyme immunoassay, high performance liquid chromatography [HPLC]), possibly due to the variability in cross-reactivity with the three estrogens that are found in milk (estradiol-17β, estrone sulfate, and estriol) [333,336,340,341,347–350,353,355–360]. Estrone sulfate is the main form of estrogen in the milk from pregnant cows, and it has been reported at up to four times the concentration blood plasma [333,336,338,355,361]. When fresh cows (days 3–5 postpartum) were treated with 4 mg ECP, the milk estradiol-17β levels exceeded those in control animals [362]. Although there is a relatively high concentration of estrogen in the system of cows in late gestation, their declining milk production contributes relatively little volume to the bulk tank in comparison with that from cows in early lactation. Thus, if cows in early lactation have been treated with exogenous estrogens, then the potential volume contribution could be far more significant. The levels of estradiol-17β, estrone, and estriol in milk are reported to be found in significantly higher concentrations in colostrum and butter [333–336]. There were no labeled ECP withholding recommendations for either meat or milk [276]. When this author treated eight ovariectomized beef heifers with 4 mg ECP, the plasma levels reached as high as 52 pg/ml, and the mean value was still over 22 pg/ml 5 days later (see Fig. 3). As in a previous report [329], there was a biphasic clearance pattern. The peaks on day 1 and day 4 may reflect redistribution of the mobilized ester, followed by an elimination phase (G.S. Frazer, unpublished observations, 2004). One has to wonder how effectively the ECP would be metabolized if hepatic function is compromised (postpartum fatty liver) [363,364]. Thus, if the product is administered to sick postpartum cows, then this author concurs with European researchers, and will argue that a milk withholding is indicated [327].

Veterinarians should be cognizant of the increasing scientific and public concern about hormone contamination of food (meat and milk) products [355,356,365–368]. It has been reported that the major source (60%–70%) of animal-derived estrogens (estradiol-17β and estrone) in the human diet is from consumption of dairy products [367,369,370]. Estradiol-17β has significantly more biopotency than most identified environmental xenoestrogens [367,371]; however, there are valid concerns about estrogens in the environment [368,371–374]. Some widely used food containers and wrappings are made from an industrial chemical (bisophenol A) that exhibits estrogenic activity. [375,376]. This author believes that estrogen therapy should be used judiciously in food-producing animals, because it may unnecessarily contribute to the overall burden of human exposure to chemical entities with estrogenic activity [187]. It is the cumulative effects of exogenous estrogens that may have a negative impact on human health, and it may be that there is wide biological and age variability in individual susceptibility to any negative effects [355,356,367]. Competitive binding to estrogen receptors in target tissue (eg, breast, prostate), perhaps prepubertal, may result in insidious, long-term effect [355,356,365,366, 377–395]. It seems prudent not to administer long-acting estrogens to postpartum dairy cows, especially because there is no convincing evidence of its efficacy [187,259].

Summary

It is now well-accepted that attention to dry cow nutrition can markedly reduce the incidence of postpartum problems. Little is known about the pathophysiology of the diseased postpartum uterus, and there is no scientifically proven therapy for toxic metritis other than supportive care (systemic antibiotics, anti-inflammatory medication, and fluid therapy). There is no scientific evidence that an IM injection of prostaglandin or estrogen will stimulate the type of rhythmic tubocervical contractions required to empty an atonic postpartum uterus. It is noteworthy that the increased frequency of uterine contractions following oxytocin administration in the postpartum cow is exactly the same phenomenon as that seen when Stage II of labor commences. The presence of the fetus in the vaginal canal is known to stimulate endogenous oxytocin release (Ferguson reflex)

[96,228]. The research by scientists such as Burton, Gajewski, Kundig, and Thun and their coworkers [16,20,24,25,90,227,232] has refuted the often-quoted view that oxytocin is only uterotonic during the first 1 to 2 days postpartum. It is unfortunate that these studies of Burton, Kundig, and Gajewski and their coauthors were not conducted using the more typical IM route of oxytocin administration. Burton [16] did confirm, however, that the myometrial response following injection of 20 to 30 USP units of oxytocin is similar following administration via the IV, IM, or SQ routes. Because a low dose of oxytocin (20 USP units) is uterotonic up to 9 days postpartum, it has the most scientific validity as a therapeutic agent. Estrogen priming is not indicated. Repeated low-dose oxytocin therapy (20 USP units every 3 hours) would ensure that the uterus remains under the influence of rhythmic contractions, although this protocol may be impractical under field conditions. Farmers should be educated to adopt early intervention practices before the cow succumbs to the systemic effects of endotoxin. Although daily monitoring of rectal temperatures in the first 7 to 10 days postpartum can help to identify high-risk animals, nothing replaces close observation that permits early recognition of a cow's changing appearance and behavior.

References

[1] Hertelendy F, Zakar T. Regulation of myometrial smooth muscle functions. Curr Pharm Des 2004;10(20):2499–517.
[2] Lye SJ. Initiation of parturition. Anim Reprod Sci 1996;42:495–503.
[3] Liggins GC, Fairclough RJ, Grieves SA, et al. The mechanism of initiation of parturition in the ewe. Recent Prog Horm Res 1973;29:111–59.
[4] Senger PL. Placentation, the endocrinology of gestation and parturition. In: Senger PL, editor. Pathways to pregnancy and parturition. 2nd edition. Pullman (WA): Current Concepts, Inc; 1999. p. 304–25.
[5] Challis JRG, Matthews SG, Gibb W, et al. Endocrine and paracrine regulation of birth at term and preterm. Endocr Rev 2000;21(5):514–50.
[6] Whittle WL, Holloway AC, Lye SJ, et al. Prostaglandin production at the onset of ovine parturition is regulated by both estrogen-independent and estrogen dependent pathways. Endocrinology 2000;141(10):3783–91.
[7] Pandey AV, Miller WL. Regulation of 17, 20 lyase activity by cytochrome b5 and by serine phosphorylation of P450c17. J Biol Chem 2005;280:13265–71.
[8] Osawa Y, Higashiyama T, Shimizu Y, et al. Multiple functions of aromatase and the active site structure; aromatase is the placental estrogen 2-hydroxylase. J Steroid Biochem Mol Biol 1993;44(4–6):469–80.
[9] Larsson K, Wagner C, Sachs M. Oestrogen synthesis by bovine foetal placenta at normal parturition. Acta Endocrinol (Copenh) 1981;98:112–8.
[10] Pimentel S, Pimentel C, Weston P, et al. Progesterone secretion by the bovine fetoplacental unit and responsiveness of corpora lutea to steroidogenic stimuli at two stages of gestation. Am J Vet Res 1986;47:1967–71.
[11] Kindahl H, Kornmatitsuk B, Gustaffson H. The cow in endocrine focus before and after calving. Reprod Domest Anim 2004;39(4):217–21.
[12] Bazar FW, First NL. Pregnancy and parturition. J Anim Sci 1983;57(Suppl 2):425–60.

[13] Schatz F, Markiewicz L, Gurpide E. Differential effects of estradiol, arachidonic acid and A-23187 on prostaglandin F_{2a} output by epithelial and stromal cells of human endometrium. Endocrinology 1987;120:1465–71.

[14] Herschman HR. Review—prostaglandin synthase 2. Biochem Biophys Acta 1996;1299: 125–40.

[15] Guilbault LA, Thatcher WW, Drost M, et al. Source of F series prostaglandins during the early postpartum period in cattle. Biol Reprod 1984;31:879–87.

[16] Burton MJ. Uterine motility in periparturient dairy cattle [PhD dissertation]. St. Paul (MN): Department of Clinical Sciences, Univeristy of Minnesota; 1986.

[17] Eiler H, Oden J, Schaub R, et al. Refraxtoriness of both uterus and mammary gland of the cow to prostaglandin F_{2a} administration: clinical impression. Am J Vet Res 1981;42(3): 314–7.

[18] Eiler H, Byrd W, Hopkins F. Uterokinetic activity of fenprostalene (a prostaglandin F_{2a} analog) in vivo and in vitro in the bovine. Theriogenology 1989;32(5):755–64.

[19] Eiler H, Hopkins F, Armstrong-Backus CS, et al. Uterotonic effect of prostaglandin F_{2a} and oxytocin on the postpartum cow. Am J Vet Res 1984;45:1011–4.

[20] Gajewski Z, Thun R, Faundez R, et al. Uterine motility in the cow during puerperium. Reprod Domest Anim 1999;34:185–91.

[21] Guilbault LA, Thatcher WW, Drost M, et al. Influence of a physiological infusion of PGF_{2a} into postpartum cows with partially suppressed endogenous production of prostaglandins. I. Uterine and ovarian morphological response. Theriogenology 1987;27(6):931–46.

[22] Guilbault LA, Villeneuve P, Dufour J. Failure of exogenous prostaglandin F_{2a} to enhance uterine involution in beef cows. Can J Anim Sci 1988;68:669–76.

[23] Kindahl H, Bekana M, Kask K, et al. Endocrine aspects of uterine involution in the cow. Reprod Domest Anim 1999;34:261–8.

[24] Kundig H, Thun R, Zerobin K, et al. Uterine motility in the cow during late pregnancy, parturition and puerperium. I. Spontaneous motility. Schweiz Arch Tierheilkd 1990;132: 77–84 [in German].

[25] Kundig H, Thun R, Zerobin K. Uterine motility in the cow during late pregnancy, parturition and puerperium. II. Drug Influence. Schweiz Arch Tierheilkd 1990;132:515–24 [in German].

[26] Lindell J, Kindahl H, Jansson L, et al. Post-partum release of prostaglandin F_{2a} and uterine involution in the cow. Theriogenology 1982;17:237–45.

[27] Lindell J, Kindahl H. Exogenous prostaglandin F_{2a} promotes uterine involution in the cow. Acta Vet Scand 1983;24:269–74.

[28] Paisley LG, Mickelsen WD, Anderson PB. Mechanisms and therapy for retained fetal membranes and uterine infections of cows: a review. Theriogenology 1986;25:353–81.

[29] Patil RK, Sinha SN, Einarsson S, et al. The effects of PGF_{2a} and oxytocin on bovine myometrium in vitro. Nord Vet Med 1980;32:474–9.

[30] Singh LP, Sadiku A, Verma OP. Prostaglandin F_{2a}-induced response of the bovine ovary, oviduct (uterine tube), and uterus. Am J Vet Res 1979;40:1789–91.

[31] Thun R, Kundig H, Zerobin K, et al. Uterine motility in the cow during late pregnancy, parturition and puerperium. III. Application of flunixin meglumine and hormonal changes. Schweiz Arch Tierheilkd 1993;135:333–4.

[32] Granstrom E, Kindahl H. Species differences in circulating prostaglandin metabolites. Relevance for the assay of prostaglandin release. Biochem Biophys Acta 1982;713:555–69.

[33] Egarter CH, Husslein P. Biochemistry of myometrial contractility. Baillieres Clin Obstet Gynaecol 1992;6(4):755–69.

[34] Fuchs A, Rust W, Fields M. Accumulation of cyclooxygenase-2 gene transcripts in uterine tissues of pregnant and parturient cows: stimulation by oxytocin. Biol Reprod 1999;60: 341–8.

[35] Malkowski MG, Ginell SL, Smith WL, et al. Productive conformation of arachidonic acid bound to prostaglandin synthase. Science 2000;289:1933–7.

[36] Beretta C, Cavalli M. A sheer pharmacologic approach to compare the contractile effects of PGF_{2a}, DL-cloprostenol and D-cloprostenol on isolated uterine, tracheal, ileal and arterial smooth muscle preparations. Theriogenology 2004;62:837–46.

[37] Dong YL, Yallampalli C. Pregnancy and exogenous steroid treatments modulate the expression of relaxant EP2 and contractile FP receptors in the rat uterus. Biol Reprod 2000; 62:533–9.

[38] Phillipe M, Saunders T, Basa A. Intracellular mechanisms underlying prostaglandin F_{2a}-stimulated phasic myometrial contractions. Am J Physiol 1997;273:E665–73.

[39] Taverne M. Physiology of parturition. Anim Reprod Sci 1992;28:433–40.

[40] Al-Matubsi HY, Eis ALW, Brodt-Eppley J, et al. Expression and localization of the contractile prostaglandin F receptor in pregnant rat myometrium in late gestation, labor, and postpartum. Biol Reprod 2001;65:1029–37.

[41] Palliser HK, Hirst JJ, Ooi GT, et al. Prostaglandin E and F receptor expression and myometrial sensitivity at labor onset in the sheep. Biol Reprod 2005;72:937–43.

[42] Olson DM. The role of prostaglandins in the initiation of parturition. Best Pract Res Clin Obstet Gynaecol 2003;17(5):717–30.

[43] Chan W. Relationship between the uterotonic action of oxytocin and prostaglandins: oxytocin addition and release of PG-activity in isolated nonpregnant and pregnant rat uteri. Biol Reprod 1977;17:541–8.

[44] Molnar M, Hertelendy E. Regulation of intracellular free calcium in human myometrial cells by prostaglandin F_{2a}: comparison with oxytocin. J Clin Endocrinol Metab 1990;71: 1243–50.

[45] Fuchs AR, Rollyson MK, Meyer MT, et al. Oxytocin induces prostaglandin F_{2a} release in pregnant cows: Influence of gestational age and oxytocin receptor concentrations. Biol Reprod 1996;54:647–53.

[46] Wu WX, Verbalis JG, Hoffman GE, et al. Characterization of oxytocin receptor expression and distribution in the pregnant sheep uterus. Endocrinology 1996;137:722–8.

[47] Schrey M, Cornford P, Read A, et al. A role for phosphoinositide hydrolysis in human uterine smooth muscle during parturition. Am J Obstet Gynecol 1988;159:964–70.

[48] McCracken JA. Update on luteolysis—receptor regulation of pulsatile secretion of PGF_{2a} from the uterus. Res Reprod 1984;16:1–2.

[49] McCracken JA. Hormone receptor control of PGF_{2a} secretion by the ovine uterus. Adv Prostaglandin Thromboxane Res 1980;8:1329–33.

[50] Mitchell MD, Flint AP, Turnbull AC. Stimulation by oxytocin of prostaglandin F levels in uterine venous effluent in pregnant and puerperal sheep. Prostaglandins 1975; 9:47–56.

[51] Chan W. Uterine and placental prostaglandins and their modulation of oxytocin sensitivity and contractility in the parturient uterus. Biol Reprod 1983;29:680–8.

[52] Fairclough RJ, Moore LG, McGowan LT, et al. Temporal relationship between plasma concentrations of 13,14-dihydro-15-keto-prostaglandin and neurophysin I/II around luteolysis in sheep. Prostaglandins 1980;20:199–204.

[53] Flint AP, Sheldrick EL. Evidence for a systemic role for ovarian oxytocin in luteal regression in sheep. J Reprod Fertil 1983;67:215–25.

[54] Gillespie A, Brummer HC, Chard T. Oxytocin release by infused prostaglandin. BMJ 1972; 1:543–4.

[55] Aiken J. Aspirin and indomethacin prolong parturition in rats. Evidence that prostaglandins contribute to expulsion of the fetus. Nature 1972;240:21–5.

[56] Mitchell MD, Flint AP. Use of meclofenamic acid to investigate the role of prostaglandin biosynthesis during induced parturition in sheep. J Endocrinol 1978;76:101–9.

[57] Challis JRG. The placenta, preterm birth, and programming. Presented at Workshop on The Equine Placenta. Lexington, KY, December 5–7, 2003. p. 108–114.

[58] Edqvist LE, Kindahl H, Stabenfeldt GH. Release of prostaglandin F_{2a} during the bovine periparturient period. Prostaglandins 1978;16(1):111–9.

[59] Eley DS, Thatcher WW, Head HH, et al. Periparturient and postpartum endocrine changes of conceptus and maternal units in jersey cows bred for milk yield. J Dairy Sci 1981;64: 312–20.

[60] Schindler D, Lewis G, Rosenberg M, et al. Vulvar electrical impedence in periparturient cows and its relation to plasma progesterone, oestradiol-17B and PGFM. Anim Reprod Sci 1990;23:283–92.

[61] Csapo AI. Progesterone "block." Am J Anat 1956;98:273–91.

[62] Janszen BPM, Bevers MM, Dieleman SJ, et al. Synchronized calvings after withdrawal of norgestomet implants from cows treated near term with prostaglandin. Vet Rec 1990;127: 405–7.

[63] Lye SJ, Ou CW, Teoh TG, et al. The molecular basis of labour and tocolysis. Fetal and Maternal Medicine Review 1998;10(3):121–36.

[64] Fuchs A, Periyasamy S, Soloff M. Systemic and local regulation of oxytocin receptors in the rat uterus, and their functional significance. Can J Biochem Cell Biol 1983;61:615–24.

[65] Soloff MS, Fernstrom MA, Periyasamy S, et al. Regulation of oxytocin receptor concentration in rat uterine explants by estrogen and progesterone. Can J Biochem Cell Biol 1983;61:625–30.

[66] Puri CP, Garfield RE. Changes in hormone levels and gap junctions in the rat uterus during pregnancy and parturition. Biol Reprod 1982;27:967–75.

[67] McKenzie LW, Garfield RE. Hormonal control of gap junctions in the myometrium. Am J Physiol 1985;248:C296–308.

[68] Taverne MAM, de Schwartz NCM, Kankofer M, et al. Uterine response to exogenous oxytocin before and after pre-partum luteolysis in the cow. Reprod Domest Anim 2001;36: 267–72.

[69] Wu WX, Ma XH, Yoshizato T, et al. Differential expression of myometrial oxytocin receptor and prostaglandin H synthase 2, but not estrogen receptor alpha and heat shock protein 90 messenger ribnucleic acid in the gravid horn and nongravid horn in sheep during betamethasone-induced labor. Endocrinology 1999;140(12):5712–8.

[70] Garfield RE, Daniell EE. The structural basis of electrical coupling (cell-to-cell contacts) in rat myometrium. Gynecol Invest 1974;5:284–300.

[71] Bengtsson B. Factors of importance for regulation of uterine contractile activity. Acta Obstet Gynecol Scand 1983;108(Suppl):13–6.

[72] Cole WC, Garfield RE. Evidence for physiological regulation of myometrial gap junction permeability. Am J Vet Res 1986;251:C411–20.

[73] Garfield RE, Rabideau S, Challis JR, et al. Ultrastructural basis for maintenance and termination of pregnancy. Am J Obstet Gynecol 1979;133:308–15.

[74] Kelly EK, Verhage HG. Hormonal effects on the contractile apparatus of the myometrium. Am J Anat 1981;161:375–82.

[75] Phaneuf S, Europe-Finner GN, Carrasco MP, et al. Oxytocin signalling in human myometrium. Adv Exp Med Biol 1995;395:453–67.

[76] Lopez Bernal A, Rivera J, Europe-Finner GN, et al. Parturition: activation of stimulatory pathways or loss of uterine quiescence? Adv Exp Med Biol 1995;395:435–51.

[77] Zerobin K, Sporri H. Motility of the bovine and porcine uterus and fallopian tube. Adv Vet Sci Comp Med 1972;16:303–54.

[78] Hanzen C. Uterine motility in cattle in cattle prior to and post parturition (preliminary reports). Current Topics in Veterinary Medicine and Animal Science 1982;20:61–6.

[79] Taverne M, van der Weyden G, Fontijne P. Preliminary observations on myometrial electrical activity before, during and after parturition in the cow. In: Sureau C, editor. Avortement et Parturition Provoques. Paris: Masson and Cie; 1974. p. 297–311 [in French].

[80] Janszen BPM, Knijn H, van der Weijden GC, et al. Flumethason induced calvings are preceded by a period of myometrial inhibition during luteolysis. Biol Reprod 1990;43: 466–71.

[81] Taverne MAM, Breeveld-Dwarkasing VNA, van Dissel-Emiliani FMF, et al. Between prepartum luteolysis and onset of expulsion. Domest Anim Endocrinol 2002;23(1–2): 329–37.

[82] Bathgate R, Balvers M, Hunt N, et al. Relaxin-like factor gene is highly expressed in the bovine ovary of the cycle and pregnancy: sequence and messenger ribonucleic acid analysis. Biol Reprod 1996;55(6):1452–7.

[83] Rao M, Sanborn B. Relaxin increases calcium efflux from rat myometrial cells in culture. Endocrinology 1986;119:435–7.

[84] Anderson LL, Perezgrovas R, O'Byrne EM, et al. Biological actions of relaxin in pigs and beef cattle. Ann N Y Acad Sci 1982;380:131–50.

[85] Eiler H, Hopkins F. Bovine retained placenta: effects of collagenase and hyaluronidase on detachment of placenta. Biol Reprod 1992;46:580–5.

[86] Gross TS, Williams WF, Manspeaker JE, et al. In vitro proteolytic activity of the late pregnant and peripartum bovine placenta. J Anim Sci 1985;61(Suppl 1):391–2.

[87] Ryan JN, Woessner JF. Mammalian collagenase: direct demonstration in homogenates of involuting rat uterus. Biochem Biophys Res Commun 1971;44:144–9.

[88] Sharpe KL, Eiler H, Hopkins FM. Changes in the proportion of type I and type III collagen in the developing and retained bovine placentome. Biol Reprod 1990;43:229–35.

[89] Miyoshi M, Sawamukai Y, Iwanga T. Reduced phagocytic activity of macrophages in the bovine retained placenta. Reprod Domest Anim 2002;37(1):53–6.

[90] Burton MJ, Dzuik HE, Fahning ML, et al. Effects of oestradiol cypionate on spontaneous and oxytocin-stimulated postpartum myometrial activity in the cow. Br Vet J 1990;146: 309–15.

[91] Gillette DD, Holm L. Prepartum to postpartum uterine and abdominal contractions in cows. Am J Physiol 1963;204:1115–21.

[92] Breeveld-Dwarkasing VNA, Struijk PC, Eijskoot F, et al. Ultrasonic cervimetry to study the dilation of the caudal cervix of the cow at parturition. Theriogenology 2002;57: 1989–2002.

[93] Berridge MJ. Inositol phosphate and diacylglycerol as second messengers. Biochem J 1984; 220:345–60.

[94] Currie W. Physiology of uterine activity. Clin Obstet Gynecol 1980;23:33–49.

[95] Ruzycky A, Crankshaw D. Role of inositol phospholipid hydrolysis in the initiation of agonist-induced contractions of rat uterus: effect of domination by 17B-estradiol and progesterone. Can J Physiol Pharmacol 1988;66:10–7.

[96] Schams D, Prokopp S. Oxytocin determination by RIA in cows around parturition. Anim Reprod Sci 1979;2:267–70.

[97] Lopez Bernal A. Mechanisms of labour—biochemical aspects. BJOG 2003;110(Suppl 20): 39–45.

[98] Olson J, Bretzlaff KN, Mortimer R, et al. The metritis-pyometra complex. In: Youngquist, editor. Current therapy in theriogenology. 2nd edition. Philadelphia: WB Saunders Co.; 1986. p. 227–36.

[99] Bekana M, Jonsson P, Kindahl H. Intrauterine bacterial findings and hormonal profiles in postpartum cows with normal puerperium. Acta Vet Scand 1996;37:251–63.

[100] Mateus L, Lopes da Costa L, Bernardo F, et al. Influence of puerperal uterine infection on uterine involution and postpartum ovarian activity in dairy cows. Reprod Domest Anim 2002;37(1):31–5.

[101] Hoedemaker M. Postpartal pathological vaginal discharge: to treat or not to treat. Reprod Domest Anim 1998;33:139–46.

[102] Mateus L, Lopes da Costa L, Carvalho H, et al. Blood and intrauterine leukocyte profile and function in dairy cows that spontaneously recovered from postpartum endometritis. Reprod Domest Anim 2002;37:176–80.

[103] Klucinski W, Targowski SP, Miernik-Degorska E, et al. The phagocytic activity of polymorphonuclear leukocytes isolated from normal uterus and that with experimentally induced inflammation in cows. Zentralbl Veterinarmed A 1990;37:506–12.

[104] Cai T, Weston P, Lund L, et al. Association between neutrophil function and periparturient disorders in cows. Am J Vet Res 1994;55:934–43.

[105] Mateus L, Lopes da Costa L, Diniz P, et al. Relationship between endotoxin and prostaglandin (PGE2 and PGFM) concentrations and ovarian function in dairy cows with puerperal endometritis. Anim Reprod Sci 2003;76:143–54.

[106] Staples CR, Thatcher WW, Clark JH. Relationship between ovarian activity and energy status during the early postpartum period of high producing dairy cows. J Dairy Sci 1990; 73:938–47.

[107] Butler WR. Nutritional interactions with reproductive performance in dairy cattle. Anim Reprod Sci 2000;60/61:449–57.

[108] Beam SW, Butler WR. Energy balance and ovarian follicle development prior to the first ovulation postpartum in dairy cows receiving three levels of dietary fat. Biol Reprod 1997; 56:133–42.

[109] Beam SW, Butler WR. Energy balance effects on follicular development and first ovulation in postpartum cows. In: Reproduction in domestic animals IV. J Reprod Fertil 1998;54: 411–24.

[110] Lucy MC, Staples CR, Thatcher WW, et al. Influence of diet composition, dry matter intake, milk production, and energy balance on time of postpartum ovulation and fertility in dairy cows. Anim Prod 1992;54:323–31.

[111] Canfield RW, Butler WR. Energy balance and pulsatile LH secretion in early postpartum dairy cattle. Domest Anim Endocrinol 1990;7(3):323–30.

[112] Jorritsma R, Wensing T, Kruip T, et al. Metabolic changes in early lactation and impaired reproductive performance in dairy cows. Vet Res 2003;34:11–26.

[113] Reist M, Erdin DK, von Euw D, et al. Postpartum reproductive function: association with energy, metabolic and endocrine status in high yielding dairy cows. Theriogenology 2003; 59(8):1707–23.

[114] Meikle A, Kulcsar M, Chilliard Y, et al. Effects of parity and body condition at parturition on endocrine and reproductive parameters of the cow. Reproduction 2004;127:727–37.

[115] Wiltbank MC, Gumen A, Sartori R. Physiological classification of anovulatory conditions in cattle. Theriogenology 2002;57:21–52.

[116] Smith GD, Jackson LM, Foster DL. Leptin regulation of reproductive function and fertility. Theriogenology 2002;57:73–86.

[117] Lents CA, Wettemann RP, White FJ, et al. Influence of nutrient intake and body fat on concentrations of insulin-like growth factor-I, insulin, thyroxine, and leptin in plasma of gestating beef cows. J Anim Sci 2005;83(3):586–96.

[118] LeBlanc SJ, Duffield TF, Leslie KE, et al. Defining and diagnosing postpartum clinical endometritis and its impact on reproductive performance in dairy cows. J Dairy Sci 2002;85: 2223–36.

[119] Janowski T, Zdunczyk S, Mwaanga ES. Combined GnRH and PGF2a application in cows with endometritis puerperalis treated with antibiotics. Reprod Domest Anim 2001;36(5): 244–6.

[120] LeBlanc S, Duffield TF, Leslie KE, et al. The effect of treatment of clinical endometritis on reproductive performance in dairy cows. J Dairy Sci 2002;85:2237–49.

[121] Seals RC, Matamoros I, Lewis GS. Relationship between postpartum changes in 13,14-dihydro-15-keto-PGF$_{2a}$ concentrations in holstein cows and their susceptibility to endometritis. J Anim Sci 2002;80:1068–73.

[122] Kaker ML, Murray RD, Dodson H. Plasma hormone changes in cows during induced or spontaneous calvings and the early postpartum period. Vet Rec 1984;115:378–82.

[123] Madej A, Kindahl H, Woyno W, et al. Blood levels of 15-keto-13, 14-dihydro-prostaglandin F_{2a} during the postpartum period in primiparous cows. Theriogenology 1984;21:279–87.

[124] Kindahl H, Odensvik K, Aiumlamai S, et al. Utero-ovarian relationships during the bovine postpartum period. Anim Reprod Sci 1992;28:363–9.

[125] Del Vecchio RP, Matsas DJ, Fortin S, et al. Spontaneous uterine infections are associated with elevated prostaglandin F_{2a} metabolite concentrations in postpartum dairy cows. Theriogenology 1994;41:413–21.

[126] Bekana M, Odensvik K, Kindahl H. Prostaglandin F_{2a} metabolite and progesterone profiles in post-partum cows with retained foetal membranes. Acta Vet Scand 1996;37: 171–85.

[127] Risco C, Drost M, Thatcher WW, et al. Effects of calving-related disorders on prostaglandin, calcium, ovarian acyivity and uterine involution in postpartum dairy cows. Theriogenology 1994;42:183.

[128] Nakao T, Gamal A, Osawa T, et al. Postpartum plasma PGF metabolite profile in cows with dystocia and/or retained placenta, and effect of fenprostalene on uterine involution and reproductive performance. J Vet Med Sci 1997;59(9):791–4.

[129] Bosu WTK, Liptrap RM, Leslie KE. Peripheral changes in plasma progesterone and 15-keto-13,14-dihydro-prostaglandin F_{2a} concentrations in Holstein cows with or without retained foetal membranes. Anim Reprod Sci 1984;7:497–510.

[130] Del Vecchio RP, Matsas DJ, Inzana TJ, et al. Effects of intrauterine bacterial infusion and subsequent endometritis on prostaglandin F_{2alpha} metabolite concentrations in postpartum beef cows. J Anim Sci 1992;70:3158–62.

[131] Odensvik K, Cort N, Basu S, et al. Effect of flunixin meglumine on prostaglandin F_{2a} synthesis and metabolism in the pig. J Vet Pharmacol Ther 1989;12:307–11.

[132] Odensvik K, Gustaffson H, Kindahl H. The effect on luteolysis by intensive oral administration of flunixin granules in heifers. Anim Reprod Sci 1998;50:35–44.

[133] Mihm M. Delayed resumption of cyclicity in postpartum dairy and beef cows. Reprod Domest Anim 1999;34:278–84.

[134] Beam SW, Butler WR. Effects of energy balance on follicular development and first ovulation in postpartum dairy cows. J Reprod Fertil Suppl 1999;54:411–24.

[135] Jolly PD, McDougall S, Fitzpatrick LA, et al. Physiological effects of undernutrition on postpartum anoestrus in cows. J Reprod Fertil Suppl 1995;49:477–92.

[136] Savio JD, Boland MP, Hynes N, et al. Resumption of follicular activity in the early postpartum period of dairy cows. J Reprod Fertil 1990;88:569–79.

[137] Sartori R, Haughian JM, Shaver RD, et al. Comparison of ovarian function and circulating steroids in estrous cycles of Holstein heifers and lactating cows. J Dairy Sci 2004;87:905–20.

[138] Hampton JH, Bader JF, Lamberson WR, et al. Gonadotropin requirements for dominant follicle selection in GnRH agonist-treated cows. Reproduction 2004;127:695–703.

[139] Sakaguchi M, Sasamoto Y, Suzuki T, et al. Postpartum ovarian follicular dynamics and estrous activity in lactating dairy cows. J Dairy Sci 2004;87:2114–21.

[140] Rhodes FM, McDougall S, Burke CR, et al. Invited review: treatment of cows with an extended postpartum anestrous interval. J Dairy Sci 2003;86:1876–94.

[141] Reist M, Koller A, Busato A, et al. First ovulation and ketone body status in the early postpartum period of dairy cows. Theriogenology 2000;54:685–701.

[142] Chilliard Y, Bocquier F, Doreau M. Digestive and metabolic adaptations of ruminants to undernutrition, and consequences on reproduction. Reprod Nutr Dev 1998;38:132–51.

[143] Zurek E, Foxcroft GR, Kennelly JJ. Metabolic status and interval to first ovulation in postpartum dairy cows. J Dairy Sci 1995;78:1909–20.

[144] Kumar Shrestha H, Nakao T, Higaki T, et al. Resumption of postpartum ovarian cyclicity in high-producing Holstein cows. Theriogenology 2004;61(4):637–49.

[145] Hirsbrunner G, Knutti B, Liu I, et al. An in vivo study on spontaneous myometrial contractility in the cow during estrus and diestrus. Anim Reprod Sci 2002;70:171–80.

[146] Ruckebusch Y, Bayard F. Motility of the oviduct and uterus of the cow during the estrous cycle. J Reprod Fertil 1975;43:23–32.

[147] Hanzen C. Electrical activity of the bovine uterus prior to and post parturition. Vet Res Commun 1981;5(2):143–50.

[148] Jordan WJ. The puerperium of the cow. A study of uterine motility. J Comp Pathol 1952;62: 54–68.

[149] Martin LR, Williams WF, Rusek E, et al. Postpartum uterine motility measurements in dairy cows retaining their fetal membranes. Theriogenology 1981;15(5):513–24.

[150] Venable JH, McDonald LE. Postparturient bovine uterine motility—normal and after experimentally produced retention of the fetal membranes. Am J Vet Res 1958;19:308–13.

[151] Chen T, McDonald M, Hawes R. Mechanical and electrical activities of the female bovine genital tract in vivo. Can J Anim Sci 1965;46:25–32.

[152] Gajewski Z, Faundez R. Characteristics and analysis of uterine electromyographic activity in pregnant cattle. Theriogenology 1992;37:1133–45.

[153] Devedeux D, Margue C, Mansour S, et al. Uterine electromyography: a critical review. Am J Obstet Gynecol 1993;169(6):1636–53.

[154] Gajewski Z, Jedruch J, Boryczko Z. Uterine contractile activity in cows during the estrus cycle. J Physiol Pharmacol 1996;47:118.

[155] Okano A, Tomizuka T. Ultrasonic observation of postpartum uterine involution in the cow. Theriogenology 1987;27:369–76.

[156] Laven RA, Peters AR. Bovine retained placenta: aetiology, pathogenesis and economic loss. Vet Rec 1996;139:465–71.

[157] Hernandez J, Risco C, Elliott J. Effect of oral administration of a calcium chloride gel on blood mineral concentrations, parturient disorders, reproductive performance and milk production of dairy cows with retained fetal membranes. J Am Vet Med Assoc 1999;215: 72–6.

[158] Curtis CR. Path analysis of dry period nutrition, postpartum metabolic and reproductive disorders, and mastitis in Holstein cows. J Dairy Sci 1985;68:2347–60.

[159] Griffin JFT, Hartigan PJ, Nunn WR. Non-specific uterine infection and bovine infertility. I. Infection patterns and endometritis during the first seven weeks post-partum. Theriogenology 1974;1(3):91–106.

[160] BonDurant RH. Inflammation in the bovine reproductive tract. J Dairy Sci 1999; 82(Suppl 2):101–10.

[161] Noakes DE, Wallace L, Smith GR. Bacterial flora of the uterus of cows after calving on two hygienically contrasting farms. Vet Rec 1991;128:440–2.

[162] Kim I-H, Suh G-H. Effect of the amount of body condition loss from the dry to near calving periods on the subsequent body condition change, occurence of postpartum diseases, metabolic parameters and reproductive performance in Hosltein dairy cows. Theriogenology 2003;60(8):1445–56.

[163] Contreras LL, Ryan CM, Overton TR. Effects of dry cow grouping strategy and prepartum body condition score on performance and health of transition dairy cows. J Dairy Sci 2004; 87:517–23.

[164] Dohmen MJW, Joop K, Sturk A, et al. Relationship between intrauterine bacterial contamination, endotoxin levels and the development of endometritis in postpartm cows with dystocia or retained placenta. Theriogenology 2000;54:1019–32.

[165] Hussain AM, Daniel RCW, O'Boyle D. Postpartum uterine flora following normal and abnormal puerperium in cows. Theriogenology 1990;34(2):291–302.

[166] Peter AT, Bosu WTK, Gilbert RO. Absorption of Escherichia coli endotoxin (lipopolysaccharide) from the uteri of postpartum dairy cows. Theriogenology 1990;33:1011–4.

[167] Anderson PH, Jarlov N, Hesselholt M, et al. Studies on in vivo endotoxin plasma disappearance times in cattle. Zentralbl Veterinarmed A 1996;43:93–101.

[168] Priesler MT, Weber PS, Tempelman RJ, et al. Glucocorticoid receptor down-regulation in neutrophils of periparturient cows. Am J Vet Res 2000;61:14–9.

[169] Slama H, Vaillancourt D, Goff A. Effect of bacterial cell wall and lipopolysaccharide on arachidonic acid metabolism by caruncular and allantochorionic tissues from cows that calved normally and those that retained fetal membranes. Theriogenology 1994; 41:923–41.

[170] Vagnoni KE, Abbruzzese SB, Christiansen ND, et al. The influence of the phase of the estrous cycle on sheep endometrial tissue response to lipopolysaccharide. J Anim Sci 2001; 79:463–9.

[171] Gross TS, Williams WF, Manspeaker JE, et al. Bovine placental prostaglandin synthesis in vitro as it relates to placental separation. Prostaglandins 1987;34:903–17.

[172] Slama H, Vaillancourt D, Goff AK. Pathophysiology of the puerperal period: Relationship between prostaglandin E_2 (PGE_2) and uterine involution in the cow. Theriogenology 1991; 36:1071–90.

[173] Lewis G. Uterine health and disorders. Symposium: health problems of the postpartum cow. J Dairy Sci 1997;80:984–94.

[174] Olson J, Ball L, Mortimer R. Aspects of bacteriology and endocrinology of cows with pyometra and retained fetal membranes. Am J Vet Res 1984;45:2251–5.

[175] Broderick R, Broderick KA. Ultrastructure and calcium stores in the myometrium. In: Miller JD, editor. Uterine function—molecular and cellular aspects. New York: Plenum Press; 1990. p. 1–33.

[176] Bretzlaff KN, Whitmore HL, Spuhr SL, et al. Incidence and treatment of postpartum reproductive problems in a dairy herd. Theriogenology 1982;17(5):527–35.

[177] Markusfeld O. Factors responsible for postpartum metritis in dairy cattle. Vet Rec 1984; 114:539–42.

[178] Smith B, Donavon G, Risco C, et al. Comparison of various antibiotic treatments for cows diagnosed with toxic puerperal metritis. J Dairy Sci 1998;81:1555–62.

[179] Melendez P, McHale J, Bartolome J, et al. Uterine involution and fertility of holstein cows subsequent to early postpartum PGF2a treatment for acute puerperal metritis. J Dairy Sci 2004;87:3238–46.

[180] Tennant B, Peddicord RG. The influence of delayed uterine involution and endometritis on bovine fertility. Cornell Vet 1968;58(2):185–92.

[181] Zamet CN, Cloenbrander VF, Erd RE, et al. Variables associated with postpartum traits in dairy cows. II. Interrelationships among disorders and their effects on intake of feed and on reproductive efficiency. Theriogenology 1979;11(3):245–60.

[182] Fredriksson G. Some reproductive and clinical aspects of endotoxins in cows with special emphasis on the role of prostaglandins. Acta Vet Scand 1984;25:365–77.

[183] Markusfeld O. Periparturient traits in seven high producing dairy herds. Incidence rates, association with parity, and interrelationships among traits. J Dairy Sci 1987; 70(1):158–66.

[184] Stevens RD, Dinsmore RP, Cattell MB. Evaluation of the use of intrauterine infusion of oxytetracycline, subcutaneous injections of fenprostalene, or a combination of both, for the treatment of retained fetal membranes in dairy cows. J Am Vet Med Assoc 1995;207: 1612–5.

[185] Laven RA, Leung ST, Cheng Z. The use of oxytocin to prevent retained placenta after induction with cloprostenol. Cattle Practice 1998;6:291–6.

[186] Studer E, Holtan A. Treatment of retained placentas in dairy cattle with prostaglandin. The Bovine Practitioner 1986;21:159–60.

[187] Frazer GS. Hormonal therapy in the postpartum cow—days 1 to 10. Paper presented at Society for Theriogenology. Vancouver, Canada, September 11, 2001.

[188] Konigsson K, Gustafsson B, Gunnarsson A, et al. Clinical and bacteriological aspects on the use of oxytetracycline and flunixin in primiparous cows with induced retained placenta and post-partal endometritis. Reprod Domest Anim 2001;36:247–56.

[189] Peeler EJ, Otte MJ, Esslemont RJ. Inter-relationships of periparturient diseases in dairy cows. Vet Rec 1994;134:129–32.

[190] Boos A, Janssen V, Mulling C. Proliferation and apoptosis in bovine placentomes during pregnancy and around induced and spontaneous parturition as well as in cows retaining the fetal membranes. Reproduction 2003;126:469–80.

[191] Williams WF, Margolis MJ, Manspeaker JE, et al. Peripartum changes in the bovine placenta related to fetal membrane retention. Theriogenology 1987;28:312–23.

[192] Grunert E. Placental separation/retention in the bovine. Paper presented at International Congress on Animal Reproduction and Artificial Insemination. Urbana, Illinois, June, 1984. p. X117–24.

[193] Grunert G. Etiology and pathogenesis of retained bovine placenta. In: Morrow DA, editor. Current therapy in theriogenology. Philadelphia: W.B. Saunders Co.; 1986. p. 237–42.

[194] Joosten I, Hensen EJ. Retained placenta: an immunological approach. Anim Reprod Sci 1992;28:451–61.

[195] Wischral A, Verreschi IT, Lima SB, et al. Pre-parturition profile of steroids and prostaglandin in cows with or without foetal membrane retention. Anim Reprod Sci 2001;67(3–4):181–8.

[196] Erb HN, Smith RD, Oltenacu PA, et al. Path model of reproductive disorders and performance, milk fever, mastitis, milk yield, and culling in Holstein cows. J Dairy Sci 1985; 68:3337–49.

[197] Stevenson JS. Reproductive disorders in the periparturient dairy cow. J Dairy Sci 1988;71: 2572–83.

[198] Goff JP, Horst RL. Physiological changes at parturition and their relationship to metabolic disorders. J Dairy Sci 1997;80:1260–8.

[199] Kamgarpour R, Daniel RC, Fenwick DC, et al. Postpartum subclinical hypocalcaemia and effects on ovarian function and uterine involution in a dairy herd. Vet J 1999;158:59–67.

[200] Bolinder A, Seguin B, Kindahl H, et al. Retained fetal membranes in cows: manual removal versus nonremoval and its effect on reproductive performance. Theriogenology 1988;30: 45–56.

[201] Peters AR, Laven RA. Treatment of bovine retained placenta and its effects. Vet Rec 1996; 139:535–9.

[202] Joosten I, Stelwagen J, Dijkhuizen AA. Economic and reproductive consequences of retained placenta in dairy cattle. Vet Rec 1988;123:53–7.

[203] Fourichon C, Seegers H, Malher X. Effect of disease on reproduction in the dairy cow: a meta-analysis. Theriogenology 2000;53:1729–59.

[204] Bartlett PC, Kirk JH, Wilke MA, et al. Metritis complex in Michigan Holstein-Fresian cattle: incidence, descriptive epidemiology, and estimated economic impact. Prev Vet Med 1986;4:235–48.

[205] Horst RL, Goff JP, Reinhardt TA, et al. Strategies for preventing milk fever in dairy cattle. J Dairy Sci 1997;80:1269–80.

[206] Sheldon I, Rycroft AN, Zhou C. Association between postpartum pyrexia and uterine bacterial infection in dairy cattle. Vet Rec 2004;154:289–93.

[207] Konigsson K, Gustafsson H, Kindahl H. 15-Ketodihydro-PGF2a, progesterone and uterine involution in primiparous cows with induced retained placenta and post partal endometritis treated with oxytetracycline and flunixin. Reprod Domest Anim 2002;37:43–51.

[208] Chenault JR, McAllister JF, Chester ST, et al. Efficacy of ceftiofur hydrochloride sterile suspension administered parenterally for the treatment of acute postpartum metritis in dairy cows. J Am Vet Med Assoc 2004;224(10):1634–9.

[209] Drillich M, Pfutzner A, Sabin H-J, et al. Comparison of two protocols for the treatment of retained fetal membranes in dairy cattle. Theriogenology 2003;59:951–60.

[210] Drillich M, Beetz O, Pfutzner A, et al. Evaluation of systemic antibiotic treatment of toxic puerperal metritis in dairy cows. J Dairy Sci 2001;84:2010–7.

[211] Risco C, Hernandez J. Comparison of ceftiofur hydrochloride and estradiol cypionate for metritis prevention and reproductive performance in dairy cows affected with retained fetal membranes. Theriogenology 2003;60:47–58.

[212] Amiridius G, Leontides L, Tassos E, et al. Flunixin meglumine accelerates uterine involution and shortens the calving-to-first-oestrus interval in cows with puerperal metritis. J Vet Pharmacol Ther 2001;24:365–7.

[213] Zhou C, Boucher JF, Dame KJ, et al. Multi-location trial of ceftiofur for treatment of postpartum cows with fever. J Am Vet Med Assoc 2001;219(6):805–8.

[214] LeBlanc SJ, Leslie KE, Duffield TF. Metabolic predictors of displaced abomasum in dairy cattle. J Dairy Sci 2005;88:159–70.

[215] Dinsmore RP, Stevens RD, Cattell MB, et al. Oxytetracycline residues in milk after intrauterine treatment of cows with retained fetal membranes. J Am Vet Med Assoc 1996; 209(10):1753–5.

[216] Gustafsson BK. Therapeutic strategies involving antimicrobial treatment of the uterus in large animals. J Am Vet Med Assoc 1984;185:1194–8.

[217] Stevens RP, Stevens RD, Cattell MB, et al. Oxytetracycline residues in milk after intrauterine treatment of cows with retained membranes. J Am Vet Med Assoc 1996; 209(10):1753–5.

[218] Plumb DC. Veterinary drug handbook. Ames (IA): Iowa State University press; 1999.

[219] Bruckmaier RM, Schams D, Blum JW. Continuously elevated concentrations of oxytocin during milking are necessary for complete milk removal in dairy cows. J Dairy Res 1994;61: 323–34.

[220] Bruckmaier RM, Schams D, Blum JW. Milk removal in familiar and unfamiliar surroundings: concentration of oxytocin, prolactin, cortisol, and beta-endorphin. J Dairy Res 1993;60:449–56.

[221] Bruckmaier R, Blum J. Oxytocin release and milk removal in ruminants. J Dairy Sci 1998; 81:939–49.

[222] Akers R, Lefcourt A. Milking- and suckling-induced secretion of oxytocin and prolactin in parturient dairy cows. Horm Behav 1982;16:87–93.

[223] Bar-Peled U, Maltz E, Bruckental I, et al. Relationship between frequent milking or suckling in early lactation and milk production of high producing dairy cows. J Dairy Sci 1995;78:2726–36.

[224] Macuhova J, Tancin V, Bruckmaier RM. Effects of oxytocin administration on oxytocin release and milk ejection. J Dairy Sci 2004;87:1236–44.

[225] Wachs EA, Gorewit RC, Currie WB. Half-life, clearance and production rate for oxytocin in cattle during lactation and mammary involution I. Domest Anim Endocrinol 1984;1(2): 121–40.

[226] Hemeida NA, Gustafsson BK, Whitmore HL. Therapy of uterine infections: alternatives to antibiotics. In: Morrow DA, editor. Current therapy in theriogenology. 2nd edition. Philadelphia: W.B. Saunders Co.; 1986. p. 45–7.

[227] Roberts SJ. Injuries and diseases of the puerperal period. In: Roberts SJ, editor. Veterinary obstetrics and genital diseases—theriogenology. 3rd edition. North Pomfret (VT): David and Charles, Inc.; 1986. p. 353–96.

[228] Ruesse M. Myometrial activity postpartum. Factors influening fertility in the postpartum cow. Current Topics in Veterinary Medicine and Animal Science 1982;20:55–60.

[229] Ehrenreich H, Ruesse M, Schams D, et al. An opiod antagonist stimulates myometrial activity in early postpartum cows. Theriogenology 1985;23:309–24.

[230] Zerobin K, Kundig H. The control of myometrial functions during parturition with Beta2-mimetic compund, Planipart. Theriogenology 1980;14:21–35.

[231] Bulbring E, Tomita T. Catecholamine action on smooth muscle. Pharmacol Rev 1987;39: 50–96.

[232] Arthur GH. Retention of the afterbirth in cattle: a review and commentary. Veterinary Annual 1979;19:26–36.

[233] Hickey GJ, White ME, Wickenden RP, et al. Effects of oxytocin or placental retention following dystocia. Vet Rec 1984;114:189–90.

[234] Miller BJ, Lodge JR. Effect of oxytocin on retained placentas [abstract]. J Anim Sci 1981; 53(Suppl):350.

[235] Miller BJ, Lodge JR. Postpartum oxytocin treatment for prevention of retained placentas. Theriogenology 1982;17:237–43.

[236] Shaw RN. Pituitary extract in cattle practice with particular reference to its use in cases of retained placenta. Vet Bull 1938;8:9.

[237] Steward R, Stevenson J. Hormonal, estral, ovulatory, and milk traits in postpartum dairy cows following multiple daily injections of oxytocin. J Anim Sci 1987;65:1584–5.

[238] Mollo A, Veronesi MC, Cairoli F, et al. The use of oxytocin for the reduction of cow placental retention, and subsequent endometritis. Anim Reprod Sci 1997;48(1): 47–51.

[239] Gustafsson B, Ott RS. Current trends in the treatment of genital infections in large animals. Compend Contin Educ Pract Vet 1981;3:S147.

[240] Gross T, Williams W, Morehead T. Prevention of the retained fetal membrane syndrome (retained placenta) during induced calving in dairy cattle. Theriogenology 1986;26:365–70.

[241] Stocker H, Waelchli R. A clinical trial on the effect of prostaglandin F_{2a} on placental expulsion in dairy cattle after caesarean operation. Vet Rec 1993;132:507–8.

[242] Archbald L, Tran T, Thomas P, et al. Apparent failure of prostaglandin F_{2a} to improve the reproductive efficiency of postpartum dairy cows that had experienced dystocia and/or retained fetal membranes. Theriogenology 1990;34:1025–34.

[243] Burton MJ, Herschler R, Dzuik H, et al. Effect of fenprostalene on postpartum myometrial activity in dairy cows with normal or delayed placental expulsion. Br Vet J 1987;143: 549–54.

[244] Garcia A, Barth A, Mapletoft R. Induction of parturition in the cow: effects of prostaglandin treatment on the incidence of retained placenta. Theriogenology 1989;31: 195.

[245] Garcia A, Barth A, Mapletoft R. The effects of treatment with cloprostenol or dinoprost within one hour of induced parturition on the incidence of retained placenta in cattle. Can Vet J 1992;33:175–83.

[246] Herschler RC, Lawrence JR. A prostaglandin analogue for therapy of retained placentae. Vet Med Small Anim Clin 1984;79:822–6.

[247] Kindahl H, Fedriksson G, Madej A, et al. Role of prostaglandins in uterine involution. Presented at International Congress on Animal Reproduction and Artificial Insemination. Urbana, Illinois, June, 1984.

[248] Ko J, McKenna D, Whitmore H, et al. Effects of estradiol cypionate and natural and synthetic prostaglandins on myometrial activity in early postpartum cows. Theriogenology 1989;32:537–43.

[249] Steffan J, Adriamanga S, Thibier M. Treatment of metritis with antibiotics or prostaglandin F_{2a} and influence of ovarian cyclicity in dairy cows. Am J Vet Res 1984; 45:1090–4.

[250] Stevens R, Dinsmore R. Treatment of dairy cows at parturition with prostaglandin F_{2a} or oxytocin for prevention of retained fetal membranes. J Am Vet Med Assoc 1997;211: 1280–4.

[251] Waelchli R, Thun R, Stocker H. Effect of flunixin meglumine on placental expulsion in dairy cattle after a caesarean. Vet Rec 1999;144:702–3.

[252] Young I, Anderson D, Plenderleith R. Increased conception rate in dairy cows after early postpartum administration of prostaglandin F_{2a} THAM. Vet Rec 1984;115:429–31.

[253] Gruys E, Obwolo MJ, Toussaint MJM. Diagnostic significance of the major acute phase proteins in veterinary clinical chemistry. Vet Bull 1994;64:1009–18.

[254] Hirvonen JG, Huszenicza G, Kulcsar M, et al. Acute-phase response in dairy cows with acute postpartum metritis. Theriogenology 1999;51:1071–83.

[255] Smith BI, Donovan GA, Risco CA, et al. Serum haptoglobulin concentrations in Holstein dairy cattle with toxic puerperal metritis. Vet Rec 1998;142:83–5.

[256] Sheldon IM, Noakes DE, Rycroft AN, et al. Acute phase protein responses to uterine bacterial contamination in cattle after calving. Vet Rec 2001;148:172–5.

[257] Eilts BE. Pregnancy termination in the bitch and queen. Clin Tech Small Anim Pract 2002; 17(3):116–23.

[258] Pena FJ, Gil MC. Mismating and abortion in bitches: the preattachment period. Compend Contin Educ Pract Vet 2002;24(5):400–7.

[259] Gilbert R, Schwark W. Pharmacologic considerations in the management of peripartum conditions in the cow. Applied pharmacology and therapeutics II. Vet Clin North Am Food Anim Pract 1992;8(1):29–56.

[260] Samuelsson B, Granstrom E, Green K, et al. Prostaglandins. Annu Rev Biochem 1975;44: 669–95.

[261] Davis AJ, Fleet IR, Harrison FA, et al. Pulmonary metabolism of prostaglandin F_{2a} in the conscious nonpregnant ewe and sow. J Physiol 1980;301:86.

[262] Chen J, Woodward DF, Yuan YD, et al. Prostanoid-induced contraction of the rabbit isolated uterus is mediated by FP receptors. Prostaglandins 1998;55:387–94.

[263] Garcia-Villar R, Marnet P, Laurentie M, et al. Fenprostalene in cattle: evaluation of oxytocic effects in ovariectomized cows and abortion potential in a 100-day pregnant cow. Theriogenology 1987;28:467–80.

[264] Rodriguez-Martinez H, Ko J, McKenna D, et al. Uterine motility in the cow during the estrous cycle. II. Comparative effects of prostaglandins F_2, E_2, and cloprostenol. Theriogenology 1987;27:349–58.

[265] Hirsbrunner G, Kupfer U, Burkhardt H, et al. Effect of different prostaglandins on intrauterine pressure and uterine motility during diestrus in experimental cows. Theriogenology 1998;50:445–55.

[266] Hirsbrunner G, Knutti B, Kupfer U, et al. Effect of prostaglandin E_2, DL-cloprostenol, and prostaglandin E_2 in combination with D-cloprostenol on uterine motility during diestrus in experimental cows. Anim Reprod Sci 2003;79:17–32.

[267] Odensvik K, Fredriksson G. The effect of intensive flunixin treatment during the postpartum period in the bovine. Zentralbl Veterinarmed A 1993;40:561–8.

[268] Razin E, Bauminger S, Globerson A. Effect of prostaglandins on phagocytosis of sheep erythrocytes by mouse peritoneal macrophages. J Reticuloendothel Soc 1978;23:237–42.

[269] Hoedemaker M, Lund LA, Wagner WC. Influence of arachidonic acid metabolites and steroids on function of bovine polymorphonuclear neutrophils. Am J Vet Res 1992;53: 1534–9.

[270] Bretzlaff KN, Ott RS. Postpartum reproductive problems in a large dairy herd. Bovine Clinics 1981;1:4.

[271] Oxenrider SL. Evaluation of various treatments for chronic uterine infections in dairy cattle. Presented at the Annual Meeting of the Society for Theriogenology. Milwaukee, WI, September 22–24, 1982.

[272] Upham GL. A practitioner's approach to management of metritis/endometritis. Early detection and supportive treatment. Presented at the 29th AGM of the American Association of Bovine Practitioners, San Diego, CA, September 14–16, 1996. p. 19–21.

[273] Callahan C, Horstman L. Treatment of early postpartum metritis in a dairy herd: response and subsequent fertility. The Bovine Practitioner 1987;22:124–8.

[274] Dialogue newsletter. Pharmacia & Upjohn Animal Health. Vol 7; 1998.

[275] Dialogue newsletter. Pharmacia & Upjohn Animal Health. Vol 8; 1999.

[276] ECP sterile solution package insert. Kalamazoo (MI): Pharmacia & Upjohn; 1998.

[277] Wagner DC, Bon Durant RH, Sischo WM. Reproductive effects of estradiol cypionate in postparturient dairy cows. J Am Vet Med Assoc 2001;219(2):220–3.

[278] Overton MW, Sischo W, Reynolds JP. Evaluation of effect of estradiol cypionate administered prophylactically to postparturient dairy cows at high risk for metritis. J Am Vet Med Assoc 2003;223(6):846–51.

[279] Haughian JM, Sartori R, Guenther JN, et al. Extending the postpartum anovulatory period in dairy cattle with estradiol cypionate. J Dairy Sci 2002;85:3238–49.

[280] Sheldon IM, Noakes DE, Rycroft AN, et al. The effect of intrauterine administration of estradiol on postpartum uterine involution in cattle. Theriogenology 2003;59:1357–71.

[281] Soloff MS. Uterine receptor for oxytocin: effects of estrogen. Biochem Biophys Res Commun 1975;65:205–12.

[282] Robinson RS, Mann GE, Lamming GE, et al. Expression of oxytocin, oestrogen and progesterone receptors in uterine biopsy samples throughout the oestrus cycle and early pregnancy in cows. Reproduction 2001;122:965–79.

[283] Zhang J, Weston PG, Hixon JE. Role of progesterone and oestradiol in the regulation of uterine oxytocin receptors in ewes. J Reprod Fertil 1992;94:395–404.

[284] Jenner LJ, Parkinson TJ, Lamming GE. Uterine oxytocin receptors in cyclic and pregnant cows. J Reprod Fertil 1991;91:49–58.

[285] Lau TM, Kerton DJ, Gow CB, et al. Increase in concentration of uterine oxytocin receptors and decrease in response to 13,14-dihydro-15-keto- prostaglandin F_{2a} in ewes after withdrawal of exogenous progesterone. J Reprod Fertil 1992;95:885–93.

[286] Rodriguez-Martinez H, Ko J, McKenna D, et al. Uterine motility in the cow during the estrous cycle. III. Effects of oxytocin, xylazine, and adrenoceptor blockers. Theriogenology 1987;27:359–68.

[287] Lamming G, Mann G. Control of endometrial oxytocin receptors and prostaglandin F_{2a} production by progesterone and oestradiol. J Reprod Fertil 1995;103:69–73.

[288] Mann G, Lamming G. Effect of the level of oestradiol on oxytocin-induced prostaglandin F_{2a} release in the cow. J Endocrinol 1995;145:175–80.

[289] Lamming GE, Mann GE. A dual role for progesterone in the control of cyclicity in ruminants. J Reprod Fertil Suppl 1995;49:561–6.

[290] Mann GE, Lamming GE. Use of repeated biopsies to monitor endometrial oxytocin receptors in cows. Vet Rec 1994;135:403–5.

[291] Vallet JL, Lamming GE, Batten M. Control of endometrial oxytocin receptor and uterine response to oxytocin by progesterone and oestradiol in the ewe. J Reprod Fertil 1990;90: 625–34.

[292] Mann GE. Hormone control of prostaglandin F_{2a} production and oxytocin receptor concentrations in bovine endometrium in explant culture. Domest Anim Endocrinol 2001; 20(3):217–26.

[293] Leung S, Wathes D. Oestradiol regulation of oxytocin receptor expression in cyclic bovine endometrium. J Reprod Fertil 2000;119:287–92.

[294] Rodriguez-Pinon M, Tasende C, Meikle A, et al. Estrogen and progesterone receptors in the ovine cervix during the postpartum period. Theriogenology 2000;53:743–50.

[295] Tasende C, Meikle A, Rubianes E, et al. Restoration of estrogen and progesterone uterine receptors during the ovine postpartum period. Theriogenology 1996;45(8):1545–51.

[296] Warren JE, Hawk HW. Effect of an intrauterine device on sperm transport and uterine motility in sheep and rabbits. J Reprod Fertil 1971;26:419–22.

[297] Croker KP, Shelton JN. Influence of stage of cycle, progestagen treatment and dose of oestrogen on uterine motility in the ewe. J Reprod Fertil 1973;32:521–4.

[298] Hawk HW. Uterine motility and sperm transport in the estrous ewe after prostaglandin induced regression of corpora lutea. J Anim Sci 1973;37:1380–5.

[299] Hawk HW, Echternkamp SE. Uterine contractions in the ewe during progestagen-regulated oestrus. J Reprod Fertil 1973;34:347–9.

[300] Hawk HW. Hormonal control of changes in the direction of uterine contractions in the estrous ewe. Biol Reprod 1975;12:423–30.

[301] Gilbert CL, Cripps PJ, Wathes DC. Effect of oxytocin on the pattern of electromyographic activity in the oviduct and uterus of the ewe around oestrus. Reprod Fertil Dev 1992;4: 193–203.

[302] Ulbrich SE, Kettler A, Einspanier R. Expression and localization of estrogen receptor alpha, estrogen receptor beta and progesterone receptor in the bovine oviduct in vivo and in vitro. J Steroid Biochem Mol Biol 2003;84:279–89.

[303] Bennett WA, Watts TL, Blair WD, et al. Patterns of oviductal motility in the cow during the oestrus cycle. J Reprod Fertil 1988;83:537–43.

[304] Wijayagunawardane MPB, Miyamoto A, Cerbito WA, et al. Local distributions of oviductal estradiol, progesterone, prostaglandins, oxytocin and endothelin-1 in the cyclic cow. Theriogenology 1998;49:607–18.

[305] Docke F. Untersuchungen zur Uteruskontraktilitat beim Rind [Investigation of uterine contractility in cattle.]. Arch Exp Vetinarmed 1962;16:1205–9 [in German].

[306] Rodriguez-Martinez H, Ko J, McKenna D, et al. Uterine motility in the cow during the estrous cycle. I. Spontaneous activity. Theriogenology 1987;27:337–48.

[307] Kotwica G, Kurowicka B, Franczak A, et al. The concentrations of catecholamines and oxytocin receptors in the oviduct and its contractile activity in cows during the estrous cycle. Theriogenology 2003;60:953–64.

[308] Einspanier R, Gabler C, Kettler A, et al. Characterization and localization of beta2-adrenergic receptors in the bovine oviduct: indication for progesterone-mediated expression. Endocrinology 1999;140:2679–84.

[309] Carson R, Wolfe D, Klesius P, et al. The effects of ovarian hormones and ACTH on uterine defense to C. Pyogenes in cows. Theriogenology 1988;30:91–7.

[310] Frank T, Anderson KL, Smith AR, et al. Phagocytosis in the uterus: a review. Theriogenology 1983;20:103–10.

[311] Hawk HW, Brinsfield T, Turner GD, et al. Effect of ovarian status on induced acute inflammatory responses in cattle uteri. Am J Vet Res 1964;25:362–6.

[312] Sheldon IM, Noakes DE, Rycroft AN, et al. Effect of intrauterine administration of oestradiol on postpartum uterine bacterial infection in cattle. Anim Reprod Sci 2004;81: 13–23.

[313] Roth J, Kaeberle M, Appel L, et al. Association of increased estradiol and progesterone blood values with altered bovine polymorphonuclear leukocyte function. Am J Vet Res 1983;44:247–53.

[314] Lamote I, Meyer E, Duchateau L, et al. Influence of 17beta-estradiol, progesterone, and dexamethasone on diapedesis and viability of bovine blood polymorphonuclear leukocytes. J Dairy Sci 2004;87:3340–9.

[315] Subandrio A, Sheldon I, Noakes D. Peripheral and intrauterine neutrophil function in the cow: the influence of endogenous and exogenous sex steroid hormones. Theriogenology 2000;53(8):1591–608.

[316] Smits E, Cifrian E, Guidry A, et al. Cell culture systems for studying bovine neutrophil diapedesis. J Dairy Sci 1996;79:1353–60.

[317] Anderson K, Hemeida N, Frank A, et al. Collection and phagocytic evaluation of uterine neutrophilic leukocytes. Theriogenology 1985;24:305–17.

[318] Lander-Chacin MF, Hansen PJ, Drost M. Effects of stage of the estrous cycle and steroid treatment on uterine immunglobulin content and polymorphonuclear leukocytes in cattle. Theriogenology 1990;34:1169–84.

[319] Slama H, Vaillancourt D, Goff A. Leukotriene B4 in cows with normal calving, and in cows with retained fetal membranes and/or uterine subinvolution. Can J Vet Res 1993;57:293–9.

[320] Slama H, Vaillancourt D, Goff A. Metabolism of arachidonic acid by caruncular and allantoic tissues in cows with retained fetal membranes (RFM). Prostaglandins 1993;45: 57–75.

[321] Broome AW, Winter AJ, McNurr SH, et al. Variation in uterine response to experimental infection due to the hormonal state of the ovaries. II. The mobilization of leukocytes and their importance in uterine bactericidal activity. Am J Vet Res 1960;21:675–82.

[322] Hawk HW, Turner GD, Sykes JF. The effect of ovarian hormones on uterine defence mechanism during the early stages of induced infection. Am J Vet Res 1960;21:644–8.

[323] Kehrli M, Nonneke B, Roth J. Alterations in bovine neutrophil function during the periparturient period. Am J Vet Res 1989;50:207–14.

[324] Ramadan AA, Johnson GL, Lewis GS. Regulation of uterine immune function during the estrous cycle and in response to infectious bacteria in sheep. J Anim Sci 1997;75:1621–32.

[325] Al-Eknah M, Noakes D. Uterine activity in cows during the oestrous cycle, after ovariectomy, and following exogenous oestradiol and progesterone. Br Vet J 1989;145: 328–36.

[326] Dielman S, Bevers M. Development of preovulatory follicles in the cow from luteolysis until ovulation. In: O'Callaghan D, editor. Follicle growth and ovulation rate in farm animals. Dordrecht (Netherlands): Martinus Nijhoff; 1987. p. 31.

[327] Vynckier L, Debackere M, De Kruif A, et al. Plasma estradiol-17β concentrations in the cow during induced estrus and after injection of estradiol-17β benzoate and estradiol-17β cypionate—a preliminary study. J Vet Pharmacol Ther 1990;13:36–42.

[328] Syncro-Mate-B Package insert. NADA No: 097–037. Iselin (NJ): Merial Ltd.

[329] Kojima N, Stumpf T, Cupp A, et al. Exogenous progesterone and progestagens as used in estrous synchrony regimens do not mimic the coprus luteum in regulation of luteinizing hormone and 17B-estradiol in circulation of cows. Biol Reprod 1992;47:1009–17.

[330] Glencross R, Pope S. Concentrations of oestradiol-17β and progesterone in the plasma of dairy heifers before and after cloprostenol induced and natural luteolysis and during early pregnancy. Anim Reprod Sci 1981;4:93–106.

[331] Schallenberger E, Schams D, Bullerman B, et al. Pulsatile secretion of gonadotrophins, ovarian steroids and ovarian oxytocin during prostaglandin-induced regression of the corpus luteum in the cow. J Reprod Fertil 1984;71:493–501.

[332] Walters D, Schalenberger E. Pulsatile secretion of gonadotropins, ovarian steroids and ovarian oxytocin during the preovulatory phase of the oestrous cycle in the cow. J Reprod Fertil 1984;71:503–12.

[333] Gyawu P, Pope GS. Oestrogens in milk. J Steroid Biochem 1983;19:877–82.

[334] Lunaas T. Bovine colostrum levels of oestrone and oestradiols. Acta Vet Scand 1964;5: 257–64.

[335] Pope GS, Roy JHB. The oestrogenci activity of bovine colostrum. Biochem J 1953;53: 427–30.

[336] Wolford ST, Argoudelis CJ. Measurement of estrogens in cow's milk, human milk, and dairy products. J Dairy Sci 1979;62:1458–63.

[337] Pandey RS, Pahwa GS, Suri AK, et al. Diurnal variations of oestradiol-17β in milk of cross-bred cows during oestrus cycle and early pregnancy. Br Vet J 1981;137:596–600.

[338] Monk EL, Erb RE, Mollett TA. Relationships between immunoreactive estrone and estradiol in milk, blood, and urine of dairy cows. J Dairy Sci 1975;58:35–9.

[339] Abeyawardene SA, Hathorn DJ, Glencross RG. Concentrations of oestradiol-17β and progesterone in bovine plasma and defatted milk during the postpartum anovulatory period. Br Vet J 1984;140:458–67.

[340] Schwalm JW, Tucker HA. Glucocorticoids in mammary secretions and blood serum during reproduction and lactation and distributions of glucocorticoids, progesterone, and estrogens in fractions of milk. J Dairy Sci 1978;61(5):550–60.

[341] Lopez H, Bunch TD, Shipka MP. Estrogen concentrations in milk at estrus and ovulation in dairy cows. Anim Reprod Sci 2002;72(1–2):37–46.

[342] Batra SK, Arora RC, Bachlaus NK, et al. Quantitative relationships between oestradiol-17beta in the milk and blood of lactating buffaloes. J Endocrinol 1980;84:205–9.

[343] Erb RE, Chew BP, Keller HF. Relative concentrations of estrogen and progesterone in milk and blood, and excretion of estrogen in urine. J Anim Sci 1977;45:617–26.

[344] Hamon M, Fleet IR, Heap RB. Comparison of oestrone sulphate concentrations in mammary secretions during lactogenesis and lactation in dairy ruminants. J Dairy Res 1990;57:419–22.

[345] Pope GS, Swinburne JK. Reviews of the progress of dairy science: hormones in milk: their physiological significance and value as diagnostic aids. J Dairy Res 1980;47:427–49.

[346] Hamon M, Fleet IR, Holdsworth RJ, et al. The time of detection of oestrone sulphate in milk and the diagnosis of pregnancy in cows. Br Vet J 1981;137:71–7.

[347] Holdsworth RJ, Heap RB, Booth JM, et al. A rapid direct radioimmunoassay for the measurement of estrone sulphate in the milk of dairy cows and its use in pregnancy diagnosis. J Endocrinol 1982;95:7–12.

[348] Henderson KM, Camberis M, Simmons MH, et al. Application of enzyme immunoassay to measure oestrone sulphate concentration in cow's milk during pregnancy. J Steroid Biochem 1994;50:189–96.

[349] Hatzidakis G, Katrakili K, Krambovitis E. Development of a direct and specific enzyme immunoassay for the measurement of estrone sulfate in bovine milk. J Reprod Fertil 1993; 98:235–40.

[350] Heap RB, Hamon M. Oestrone sulphate in milk as an indicator of a viable conceptus in cows. Br Vet J 1979;135:355–63.

[351] Lunaas T. Transfer of oestradiol-17beta to milk in cattle. Nature 1963;198:288–9.

[352] Glencross RG, Abeywardene SA. Concentrations of oestradiol-17beta and progesterone in plasma and defatted milk of cattle during the oestrous cycle. Br Vet J 1983;139:49–51.

[353] Glencross RG, Abeyawardene SA, Corney SJ, et al. The use of oestradiol-17beta antiserum covalently coupled to Sepharose to extract oestradiol-17beta from biological fluids. J Chromatogr 1981;233:193–7.

[354] Meisterling EM, Dailey RA. Use of concentrations of progesterone and estradiol-17beta in milk in monitoring postpartum ovarian function in dairy cows. J Dairy Sci 1987;70(10): 2154–61.

[355] Qin LQ, Wang PY, Kaneko T, et al. Estrogen: one of the risk factors in milk for prostate cancer. Med Hypotheses 2004;62(1):133–42.

[356] Ganmaa D, Wang PY, Qin LQ, et al. Is milk responsible for male reproductive disorders? Med Hypotheses 2001;57(4):510–4.

[357] Richards RC. Milk secretion: with special reference to its content of hormones, enzymes and immunoreactive components. In: Finn CA, editor. Oxford reviews of reproductive biology, vol. 1. Oxford (England): Claredon Press; 1979. p. 262–82.

[358] Coulson WF, Hamon M, Heap RB, et al. Pregnancy diagnosis in cows by the measurement of oestrone sulphate in milk. J Physiol 1981;319:19.

[359] Bloomfield GA, Morant SV, Ducker MJ. Oestrone sulphate in milk of pregnant dairy cows. Br Vet J 1982;138:545.

[360] MacDonald BJ, Sauer MJ, Watson ED, et al. Direct radioimmunoassay of estradiol-17beta in defatted bovine milk. Steroids 1982;639:711–72.

[361] Eley RM, Thatcher WW, Bazer FW. Hormonal and physical changes associated with bovine conceptus development. J Reprod Fertil 1979;55:181–90.

[362] Henricks DM, Owenby JJ, Gray SL. Concentration of estradiol-17β (E$_2$) in milk of dairy cows; effect of injection of E$_2$ cypionate. J Anim Sci 2003;81(Suppl 1):181.

[363] Jorritsma R, Jorritsma H, Schukken YH, et al. Relationships between fatty liver and fertility and some periparturient diseases in commercial Dutch dairy herds. Theriogenology 2000;54(7):1065–74.

[364] Bobe G, Young JW, Beitz DC. Pathology, etiology, prevention, and treatment of fatty liver in dairy cows. J Dairy Sci 2004;87:3105–24.

[365] Liu SL, Lin YC. Transformation of MCF-10A human breast epithelial cells by zeranol and estradiol-17beta. Breast J 2004;10(6):514–21.

[366] Irshaid F, Kulp SK, Sugimoto Y, et al. Zeranol stimulated estrogen-regulated gene expression on MCF-7 human breast cancer cells and normal human breast epithelial cells. Biol Reprod 1999;60(Suppl 1):234–5.

[367] Anderson AM, Skakkebaek NE. Exposure to exogenous estrogens in food: possible impact on human development and health. Eur J Endocrinol 1999;140:477–85.

[368] Kolpin DW, Furlong ET, Meyer MT, et al. Pharmaceuticals, hormones, and other organic wastewater contaminants in US streams, 1999–2000: a national reconnaissance. Environ Sci Technol 2002;36:1202–11.

[369] Hartmann S, Lacorn M, Steinhart H. Natural occurrence of steroid hormones in food. Food Chemistry 1998;62:7–20.

[370] Remesar X, Tang V, Ferrer E, et al. Estrone in food: a factor influencing the development of obesity. Eur J Nutr 1999;38:247–53.

[371] Sumpter JP. Reproductive effect from oestrogen activity in polluted water. Arch Toxicol 1998;20:143–50.

[372] Safe SH. Environmental and dietary estrogens and human health: is there a problem? Environ Health Perspect 1995;103:346–51.

[373] Hill P, Wynder EL, Garnes H, et al. Environmental factors, hormones, and prostatic cancer. Prev Med 1980;9:657–66.

[374] Fisher JS. Environmental anti-androgens and male reproductive health: focus on phthalates and testicular dysgenesis syndrome. Reproduction 2004;127:305–15.

[375] Wetherill YB, Fisher NL, Staubach A, et al. Xenoestrogen action in prostate cancer: pleiotropic effects dependent on androgen receptor status. Cancer Res 2005;65:54–65.

[376] Wetherill YB, Petre CE, Monk KR, et al. The xenoestrogen bisphenol A induces inappropriate androgen receptor activation and mitogenesis in prostate adenocarcinoma cells. Mol Cancer Ther 2002;1:515–24.

[377] Hollinger R, Ekperigin H. Mycotoxins in food producing animals. Chemical food borne hazards and their control. Vet Clin North Am Food Anim Pract 1999;15(1):133–65.

[378] Liu SL, Sugimoto Y, Kulp SK, et al. Estrogenic down-regulation of protein tyrosine phosphatase y (PTPy) in human breast is associated with estrogen receptor a. Anticancer Res 2002;22:3917–24.

[379] Henderson BE, Rose R, Bernstein L. Estrogen as a cause of human cancer. Cancer Res 1988;48:246–53.

[380] Colditz GA. The benefits of hormone replacement therapy do not outweigh the increased risk of breast cancer. J NIH Res 1996;8:41–4.

[381] Ho SM. Estrogens and anti-estrogens: key mediators of prostate carcinogenesis and new therapeutic candidates. J Cell Biochem 2004;91(3):491–503.

[382] Davies TW, Palmer CR, Ruja E, et al. Adolescent milk, dairy product and fruit consumption and testicular cancer. Br J Cancer 1996;74:657–60.

[383] Ganmaa D, Li XM, Wang J, et al. Incidence and mortality of testicular and prostatic cancer in relation to world dietary practices. Int J Cancer 2002;98:262–7.

[384] Sharpe RM, Skakkebaek NE. Are oestrogens involved in falling sperm counts and disorders of the male reproductive tracts? Lancet 1993;340:1392–5.

[385] Vecchia C, Negri E, D'Avanzo B, et al. Dairy products and the risk of prostatic cancer. Oncology 1991;48:406–10.

[386] Tzonou A, Signorello LB, Lagiou P, et al. Diet and cancer of the prostate: a case-control study in Greece. Int J Cancer 1999;80:704–8.

[387] Chan JM, Giovanucci E, Andersson SO, et al. Dairy products, calcium, phosphorous, vitamin D and risk of prostate cancer (Sweden). Cancer Causes Control 1998;9:559–66.

[388] Talamini R, Franceschi S, Vecchia CL, et al. Diet and prostate cancer: a case-control study in Northern Italy. Nutr Cancer 1992;18:277–86.

[389] Snowdon DA, Phillips RL, Choi W. Diet, obesity and risk of fatal prostate cancer. Am J Epidemiol 1984;120:244–50.

[390] Marchand LL, Kolonel LN, Wilkens LR, et al. Animal fat consumption and prostate cancer: a prospective study in Hawaii. Epidemiology 1994;5:276–82.

[391] Chan JM, Stampfer MJ, Ma J, et al. Dairy products, calcium, and prostate cancer risk in the Physicians Health Study. Am J Clin Nutr 2001;74:549–54.

[392] Tavani A, Gallus S, Franceschi S, et al. Calcium, dairy products, and the risk of prostate cancer. Prostate 2001;48:118–21.

[393] Mettlin CJ, Schoenfeld ER, Natarajan N. Patterns of milk consumption and risk of cancer. Nutr Cancer 1990;13:89–99.

[394] Wu AH, Pike MC, Stram DO. Meta-analysis: dietary fat intake, serum estrogen levels, and the risk of breast cancer. J Natl Cancer Inst 1999;91:529–34.

[395] International prostate health council study group. Estrogens and prostatic disease. Prostate 2000;45:87–100.

VETERINARY
CLINICS
Food Animal Practice

ELSEVIER
SAUNDERS

Vet Clin Food Anim 21 (2005) 569–584

Reducing Calf Losses in Beef Herds

Robert L. Larson, DVM, PhD*,
Jeff W. Tyler, DVM, PhD

*Department of Veterinary Medicine and Surgery, College of Veterinary Medicine,
University of Missouri, 379 East Campus Drive, Columbia, Columbia, MO 65211, USA*

Neonatal mortality is a major cause of economic loss in beef cattle herds [1–3]. The foundation for a comprehensive herd management plan to decrease preweaning mortality is sound reproductive management that ensures that a herd calves during a predetermined period of time, with a concentrated distribution of births, and with a controlled incidence of dystocia.

An important concept that must be addressed in development of plans to reduce neonatal calf mortality is the role of the calf as a biological incubator and amplifier. The pathogens responsible for most neonatal calf disease are common, if not ubiquitous [4,5]. Infectious bacteria, viruses, and protozoa are shed by clinically ill calves, healthy adult cattle, and subclinically infected calves [6–10]. Calves exposed to low concentrations of pathogens generally have occult or mild clinical signs; however, these same calves will shed pathogens in large quantities, causing considerable environmental contamination [7–9]. Consequently, control strategies for neonatal health place a premium on limiting the exposure of young calves to older calves, which serve as reservoirs and amplifiers of infectious disease agents, and on dispersing young calves in order to maximize hygiene. The percentage of a herd that calves early in the calving season is a major determinant of the amount and duration of environmental exposure to enteric pathogens in a herd.

Beef cattle reproduction is a continuum rather than a series of unrelated breeding seasons. The percentage of a herd breeding early in one breeding season strongly influences the likelihood for a similar percentage of the herd breeding early in the next breeding season. Tools such as breeding soundness examinations (BSE) of bulls, body condition scores (BCS) of cows, and reproductive tract scoring of heifers are used before the breeding

* Corresponding author.
  E-mail address: LarsonR@missouri.edu (R.L. Larson).

season to ensure that a high percentage of females are expressing estrus and ovulating viable oocytes before the start of the breeding season, and that bulls are able to deliver fertile sperm. Tools such as estimation of fetal age via transrectal uterine palpation or ultrasound to predict calving distributions are used to monitor the success of heifer development, cow management pre- and postcalving, and mating ability of bulls in the immediately proceeding breeding season. Results of monitoring allow targeted adjustments in herd management to support continued desirable reproductive outcome, or to return the herd to a more optimum percentage of females conceiving early in the next breeding season.

To reduce calf losses in beef herds, management strategies should improve host defenses and environmental hygiene. Specific attention is focused on preventing dystocia to directly reduce calf losses, on improving passive transfer of colostral immunoglobulins (IgG), and on limiting environmental contamination via calving season management. Rigorous implementation of these management strategies should reduce neonatal mortality, regardless of the specific pathogen or syndrome.

Ensuring adequate transfer of colostral immunoglobulins

The importance of early colostrum intake on calf health is well-documented [11–15]. Cattle do not pass antibodies from the dam to the fetus before birth; therefore, calves rely on antibodies in colostrum to provide protection against disease [16,17]. Calves absorb colostral antibodies for only a short time after birth [18]. By 12 hours after birth, the ability to absorb antibodies decreases drastically, eventually ceasing between 1 and 2 days of age [16,17]. Calf serum IgG concentrations less than 1000 mg/dL are associated with increased morbidity, increased mortality, and decreased performance [14,16,19].

For a beef calf to consume adequate amounts of colostrum, it must be able to stand, walk, find the dam's teats, and suckle. Consequently, the dam must stand, bond with the calf, produce colostrum with adequate concentrations of immunoglobulin, and have teats that can be grasped by the calf. Problems in any of these areas can lead to inadequate colostrum intake and low calf serum IgG concentrations. Delayed suckling appears to be the most common cause of failure of passive transfer (FPT) of antibodies in beef cattle [20,21].

Calves born unassisted have a shorter interval from birth to standing, decreased risk of poor bonding with their dams, and greater antibody absorption, compared with calves that required assistance during birth [22]. Calves requiring minimal assistance during delivery are at a substantial advantage for the aforementioned factors, compared with calves requiring greater assistance during delivery [22]. Timely assistance is necessary to minimize the negative effects of dystocia, but according to a survey of 4092 beef farms in the United States [23], only 60.7% of operations intervened after 2 hours or less of labor in heifers, and 45.5% of operations intervened after 2 hours or less in cows. A difficult birth that does not result in calf death, but prevents either the cow or calf from standing in a timely manner, can serve as an additional negative result of dystocia. Even when fresh colostrum is obtained from the dam and administered by bottle to calves that survive a difficult birth, the amount of absorbed antibodies may be decreased [22].

The mass of IgG available for absorption by the calf is determined by the IgG content and amount of colostrum produced by the dam. Several maternal factors, including age of the dam and nutritional plane, affect colostrum IgG concentration. Older cows tend to produce colostrum that contains higher concentrations of IgG than do younger cows [24]. And, calves born to heifers have lower ($P < 0.05$) mean serum IgG concentrations at 1 to 7 days of age than do calves born to cows [25]; however, it should be noted that the magnitude of this difference may not be great. In one recent study [24], Holstein cows in their first and second lactation produced colostrum with an IgG concentration of 66 and 75 g/L, whereas older cows produced colostrum with an IgG concentration of 97 g/L. Colostrum from first-calf heifers is acceptable if an adequate volume is ingested in a timely manner. In general, heifers and cows that are in good body condition at parturition are more likely to have calves that have adequate passive transfer than are thin or obese heifers or cows. If a dam's diet is deficient in protein before parturition, it will result in a selective decrease in the absorption of IgG_1 and IgG_2 by the calf [26].

Prevention of dystocia—general considerations

The two major causes of dystocia, and hence FPT, are disproportionately large calves and inadequate heifer or cow pelvic area [27–30]. Of these two factors, calf birth weight is more closely associated with calving difficulty (0.47 versus -0.07 for pelvic area) [28,30]. Dystocia can directly cause calf mortality. Dystocia also has an indirect role in many deaths attributed to infectious disease. Calves that survive dystocia are 2.4 [31] to 6 [32] times more likely to become sick soon after birth. At least a portion of this effect results from inadequate passive transfer of colostral IgG. Not only are calves less likely to stand and nurse in a timely fashion following a difficult birth, but some studies also suggest that dystocic calves are less able to absorb colostral IgG [33–35]. Prevention of dystocia centers on two issues. First, efforts should be made to limit calf size. Second, dams should be selected for adequate size and adequate pelvic area.

Parity is an important risk factor for dystocia. Beef heifers have a higher number of calves that die by 3 weeks of age than do cows (3.8% versus 1.8%) [36]. This effect is primarily attributable to the higher incidence of dystocia in heifers, an expected consequence of the smaller size of first-calf heifers when compared with mature cows. Concerns regarding the potential for dystocia should not be restricted to first calf heifers, however. Herds that are in the midst of rapid phenotype change, shifting from small- to large-framed cattle, may experience high dystocia proportions when small-framed cows who have small pelvic areas are being bred to bulls who have greater growth potential. Unfortunately, most growth traits, including weaning, yearling, and mature weight, are positively correlated with calf birth weight [37]. Consequently, attempts to increase calf growth rate will likely cause an increased incidence of dystocia unless concerted efforts are made to simultaneously select for acceptable birth weight. On the other hand, overly aggressive and persistent selection for low birth can result in smaller mature size and smaller pelvic area, leading to dystocia problems in subsequent generations.

In the face of disease outbreaks, adequacy of passive transfer should be assessed using refractometry or the sodium sulfite test. Ideally, serum samples should be collected from a representative sample of both sick and overtly healthy calves less than two weeks of age. If the FPT (<1000 mg/dL IgG) proportion exceeds 15%, FPT may be an important contributing factor to a calf health problem. Although poor colostrum quality (low IgG concentration) may be a contributing factor to a herd that has a high percentage of FPT calves, inadequate colostral intake is more likely and common in beef cattle [20,21].

Prevention of dystocia—limiting calf size

The best predictor of dystocia is a comparison of expected birth weight or calving ease of offspring by a calculation called expected progeny differences (EPD). Expected progeny differences are a prediction of the transmitting ability of a parent animal, or how a bull's or cow's progeny will compare with other animals' progeny for various traits [38,39]. All breeds report a birth weight EPD, which is expressed in pounds of birth weight. Several breeds also report direct and maternal calving-ease EPD (usually as a ratio). Sires with higher direct calving-ease ratios will have less dystocia than lower EPD bulls. Maternal calving-ease EPD is an indication of how easily a sire's daughters will calve. Calculation of EPD considers the performance data of the animal, its relatives, and its offspring compared with other members of that animal's contemporary group. As the amount of information on an animal, its ancestors, and its progeny increases, the accuracy of these predictions increases. Consequently, young bulls and bulls sired by bulls with low-accuracy EPD have less accurate EPD. The accuracy of EPD estimates will improve as performance data are acquired from larger numbers of progeny.

It should be noted that EPDs are valid only within a given breed, and that the estimated differences are calculated relative to a base year, which was set several years in the past. In most cattle breeds, birth weights have increased over time. Consequently, a bull may have a positive EPD for birth weight and still produce calves that are smaller than his breed average. When bulls are selected to breed to heifers of the same breed or similar breed type, an upper percentile ranking should be established that results in an acceptable proportion of difficult births. For example, one may limit breeding heifers to bulls that rank within the lowest 30% of their breed with regards to calf size (lowest 30% of birth weight EPD). When Continental breed bulls are bred to English breed heifers, a practice that we strongly discourage, a much lower percentile limit (ie, tenth percentile) should be used. Bulls that produce exceptionally large calves should be avoided, even in older cows. When assisting producers making selections based on EPD, it is important to realize that simultaneous selection for all traits of economic importance in beef production is not feasible, because some positive traits are genetically antagonistic. The antagonism between growth rate and calving ease is noteworthy; however, sires do exist that produce progeny with both acceptable calving ease and acceptable pre- and postweaning growth [40].

Prevention of dystocia—ensuring adequate dam pelvic diameter

Although of less importance than calf weight, insufficient pelvic area can also explain dystocia in some herds. The use of pelvic measurement at 1 year of age as a tool to decrease the incidence of dystocia has been described extensively since the middle 1970s [41–43]. The correlation between yearling and 2-year-old pelvic areas is 0.70; therefore, measuring heifers' pelvic area as yearlings is beneficial for predicting pelvic size at the time of parturition [43]. Pelvic area is moderately to highly heritable (.44 to .61), so after a few years of measuring replacement heifers and bulls used to produce replacements, producers can increase average pelvic size of the herd [42,44].

Critics of using pelvic area measurements to decrease dystocia point out that pelvic area is positively correlated to mature cow size and calf birth weight [29,41]. If producers select for larger pelvic area, calf birth weight will increase and the proportion of dystocia may remain static [45]. This hypothesis has been confirmed by several studies [28,46,47]. Rather than using pelvic area measurement to select for maximum pelvic size, pelvimetry should be used to set a minimum pelvic size as a culling criterion (such as 140 to 170 cm^2 at a year of age, depending on breed and other factors) without assigning preference for heifers that exceed the minimum [28]. Based on available data, pelvic area measurements have limited usefulness in predicting dystocia on an individual basis, but can predict herd problems [44–46,48].

Pelvic area at the time of calving is influenced both by the genetic potential for the skeletal size of the pelvis and by the nutrient intake from birth to first calving, and especially from birth through the attainment of puberty. Because the correlations between body weight and dystocia incidence are generally stronger than those between pelvic area and dystocia incidence, it appears that nutritional management of heifers is more important than the genetic potential for skeletal size of the pelvis when managing dystocia [30,45,46]. To assure that heifers have received adequate nutrition for proper growth and development, replacements should weigh 65% to 70% of mature weight at the time of breeding, and should reach 85% to 90% of mature weight by the time they calve.

Limiting environmental contamination and exposure of neonatal calves to pathogens

Despite the importance of adequate antibody protection, colostral intake is not the only factor that determines morbidity and mortality of calves. Not all calves who have poor antibody protection become sick [11]. In fact, investigators often find healthy, rapidly growing calves who have evidence of poor transfer of maternal antibodies [47]. The other important factor that determines morbidity and mortality is the amount of pathogen exposure. Sanitation, protection from inclement weather and other stressors, and separation from sick calves will decrease the risk of morbidity and mortality of calves.

Control timing of heifer parturition

Beef producers should plan to have their heifers give birth 2 or more weeks earlier than mature cows in the herd. Limiting the breeding, and therefore the calving season, to 45 days or fewer for heifers also offers several advantages. From a labor standpoint, an early, short, calving season prevents overlap between increased labor needed to monitor and assist heifers and to care for their calves, and labor needed to monitor and assist mature cows. In addition, the length of time from calving to the resumption of cycling is longer in heifers than in cows [49]. Therefore, calving heifers earlier than mature cows gives the heifers the extra time they need to return to estrus and be cycling at the start of the subsequent breeding season.

Scheduling parturition of heifers earlier than the mature cows in the herd should result in less exposure of their calves to pathogens. As noted previously, heifers produce less colostrum, with a lower concentration of antibodies than that of mature cows [22]. Poorer quality and quantity of colostrum, coupled with the higher proportion of dystocia and mismothering for heifers, results in calves born to heifers that have less passively acquired immune protection against disease than calves born to mature cows. The primary reservoirs for pathogens that cause diarrhea in young calves are calves that have diarrhea, clinically normal calves that have subclinical infection, and adult cattle [50]. Calves that recover from diarrhea may continue to shed pathogens for several months [6,8–10]. Cattle (calves or adults) that become infected with diarrhea-causing pathogens will shed a large number of the pathogens, regardless of whether they become ill [5–10]. Because of this multiplication effect, exposure to infectious agents increases as the calving season progresses. By limiting the period during which heifers are scheduled to give birth to the early part of the calving season, their more poorly protected calves do not come into contact with as many pathogens as better-protected calves from mature cows that are born later during the calving season.

Shorten the calving season and concentrate most births early in the calving season

The incidence and severity of neonatal disease will typically increase and the age at disease onset will decrease as the calving season progresses [25]. This phenomenon is common in beef herds because of the previously noted role of the calf as a biological amplifier. Calves that are exposed to low pathogen doses early in the calving season will typically have occult or asymptomatic disease. Unfortunately, these calves will shed pathogens in much higher concentrations than were necessary to infect them. Calves born later in the calving season are exposed to escalating doses of pathogens, and will experience more severe clinical signs and shed massive doses of infectious organisms. The more the calving season is shortened, the more this biological amplification effect is negated. In the United States, however, most producers (53.6%) had no set breeding season, meaning that many producers and their veterinarians have the potential to decrease the risks of neonatal infectious disease and death by instituting a planned breeding season [23].

To ensure that most calves are born early in the calving season (ie, the first 21 days; Fig. 1), thereby limiting their exposure to amplified pathogen numbers, 65% of the herd should be 60 days or more postpartum at the start of the breeding season. If less than 55% of the herd is 60 days or more

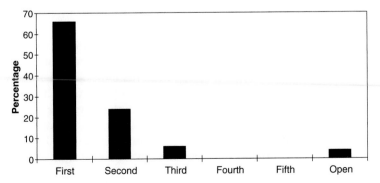

Fig. 1. Example of concentrating most births early in the calving season to ensure that a high percentage of the calf crop is not exposed to older calves and amplified pathogen populations.

postpartum, then last year's calving distribution or the date of the start of this year's breeding season become limiting factors in achieving a high percentage of conceptions early in the breeding season.

One common reason a herd has a less than an ideal number of calves born early in the calving season is the previous year's calving distribution. Without implementing culling, nutrition, and heifer development changes on such a farm, it is very difficult to positively impact the percentage of the herd pregnant in the first 21 days of the breeding season. Reasons that a herd with a previously ideal calving distribution can deteriorate to a less than ideal situation include females too thin at calving, poor postpartum cow herd nutrition, subfertile bulls, or infectious or noninfectious disease [51–54].

Because the average bovine pregnancy lasts 283 days, one can calculate that a cow/heifer must rebreed within 82 days after calving to maintain a yearly (365-day) calving interval. The typical amount of time from calving to the resumption of cycling (postpartum period) for mature cows is 40 to 60 days [55]. For first-calf heifers, the postpartum period is closer to 80 days [49]. If the breeding season begins on the same date as the previous year, the breeding season will commence 63 to 82 days postpartum and end 123 to 142 days postpartum for cows calving in the first 20-day period of the previous calving season. This time period should allow all cows, including first-calf heifers, to have the opportunity to cycle and be bred several times during the breeding season. Cows calving in the second 20-day period will be 43 to 62 days postpartum at the start of the breeding season and 103 to 122 days past calving at the end of the breeding season. Once again, this timing should allow the mature cows to resume cycling and have the opportunity to be bred several times during the breeding season. First-calf heifers should also resume cycling early enough in the breeding season to have at least two opportunities to be bred. In contrast, for those cows that calve in the fourth 20-day period, calving has just finished as the breeding season begins, and for those in the fifth 20-day period, the breeding season has begun before the time they calve. Limited (or nonexistent) time from calving until the start of the breeding season essentially eliminates the potential for nursing cows, and even more so for first-calf heifers, to rebreed early in the breeding season, if at all.

To ensure a high rate of cyclicity, mature cows should have a minimum BCS of 5 (using a 9-point scale) at the start of the breeding season [56,57], Heifers should have a BCS of 6 [51,58]. If records indicate that BCSs were below these levels, then energy-reserve status at the start of the breeding season becomes a limiting factor in achieving a high percentage of conceptions early in the breeding season. If farm records are inadequate to supply this information, nutritional status at the start of the breeding season remains an unknown variable, and veterinary involvement in capturing this data in following years is warranted.

Higher BCS or greater levels of supplemental energy during late gestation improved the percentage of heifers and cows showing estrus by 60 days after calving, and subsequent pregnancy proportion [59–63]. Females that calve in poor body condition (<4–5 on a 9-point body condition scale) have lighter birth weight calves, a longer postpartum interval to return to estrus, and lower pregnancy proportion during the following breeding season [59–63]. The appreciably higher energy and protein requirements postcalving, which greatly exceed those of even late-gestation females, make it difficult to add body condition to cows and heifers once they begin lactation [63]. Because postcalving condition score and energy balance control ovulation [61] and condition scores of 5 to 6 (9-point body condition scale) are required for high conception success, both body condition at calving and level of nutrition postpartum are critical control points affecting pregnancy proportion [59–62].

Practitioners can evaluate the reproductive potential for a herd approximately 2 weeks before the start of the breeding season by examining a random portion (ie, 30%) of the herd for BCS and presence of a corpus luteum (CL). Because a CL is generally palpable from about day 6 to 7 to day 17 of a 21 day cycle (ie, 55% of the days of a 21-day cycle), from a single reproductive tract evaluation, percent cycling can be estimated by dividing the percentage of examined cows that have a palpable CL by 0.55 (55%). Therefore, if 30% of a herd subset has a palpable CL, one can estimate that approximately 55% of the herd is cycling. If the percent cycling is lower than desired, interventions such as 48-hour weaning of calves and increased caloric intake may be implemented before the start of the breeding season.

In the presence of adequate body condition and days postpartum, estrous synchronization systems can be used to increase the percentage of calves born early in the calving season. A feed-grade progestogen, a progesterone intravaginal device, and injectable prostaglandin have all been used successfully in both heifers and cows. A herd that successfully synchronizes estrus of 80% of the breeding females and achieves a 60% conception proportion would have nearly 50% of the herd conceive during the first week of the breeding season, thereby ensuring that a high percentage of calves will not be exposed to older calves during the subsequent calving season.

In any breeding situation, but especially when concentrating the number of cows exhibiting estrus early in the breeding season with estrous synchronization, having an adequate number of fertile bulls to breed the females is essential to having high conception rates. At this time, the best on-ranch predictors of bull fertility are the breeding soundness evaluation of bulls (BSEB) and careful observation of mating ability during natural service. The BSEB is a relatively quick and economic procedure for screening bulls before the breeding season. It is intended for wide application with a variety of breeds in different environments, and it is simple, repeatable, and unambiguous. The evaluation is most effective in identifying bulls at the lower end of the potential fertility spectrum, and it is relatively less effective in predicting individual bull performance at the upper end of the fertility spectrum [63]. The limitations of the BSEB are due to the fact that it is relatively quick and inexpensive, and therefore does not comprehensively assess all aspects of male fertility; in addition, the complex trait of fertility is influenced by female traits and extraneous factors as well as by male traits. The importance of a BSEB, however, is demonstrated in a resent large-scale study [64] that found that highest calf crops were obtained from bulls that have >70% normal sperm, whereas bulls that have <50% normal sperm sired relatively few calves.

When evaluating nonsynchronized breeding situations, a bull-to-female ratio of 1:60 resulted in the same estrus detection and pregnancy rates as bull-to-female ratios of 1:25 and 1:44 in both single- and multisire breeding systems [65]. If a synchronization system effectively doubles to triples the number of cows expressing estrus per day early in the breeding season, a logical mature bull-to-female ratio would be 1:20 to 1:30, with a lower ratio for yearling bulls—if the bulls have passed a thorough BSEB and have been observed to successfully mate in natural situations.

Group assortment strategies

Beef herd managers need to have a plan for cattle movement throughout the calving season. Such a plan generally requires a minimum of four, and preferably five, separate pastures. These include a gestation pasture, a calving pasture and a series of nursery pastures. To ensure that beef calves are born in a sanitary environment, the herd should not be fed throughout the winter in the same pasture or area in which calves will be born, or to which neonatal calves will be moved. Cattle are moved from the gestation pasture to the calving pasture 1 to 2 weeks before calving. Within one day of parturition, a cow or heifer and her calf should be moved from the calving pasture to a nursery pasture. Cow-calf pairs are added to a single nursery pasture until the goal number of pairs has been reached. Thereafter, the farmer or rancher begins adding pairs to a second pasture. The age spread from the oldest to the youngest calf in a nursery pasture should never exceed 30 days, and more compact calf-age distributions are preferable. This process of age assortment in calves effectively negates the biologic amplification effect. If neonatal calves are not exposed to older calves shedding high concentrations of infectious pathogens, they will probably remain healthy. The longer the calving season, the greater the need for a large number of nursery pastures. Calves that develop diarrhea should be moved immediately to an area away from healthy calves and treated, and not returned until all the calves in the group are at low risk for developing diarrhea (ie, >30 days of age, or at time of summer turn-out).

Breeding records in herds in which artificial insemination is used will permit accurate prediction of calving dates, facilitating timely movement of cows from gestation to calving pastures. In naturally serviced herds, practitioners should consider adopting herd health programs that incorporate early pregnancy diagnosis and estimation of fetal age, in order to improve accuracy of calving date prediction. Most traditional herd health programs schedule pregnancy diagnosis of cows coincidental with weaning. In these circumstances, some cows may be as much as 6 months pregnant. More accurate prediction of stage of pregnancy can be attained if cows are examined earlier in gestation. Consequently, pregnancy diagnosis should be scheduled 35 to 40 days after the end of a 65-day or shorter breeding season, or 95 to 105 days after the initiation of a longer breeding season. By changing the purpose of pregnancy examination from identifying cows to cull to save feed costs to a tool to monitor the success of a breeding plan to concentrate conceptions early in the breeding season, veterinarians can use an old procedure to influence calf health and herd reproductive efficiency in new ways.

Calving site selection

The most common system of calving is pasture calving. Alternatives include more intensive systems, such as barn or dry lot calving. It should be noted that any procedure that concentrates large numbers of cattle in a small area increases environmental contamination, and consequently, increases the potential for fulminant outbreaks of neonatal disease. Consequently, extensive systems in which calving cows are dispersed in large calving pastures are generally considered optimal from the perspective of reduced disease transmission between neonatal calves. The factors that most often force farmers and ranchers to opt for intensive calving systems is the need to assist cows experiencing dystocia in herds with a high prevalence of difficult births, and the need to avoid harsh environmental conditions.

Size of calving pasture is not a direct measure of cow concentration, and hence environmental contamination. Cows tend to congregate around feed and water sources, and these areas may become heavily contaminated. If supplemental hay and grain are fed, these should be provided at locations that are both separate and distant from water sources. This practice will encourage cow dispersal and minimize contamination. If feed bunks or bale feeders are used, they should be moved frequently. Alternatively, bales can be spread over the calving pasture and the feeding location changed daily. In areas of the country with minimal snowfall, winter pasture can be stockpiled. Cool season grasses, such as tall fescue, are permitted to grow in the fall, and access to these pastures is restricted until calving season. Use of pasture grasses encourages cow dispersal and minimizes contamination. If the herd forage plan includes feeding hay, consider feeding hay in early to midgestational and saving stockpiled pasture for the actual calving season.

The calving area should be free of mud and should be protected from the wind. A large pasture with good drainage, southern exposure, and a natural windbreak that will block prevailing winds is probably adequate for many mature herds. Inexpensive windbreaks can be constructed when natural protection is lacking. Windbreaks should be sufficiently large to avoid concentrating cattle. In addition, it is reasonable to have an area that is sheltered from the weather and that has a chute, stall, or other restraint area so that dystocia can be corrected.

When producers schedule calving to occur in the fall, late spring, or early summer to avoid periods of low ambient temperatures and inclement weather, and parturition takes place on pastures, morbidity and mortality that result from exposure to cold temperatures and infectious disease are greatly reduced. Should the calving season be scheduled for late winter or early spring, however, additional facilities may be required. The ability to dry and warm calves that have been born during inclement weather becomes critical for high survival proportions during snowstorms or rainstorms accompanied by low temperatures. Only those heifers and, less frequently, cows that require assistance during parturition or to establish a bond with their calf, should be confined to a calving barn or small pen; all other cattle should be housed in a calving pasture.

In the face of a calf mortality outbreak, the single most powerful intervention strategy is often the decision to move cows that have yet to calve to a distant, clean pasture setting. In herds that have a low dystocia incidence, this decision has few obvious drawbacks. In herds that have moderate dystocia incidence, the potential costs associated with calf mortality must be weighed against the potential for cow and calf losses associated with dystocia. Accurate records will permit practitioners and producers to base these decisions on fact rather than perception.

Summary

The core components of an effective program to prevent calf mortality are minimizing dystocia, enforcing age segregation of neonatal calves, and dispersing livestock to maximize hygiene. Intervention strategies for calf mortality problems can be readily categorized into immediate and long-term intervention strategies. Immediate intervention strategies include decreasing livestock density, designation of a clean hygienic calving pasture, and creation of multiple nursery pastures. This may entail changes in feed delivery systems, construction of temporary pastures, and a shift from intensive to extensive calving systems. Long-term intervention will require development of a cohesive plan that addresses cow nutrition, herd reproduction, and identification and designation of committed calving and nursery pastures.

A complete and comprehensive neonatal disease control program uses estrous synchronization and artificial insemination to breed a high percentage of replacement heifers to bulls that have high-accuracy EPD for acceptable birth weight. By reducing the incidence of dystocia, heifers have improved passive transfer of antibodies to their calves and reduced likelihood of a prolonged postpartum interval to the resumption of cycling, allowing first-calf heifers to be bred early in the subsequent breeding season. Use of mature cow-herd estrous synchronization systems, nutritional management to provide optimum body condition at the start of the breeding season, heifer development plans that assure that heifers are cycling before breeding, and BSE of bulls ensures that a high percentage of the herd can conceive early in each breeding season, thereby reducing the percentage of calves that are exposed to significantly older calves during the neonatal period. The best tool to monitor the effectiveness of the herd reproductive plan and to plan effective interventions is early estimation of fetal age via uterine palpation or transrectal ultrasound.

Fortunately, many of the changes required to maximize calf survival will have appreciable positive impact on herd reproduction and uniformity of weaned calves. These intervention strategies are best viewed as part and parcel of a comprehensive and cohesive herd management plan.

References

[1] Bakheit HA, Greene HJ. Control of bovine neonatal diarrhea by management techniques. Vet Rec 1981;108:455–8.
[2] Whittier WD. Management considerations to control calf diarrhea. In: Smith RA, editor. Proceedings. 32nd Convention American Association of Bovine Practitioners. Rome (GA): American Association of Bovine Practitioners; 1999. p. 123–7.
[3] National Animal Health Monitoring System (NAHMS) beef cow/calf health and productivity audit, Part II: reference of 1997 beef cow-calf health and health management practices. Fort Collins (CO): Center for Animal Health Monitoring, United States Department of Agriculture, Animal and Plant Health Inspection Service, Veterinary Services; 1997.
[4] Waltner-Toews D, Martin SW, Meek AH. An epidemiological study of selected calf pathogens on Holstein dairy farms in southwestern Ontario. Can J Vet Res 1986;50: 307–13.
[5] DeRycke J, Bernard S, Laporte J, et al. Prevalence of various enteropathogens in the feces of diarrheic and healthy calves. Ann Rech Vet 1986;17:159–68.
[6] Crouch CF, Acres SD. Prevalence of rotavirus and coronavirus antigens in the feces of normal cows. Can J Comp Med 1984;48:340–2.
[7] McLaren IM, Wray C. Epidemiology of Salmonella typhimurium infection in calves: Persistence of salmonellae on calf units. Vet Rec 1991;129:461–2.
[8] Ongerth JE, Stibbs HH. Prevalence of Crytposporidium infection in dairy calves in western Washington. Am J Vet Res 1989;50:1069–70.
[9] Lucchelli A, Lance SE, Bartlett PB, et al. Prevalence of bovine group A rotavirus shedding among dairy calves in Ohio. Am J Vet Res 1992;53:169–74.
[10] Collins JK, Riegel CA, Olson JD, et al. Shedding of enteric coronavirus in adult cattle. Am J Vet Res 1987;48:361–5.
[11] Tyler JW, Hancock DD, Wicksie SE, et al. Use of serum total protein concentration to predict mortality in mixed-source dairy replacement heifers. J Vet Intern Med 1998;12:79–83.
[12] Weaver DM, Tyler JW, VanMetre DC, et al. Passive transfer of colostral immunoglobulin in calves. J Vet Intern Med 2000;14:569–87.
[13] Virtala AMK, Grohn YT, Mechor GD, et al. The effect of maternally acquired immunoglobulin G on the risk of respiratory disease in heifers during the first 3 months of life. Prev Vet Med 1999;39:25–37.
[14] Robison JD, Stott GH, DeNise SK. Effects of passive immunity on growth and survival in the dairy heifer. J Dairy Sci 1988;71:1283–7.
[15] Irwin VCR. Incidence of disease in colostrum deprived calves. Vet Rec 1974;94:105–6.

[16] Stott GH, Marx DB, Menefee BE, et al. Colostral immunoglobulin transfer in calves I. Period of absorption. J Dairy Sci 1979;62:1632–8.

[17] Osburn BI, MacLachlan NJ, Terrell TG. Ontogeny of immune system. J Am Vet Med Assoc 1984;181:1049–52.

[18] Matte JJ, Girard CL, Seoane JR, et al. Absorption of colostral immunoglobulin G in the newborn dairy calf. J Dairy Sci 1982;65:1765–70.

[19] McGuire TC, Pfeiffer NE, Weikel JM, et al. Failure of colostral immunoglobulin transfer in calves dying from infectious disease. J Am Vet Med Assoc 1976;169:713–8.

[20] Kuse V. Absorption of immunoglobulin from colostrum in newborn calves. Anim Prod 1970;12:627–38.

[21] Selman IE, McEwan AD, Fisher EW. Serum immune globulin concentrations in calves left with their dams for the first two days of life. J Comp Pathol 1970;80:419–27.

[22] Odde KG. Survival of the neonatal calf. Vet Clin North Am Food Anim Pract 1988;4: 501–8.

[23] Dargatz DA, Dewell GA, Mortimer RG. Calving and calving management of beef cows and heifers on cow-calf operations in the United States. Theriogenology 2004;61: 997–1007.

[24] Tyler JW, Steevens BJ, Hostetler DE, et al. Colostral IgG concentrations in Holstein and Guernsey cows. Am J Vet Res 1999;60:1136–9.

[25] Clement JC, King ME, Salman MD, et al. Use of epidemiologic principles to identify risk factors associated with the development of diarrhea in calves in five beef herds. J Am Vet Med Assoc 1995;207:1334–8.

[26] Blecha F, Bull RC, Olson DP, et al. Effects of prepartum protein restriction in the beef cow on immunoglobulin content in blood and colostral whey and subsequent immunoglobulin absorption by the neonatal calf. J Anim Sci 1981;53:1174–80.

[27] Andersen KJ, Brinks JS, Lefever DG, et al. The factors associated with dystocia in cattle. Vet Med (Praha) 1993;88:764–76.

[28] Naazie A, Makarechian M, Berg RT. Factors influencing calving difficulty in beef heifers. J Anim Sci 1989;67:3243–9.

[29] Price TD, Wiltbank JN. Predicting dystocia in heifers. Theriogenology 1978;9:221–49.

[30] King BD, Cohen RDH, McCormac S, et al. Marked maternal factors and the prediction of dystocia in beef heifers. Can J Anim Sci 1993;73:431–5.

[31] Toombs RE, Wikse SE, Kasari TR. The incidence, causes, and financial impact of perinatal mortality in North American beef herds. Vet Clin North Am Food Anim Pract 1994;10:137–46.

[32] Wittum TE, Perino LJ. Passive immune status at postpartum hour 24 and long-term health and performance of calves. Am J Vet Res 1995;56:1149–54.

[33] Besser TE, Szenci O, Gay CC. Decreased colostral immunoglobulin absorption in calves with postnatal respiratory acidosis. J Am Vet Med Assoc 1990;196:1239–43.

[34] Tyler H, Ramsey H. Hypoxia in neonatal calves: effect on intestinal transport of immunoglobulins. J Dairy Sci 1991;74:1953–6.

[35] Drewery JJ, Quigley JD, Geiser DR, et al. Effect of high arterial carbon dioxide tension on efficiency of immunoglobulin G absorption in calves. Am J Vet Res 1999;60:609–14.

[36] National Animal Health Monitoring System (NAHMS) beef cow/calf health and productivity audit, Part I: beef cow/calf herd management practices in the United States. Fort Collins (CO): Center for Animal Health Monitoring, United States Department of Agriculture, Animal and Plant Health Inspection Service, Veterinary Services; 1993.

[37] Morrison DG, Williamson WD, Humes PE. Heritabilities and correlations of traits associated with pelvic area in beef cattle [abstract]. J Anim Sci 1984;59(Suppl 1):160.

[38] Pollack EJ. Expected progeny differences (within breed comparisons). In: Proceedings of Symposium on Application of Expected Progeny Differences to Livestock Improvement. Savoy (IL): American Society of Animal Science; 1992. p. 17–23.

[39] Beef Improvement Federation Guidelines for uniform beef improvement programs. 7th edition. Reno (NV): Writing & Business Support; 1996.

[40] MacNeil MD, Urick JJ, Decoudu G. Characteristics of line 1 Hereford females resulting from selection by independent culling levels for below-average birth weight and high yearling weight or by mass selection for high yearling weight. J Anim Sci 2000;78:2292–8.

[41] Laster DB. Factors affecting pelvic size and dystocia in beef cattle. J Anim Sci 1974;38: 496–503.

[42] Holtzer ALJ, Schlote W. Investigations on interior pelvic size of Simmental heifers [abstract]. J Anim Sci 1984;59(Suppl 1):174.

[43] Neville WE, Mullinix BG, Smith JB, et al. Growth patterns for pelvic dimensions and other body measurements of beef females. J Anim Sci 1978;47:1080–8.

[44] Benyshek LL, Little DE. Estimate of genetic and phenotypic parameters associated with pelvic area in Simmental cattle. J Anim Sci 1982;54:258–63.

[45] Basarab JA, Rutter LM, Day PA. The efficacy of predicting dystocia in yearling beef heifers: I. Using ratios of pelvic area to birth weight or pelvic area to heifer weight. J Anim Sci 1993; 71:1359–71.

[46] Van Donkersgoed J, Ribble CS, Townsend HGG, et al. The usefulness of pelvic measurements as an on-farm test for predicting calving difficulty in beef heifers. Can Vet J 1990;31:190–3.

[47] Barber DML. Assessment of immune globulin status. Vet Rec 1976;98:121.

[48] Whittier WD, Eller AL, Beal WE. Management changes to reduce dystocia in virgin beef heifers. Agri-Practice 1994;15:26–32.

[49] Short RE, Bellows RA, Staigmiller RB, et al. Physiological mechanisms controlling anestrus and infertility in postpartum beef cattle. J Anim Sci 1990;68:799–816.

[50] Radostis OM. Neonatal diarrhea in ruminants (calves, lambs and kids). In: Howard JL, editor. Current veterinary therapy: food animal practice 2. Philadelphia: WB Saunders; 1986. p. 105–13.

[51] Richards MW, Spitzer JC, Warner MB. Effect of varying levels of postpartum nutrition and body condition at calving on subsequent reproductive performance in beef cattle. J Anim Sci 1986;62:300–6.

[52] Selk GE, Wetteman RP, Lusby KS, et al. Relationships among weight change, body condition and reproductive performance of range beef cows. J Anim Sci 1988;66: 3153–9.

[53] Spitzer JC, Morrison DG, Wettemann RP, et al. Reproductive response and calf birth and weaning weights as affected by body condition at parturition and postpartum weight gain in primiparous beef cows. J Anim Sci 1995;73:1251–7.

[54] Utter SD, Houghton PL, Corah LR, et al. Factors influencing first-service conception and overall pregnancy rates in commercial beef heifers. Ks Agri Exp Sta Contribution No. 94–373-S. Manhattan (KS): Kansas State University; 1994. p. 107–110.

[55] Spire MF. Breeding season evaluation of beef herds. In: Howard JF, editor. Current veterinary therapy. 2nd edition. Philadelphia: WB Saunders; 1986. p. 808.

[56] Bretzlaff K. A pictorial guide to bovine pregnancy diagnosis. Vet Med (Praha) 1987;82: 295–304.

[57] Kasari T, Gleason D. Herd management practices that influence total beef calf production—Part I. Comp Cont Ed Pract Vet 1996;18:823–32.

[58] Bellows RA, Short RE. Effects of precalving feed level on birthweight, calving difficulty and subsequent fertility. J Anim Sci 1978;46:1522–8.

[59] Selk GE, Wettemann RP, Lusby KS, et al. Relationships among weight change, body condition and reproductive performance of range beef cows. J Anim Sci 1988;66:3153–9.

[60] Wright IA, Rhind SM, Whyte TK, et al. Effects of body condition at calving and feeding level after calving on LH profiles and the duration of the post-partum anoestrous period in beef cows. Anim Prod 1992;55:41–6.

[61] DeRouen SM, Franke DE, Morrison DG, et al. Prepartum body condition and weight influences on reproductive performance of first-calf beef cows. J Anim Sci 1994;72:1119–25.

[62] Marston TT, Lusby KS, Wettemann RP, et al. Effects of feeding energy or protein supplements before or after calving on performance of spring-calving cows grazing native range. J Anim Sci 1995;73:657–64.

[63] Chenoweth PJ, Spitzer JC, Hopkins FM. A new bull breeding soundness evaluation form. Proceedings Society for Theriogenology AGM. Montgomery (AL): Society for Theriogenology; 1992. p. 63–70.

[64] Fitzpatrick LA, Fordyce G, McGowan MR, et al. Bull selection and use in northern Australia. Part 2. Semen traits. Anim Reprod Sci 2002;71:39–49.

[65] Rupp GP, Ball L, Shoop MC, et al. Reproductive efficiency of bulls in natural service: effects of bull to female ratio and single vs multiple sire breeding groups. JAVMA 1977;171:639–42.

ELSEVIER
SAUNDERS

VETERINARY
CLINICS
Food Animal Practice

Vet Clin Food Anim 21 (2005) 585–593

Index

Note: Page numbers of article titles are in **boldface** type.

Doi:10.1016/S0749-0720(05)00050-2
vetfood.theclinics.com